PRION - AN OVERVIEW

Edited by **Yusuf Tutar**

Prion - An Overview
http://dx.doi.org/10.5772/63289
Edited by Yusuf Tutar

Contributors

Cemal Ün, Yalçın Yaman, Pamela J. Skinner, Davis Seelig, Gwonchan Yoon, Myeongsang Lee, Sungsoo Na, Hyunsung Choi, Jae In Kim, Damani Bryant, Michael Benneyworth, Michael Reidy, Masahiro Kawahara, Ken-Ichiro Tanaka, Dai Mizuno, Gianluigi Zanusso, Michele Fiorini, Matilde Bongianni, Cristina Casalone, Elena Vallino Costassa, Barbara Iulini, Cristiano Corona, Daniela Meloni, Alessandra Favole, Maria Mazza, Cristiana Maurella, Maria Caramelli, Theodoros Sklaviadis, Konstantinos Xanthopoulos, Eirini Kanata, Dimitra Dafou, Suzanne Sindi

Published by InTech

Janeza Trdine 9, 51000 Rijeka, Croatia

Publishing Process Manager Iva Simcic
Technical Editor SPi Global
Cover InTech Design team

First published March, 2017
Printed in Croatia
Legal deposit, Croatia: National and University Library in Zagreb

Additional hard copies can be obtained from orders@intechopen.com

Prion - An Overview, Edited by Yusuf Tutar
p. cm.
Print ISBN 978-953-51-3001-7
Online ISBN 978-953-51-3002-4

For EU product safety concerns:
IN TECH d.o.o., Prolaz Marije Krucifikse Kozulić 3, 51000 Rijeka, Croatia,
info@intechopen.com or visit our website at intechopen.com.

Meet the editor

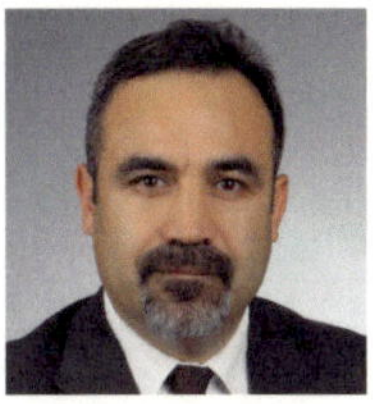

Prof. Dr. Yusuf Tutar is the head of Basic Pharmaceutical Sciences Department and the head of Biochemistry Division at the Faculty of Pharmacy, Cumhuriyet University, Sivas, Turkey. Dr. Tutar is also an adjunct faculty at Biomedical Engineering Program at the same university. He obtained his MSc and PhD degrees at Oregon State University and Texas Tech University, respectively. He pursued his postdoctoral studies at Rutgers University Medical School and National Institutes of Health (NIH/NIDDK), USA. Dr. Tutar's research is mainly focused on biochemistry, biophysics, genetics, and molecular biology with specialization in the fields of prion, drug design, cancer, protein structure-function, protein folding, microRNA, pseudogenes, molecular cancer, proteomics, genomics, and protein expression and characterization by spectroscopic and calorimetric methods.

Contents

Preface

Proteinaceous infectious particles namely prions cause neurodegenerative diseases in animals and humans. Infectious protein form (misfolded form) changes conformation of the normal proteins. This conversion leads to accumulation and propagation of certain proteins. Self-perpetuating misfolded conformations cause infectious neurodegenerative diseases. Aggregation starts with a seed occurrence, and this transforms the structure into amyloid fibrils. In this form, the protein in beta sheet structure polymerizes on top of each other. The stable prion aggregates in infected tissue cause tissue damage and cell death. Mechanisms of variety of neurodegenerative disorders depend on nonnative protein polymerization and cause Creutzfeldt-Jakob disease, kuru, and transmissible encephalopathies. Similar prion-like, self-templating mechanism causes amyotrophic lateral sclerosis, Alzheimer's disease, and Huntington's disease.

The book overviews all current aspects of protein aggregation. The content covers immunobiology, genetics, structure-activity relationship, neurobehavioral aspects, metals, molecular mechanism, and prion dynamic topics. The chapters provide an up-to-date revision of the current literature reports to the researchers in this field.

Prof. Dr. Yusuf Tutar
Cumhuriyet University, Faculty of Pharmacy
Department of Basic Pharmaceutical Sciences
Division of Pharmaceutical Biochemistry
Sivas, Turkey

Section 1

Introduction to Prion

Chapter 1

Classical and Atypical Bovine Spongiform Encephalopathy: Epidemiology, Pathogenesis and Diagnosis

Barbara Iulini, Elena Vallino Costassa,
Cristiano Corona, Daniela Meloni,
Alessandra Favole, Maria Mazza, Maria Caramelli,
Cristiana Maurella and Cristina Casalone

Additional information is available at the end of the chapter

http://dx.doi.org/10.5772/67332

Abstract

Classical bovine spongiform encephalopathy (C-BSE) is a fatal neurodegenerative disease of cattle, detected in the United Kingdom and many other countries since the 1980s. The origin of C-BSE is uncertain, but epidemiological studies suggest that the source of this disease was cattle feed prepared from prion-infected animal tissues. To date, cattle populations have been monitored through passive and active surveillance programs. From 2004, two different forms of BSE termed as L-BSE, also known as bovine amyloidotic spongiform encephalopathy (BASE), and H-BSE have been discovered in Italy and France. All these atypical cases have been detected in animals over 8 years of age. To date, there is no comprehensive information about the origin of the atypical BSEs (sporadic vs. acquired). Moreover, there are only very limited data available, concerning the pathogenesis of both atypical forms, as compared to C-BSE. This chapter provides a well-organized overview of what is known about classical and atypical BSE. It will review information on the main epidemiological features, pathogenesis, and the criteria for the routine diagnosis based on rapid tests, histological, immunohistochemical, and Western blot examinations.

Keywords: brainstem, C-BSE, atypical BSE, neurodegenerative diseases, surveillance, rapid tests, confirmatory tests

1. Introduction

Classical bovine spongiform encephalopathy (C-BSE) is a fatal neurodegenerative disorder of cattle that belongs to a group of diseases known as transmissible spongiform encephalopathies (TSEs). C-BSE is characterized by the accumulation of a disease-associated abnormal form of prion protein (PrPSc) in the central nervous system (CNS). PrPSc is commonly accepted as the pathological agent of TSEs and may be a post-translationally modified form of a normal cellular prion protein (PrPC). C-BSE has a long incubation period, about 2.5–8 years, with clinical disease usually affecting adult cattle at a peak age onset of 4–5 years, and with all breeds being equally susceptible. C-BSE is characterized by altered behavior and uncoordinated movement; histopathologic features include neuronal and neuropil vacuolization, glial reaction, and the complete absence of inflammatory lesions. BSE was first described in the United Kingdom (UK) in 1986 and is now classified as a potentially lethal zoonotic disease acquired via contaminated food [1–3], although the definite origin of BSE is still unknown. In 1996, the evidence of the pathogenetic relationship between BSE and a fatal neurodegenerative disorder in human (now known as the variant Creutzfeldt-Jakob disease) emerged and attracted the concern of the public.

From the UK, C-BSE spread to at least 28 other countries, mostly in Europe, with occasional cases also confirmed in Asia (Japan), the Middle East (Israel), and North America. To date, more than 112,000,000 animals have been examined in Europe, and more than 184,500 cases of BSE have been confirmed in the United Kingdom, 5,500 in Europe, and 60 cases in the rest of the world (Brazil, Canada, Israel, and Japan). The World Organisation for Animal Health (OIE) reported only 5 cases of BSE worldwide in 2015, 3 of which for Europe, 1 for Norway and 1 for Canada; in 2016 only 2 cases, in France and in Spain and in the current year, only one BSE case has been reported for Ireland.

Two different atypical BSE strains in cattle were discovered in 2004 in Italy and in France, respectively [4, 5]. However, these strains have been also identified in others European countries, Japan, and the Americas. They were designated L-type and H-type due to the molecular weight of PrPSc after protease degradation and Western blot (WB) analysis. The L-type is also known as bovine amyloidotic spongiform encephalopathy (BASE) because of the presence of PrP-positive amyloid plaques in the brain.

The origins of atypical BSEs remain obscure, and it has, therefore, been postulated that they represent a spontaneous TSE in cattle, comparable to most of sporadic CJDs cases in man. They are mainly detected in cattle that are 8 years of age or older. Most cases were identified in fallen stock and none were reported as clinical suspect, which suggested that the clinical presentation is unlike C-BSE.

Data on atypical BSE cases reported in the EU BSE databases since 2001 show that a total of 44 cases of L-type and 60 of H-type BSE have been identified in Europe. The prevalence of atypical BSE cases in the rest of the world is unknown because there are no official surveillance requirements or systematic reports from different countries.

2. Epidemiology

Epidemiology played a key role in deepening the knowledge of the dynamics and features of the disease and represented the foundations on which the initial control measures were built, in the early stages of the BSE epidemic. Epidemiological data established the following: dairy cows had a higher risk of BSE compared to beef cows, as demonstrated later [6–9]; BSE has an aetiological similarity with scrapie; the cases were geographically scattered in the UK, except for Scotland (it was later found that the rendering system procedures remained unchanged) where no cases were reported in the first period of the epidemic; all sick animals were index cases—that is there was usually one case per herd; a shape typical of an extended common source [10].

In the 1986–1996 decade, the British trade in livestock and animal by-products dropped sharply and the question as to whether BSE could be present in other countries arose. Shortly after reports of BSE cases appeared throughout Europe.

Following the BSE crisis, the European Parliament requested the European Commission (EC) to review its advisory system for public and animal health issues, especially those related to agricultural production and food. The EU Scientific Steering Committee (SSC) was appointed to supervise eight other specialized scientific committees dealing with food safety and public and animal health [11]. The SSC appointed a working group on TSEs to assess the risk that a country could have undetected BSE cases within its own bovine population. The outcome was the Geographical BSE-risk assessment (GBR).

2.1. Geographical risk assessment

The Geographical BSE-risk assessment (GBR) is an indicator of the likelihood in the presence of one or more bovines being infected with BSE, preclinically as well as clinically, at a given point in time, in a country/region. It is based on a semiquantitative analysis of the likelihood that the BSE agent was introduced into a country/region and if so when and to what extent and the potential of it being recycled and potentially amplified or eliminated [12].

The BSE/cattle system model is influenced by the external challenge by import of BSE contaminated meat and bone meal (MBM) and/or BSE incubating cattle. If this cattle system is unstable, allowing recycling and amplification of the infectious agent, the epidemic will grow. The system is characterized by its capability to prevent an external threat (challenge) and its ability to remove BSE infected cattle and/or MBM before processing (stability).

2.2. Risk factors

The assessment of the risk factors was biased in the early stages of the epidemics, due to the lack of an accurate surveillance. Subsequently, an enforced active surveillance system was put in place in 2001 in the majority of the European countries in order to carry out a more reliable analysis.

The main risks factors can be summarized as follows:

Production type and herd size play an important role in the spreading of the infection, albeit inconsistently across countries [8, 13–15].

A higher amount of compound feed leads to a higher risk of infection; the risk is higher in very large dairy farms because of the greater use of such feed.

Some studies demonstrated a higher incidence of the disease in autumn-born cattle compared to spring-born ones [16–18].

The relationship between milk yield and the risk of BSE was studied [7]; however, milk yield is only an approximation of the amount of concentrates given to cattle.

Dairy cattle have a higher risk than beef suckler herds [8, 18].

In July 1988, the ban on feeding ruminant-derived MBM to ruminants was introduced; a study on a cohort of cattle born after the ban, the area-level BSE risk was additionally associated with greater numbers of pigs per area relative to cattle [19]. These findings supported the influential role of low-level cross-contamination of cattle feed by pig feed in BSE incidence as the epidemic evolved.

2.3. Epidemiologic surveillance

The OIE established the criteria by which the BSE status of a country should be determined. These criteria are: the result of risk assessment, the implemented measures to manage the BSE risk, and the reported incidence rates (the OIE recommended an intensive passive surveillance approach).

An updated version of the BSE chapter was approved by the 68th OIE General Session in May 2000; this states that the presence of the disease can only be determined on the basis of the following criteria:

- Risk assessment that includes MBM consumption, importation of MBM, importation of potentially infected animals or ova/embryos, epidemiological situation of TSEs in a country, level of knowledge of the livestock structure, and source of animal waste, parameters of treatment and methods of production;
- Continuous awareness programs for veterinarians, farmers, and any other involved professional;
- Mandatory notification and diagnostic testing of all cattle showing clinical signs consistent with BSE;
- Continuous monitoring systems that take into account the risk factors listed and meet the criteria defined in a special appendix to the text;
- Diagnostic examination of the sample in an approved laboratory.

In January 1999, Switzerland enforced a targeted active surveillance program for BSE, performing a specific Western blot test [20] on all emergency slaughtered adult cows and on all fallen stocks. The newly enforced plan allowed us to identify a higher number of cases,

50% of which would have been missed with passive surveillance alone. This finding led the European Commission (EC) to quickly approve the use of various rapid tests to detect the PrPSc protein in CNS tissue samples.

Over the past decade, European legislation setting the minimum age of cattle at which rapid testing is to be performed reflects, in part, the dynamics of the BSE epidemic, with a progressive extension of the cutoff age.

Regulation (EC) 999/2001 [21] is the legislative response to the BSE crisis to prevent, control, and eradicate the disease and became a legal instrument in 2001. It provides a harmonized set of rules to be implemented in all member states. The rules are very strict because that what was necessary to get on top of the disease. The regulation is built on two main pillars, (i) a total feed ban which outlawed the feeding of animal proteins to all farmed animals and (ii) removal of specified risk material (SRM) from all slaughtered animals (bovines and small ruminants). Other prevention and control measures contained in the regulation are the surveillance measures:

- Before 2001: only passive surveillance (notification of cattle showing clinical symptoms consistent with BSE).
- From 1 January, 2001 [21] mandatory testing in healthy slaughtered animals aged above 30 months and in animals at risk above 24 months of age (fallen stock, emergency slaughter and animals with clinical signs at the ante mortem).
- From 1 January, 2009 [21]: all animals above 48 months (for 17 member states).
- From 1 July, 2011 [21]: healthy slaughtered animals above 72 months; animals at risk above 48 months (for 25 member states).

As of July 2013, the rapid tests for the detection of BSE cases have been suspended for the animals regularly slaughtered, and maintained for the animals above 48 months of age in at risk streams (fallen stock, emergency slaughtered and with clinical sign at *ante mortem*).

The introduction of the comprehensive active surveillance plan in 2001 marked a turning point in the capability to accurately describe the geographical distribution of BSE and the trend of the epidemic across Europe. Within a few months, the epidemiological BSE pattern (previously based on data only from passive surveillance) radically changed shape when reports of the disease unexpectedly arrived from countries other than the UK. Contrary to what was happening in Britain, where the number of BSE cases decreased by one-third (from 2301 to 1443) between 2000 and 2001, the total number of cases doubled (from 515 to 1012) in the rest of Europe and Japan also reported its first three cases. However, at least in Western Europe, 2001 also marked the beginning of the slow decline of BSE, demonstrating the efficacy of the control measures put in place since the mid-1990s: the MBM ban and the exclusion of specified risk material (SRM) from food and feed chains to mitigate the risk of exposure to infection.

Active surveillance subsequently allowed the identification of atypical forms which are probably very rare, different diseases, with epidemiological features different from those of classical BSE.

In the years to follow, the trend of C-BSE and, thus, the effectiveness of enforcement, would be monitored through the testing of huge numbers of cattle (10 million cows per year on average in the European Union). Now, some 15 years later, the problem seems to be solved, and since 2005 the European Union has been setting up an exit strategy from the crisis [22], providing for the gradual easing of the measures.

On the basis of the data collected from the information systems in place, and available from the annual reports the European Commission published between 2002 and 2014, detailed information can be gleaned about the prevalence and incidence of BSE in Europe and the temporal and geographical distribution of the disease.

3. Pathogenesis of classical and atypical BSE

The pathogenesis of C-BSE in cattle has been extensively studied, although there are still a number of knowledge gaps. After oral exposure to infective material, how prion agent crosses the epithelium is not exactly defined, but the most likely mechanism is via M-cells, a cell type present in the follicle-associated epithelium of the gut and tonsil which specializes in the transport of macromolecules across the epithelium [23]. These cells are capable of transcytosing the prion protein from the lumen of the gut into the epithelium. During the first 8 months post-infection (mpi), the earliest PrPSc accumulation is displayed by tingible body macrophages (TBM) in gut-associated lymphoid tissue (GALT) of the ileocaecal junction and the jejunum and in Peyer's patches of the ileum [24].

Moreover, at 6–10 mpi the infectivity is also located in palatine tonsils [25]. At 12 mpi, a peak of infectivity in the distal ileum is related to the number of follicles involved and the amount of PrPSc detectable in the follicular dendritic cells (FDC) and TBM, indicating an increased clearance activity of these cells. There is a second peak of infectivity at 24 mpi, where PrPSc is mainly located in TBM and FDC of jejunum and ileum and, later, a third peak of PrPSc accumulation between 32 and 40 mpi [26].

During the infection of the gut, the TSE agent can come into contact with the fine nerve fibers of the mucosal plexus of the enteric nervous system [27]. Then, through mesenteric nerves, prion proteins accumulate in the cranial coeliaco mesenteric ganglion complex and then ascend to the thoracic spinal cord via the sympathetic nervous system (e.g. splanchnic nerves) and to the brainstem and the brain via the parasympathetic nervous system (e.g. vagus nerve) and nodose ganglion.

From the thoracic spinal cord, PrPSc spreads rostrally to the cranial medulla and caudally to the cauda equine [28]. From the spinal cord, PrPSc then accumulates in the dorsal root ganglia, trigeminal, and cervical ganglia [29] and the adrenal glands and sciatic nerve have also been described as positive tissues with demonstrable prion protein accumulation [30]. Between 42 and 84 mpi PrPSc spreads to the spindles of various muscles such as the masseter, the triceps brachii, intercostal muscles, and the semitendinosus [31].

Currently, it is very difficult to hypothesize about the pathogenesis of atypical BSE, because information on the tissue distribution of PrPSc in cattle affected by atypical BSE is limited, and largely confined to experimental animals at clinical endpoint. According to experimental transmission studies, PrPSc has been reported in CNS tissues, peripheral ganglia and nerves, muscles (muscle spindles), adrenal glands, and retina for both H-BSE and L-BSE [32]. No lymphoid tissues or gastrointestinal tissues have tested positive in atypical cases. Furthermore, a study of intraspecies transmission of a case of L-type BSE suggested the possibility that prions propagated in the CNS and were spread centrifugally by nerve pathways [33].

4. Diagnosis

Historically, BSE diagnosis has always been made by the detection of characteristic vacuolation in certain anatomical regions of the formalin-fixed brain [34] by histopathological examination. In the early 1980, the discovery of scrapie-associated fibrils (SAF) and the production of antibody against SAFs were the first steps of the revolution in TSE investigations [35, 36]. At the moment, cattle populations are monitored through passive and active surveillance programs. Under passive surveillance, cattle are tested for the disease with confirmatory tests: histopathology (H&E), immunohistochemistry (IHC), Western blot (WB), or demonstration of characteristic fibrils (SAF) by electron microscopy. If a brainstem sample tests negative, the OIE manual requires that the entire brain of the animal be tested to establish differential diagnosis. Samples collected in active BSE surveillance are screened with approved rapid tests, in accordance with Regulation (EC) No. 999/2001 (European Commission, 2001) on the prevention, control, and eradication of certain TSEs. In inconclusive or positive cases, the sample is submitted to confirmatory tests.

5. Sampling

The first stage of all the current TSE diagnostic or screening tests involves the sampling of the CNS and the subsequent examination of the sampled tissue for the presence of PrPSc. In particular, the minimum sampling requirement is the brainstem, at the level of the obex [37]. This area can be accessed through the foramen magnum using a proprietary sampling spoon (**Figure 1**).

The quantity of tissue taken for testing (**Figure 2**) should be sufficient to provide the following:

A hemisection of fresh obex, for the initial rapid test.

A fixed cross-section, or hemi-section of obex for confirmatory IHC and H&E.

Sufficient remaining fresh-frozen medullary tissue (adjacent to the obex) for primary molecular testing (discriminatory WB) and possibly a range of secondary and tertiary testing (5–10 g whenever possible).

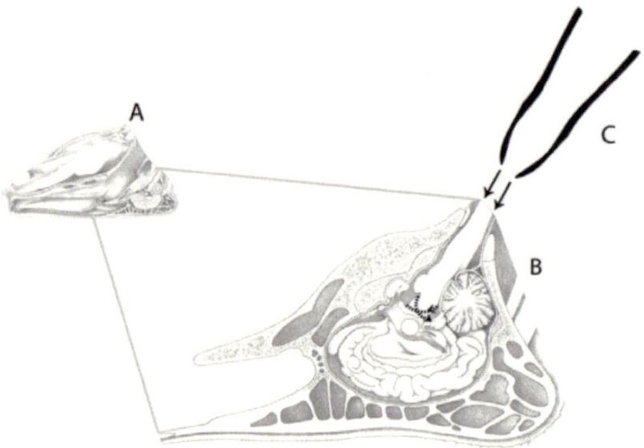

Figure 1. A) Place the disarticulated head upside down and C) using the forceps, B) insert it to the level of the foramen magnum.(http://www.oie.int/fileadmin/Home/eng/Animal_Health_in_the_World/docs/pdf/2.04.06_BSE.pdf)

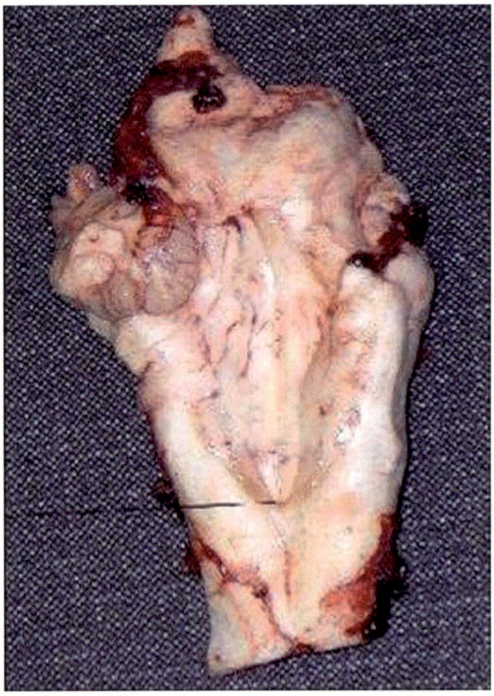

Figure 2. Fresh brainstem, at the level of the obex.

6. Rapid tests

Rapid molecular diagnostic assays became officially available in the late 1990s. With the enforcement of Regulation (EC) No. 999/2001 [21] the use of rapid tests became mandatory: many countries subsequently detected the first BSE cases. To provide dependable tools for

http://dx.doi.org/10.5772/67332

an active surveillance system, in 1999 the EC carried out the first scientific evaluation of four new rapid *post mortem* BSE tests to assess their diagnostic accuracy and analytical sensitivity on brain tissue from clinically affected bovines [38]. Subsequent EU validation exercises enhanced the estimating parameters, including test robustness on autolyzed samples and testing of negative field samples to address the test specificity and to simulate routine activity [39–41]. To date, the EC has assessed 19 rapid tests in the frame of 3 "successive" evaluations and approved 9 for survey purposes [42]. In 2009 the Community Reference Laboratory for TSEs assessed the analytical sensitivity of all the currently approved TSE rapid tests to determine their continued suitability for active surveillance plans [43]. The analytical sensitivity study was then evaluated by the European Food Safety Authority (EFSA) [44, 45] on the basis of current EFSA requirements for the evaluation of TSE rapid *post mortem* tests [46]. In that context, the lowest limit of detection (LOD) of rapid tests approved for the diagnosis of classical BSE in bovines was assessed. The rapid tests with an LOD poorer than $2\log_{10}$ as compared to the best-performing assay could not be recommended for use in the frame of BSE monitoring in cattle within the EU. Recent studies [47] demonstrate the suitability of BSE EU-approved rapid tests also for the detection of both L- and H-type BSE. Despite the evidence of clear differences in relative analytical sensitivity, the LOD of rapid tests applied on BSE atypical nervous tissues meets EFSA criteria for BSE monitoring purposes.

According to EU Regulation 999/2001, for the purposes of carrying out the active only the following methods shall be used as rapid tests for the monitoring of BSE in bovine animals:

The immuno-blotting test based on a Western blotting procedure for the detection of the Proteinase K-resistant fragment PrPSc (Prionics®—Check WESTERN Prionics AG, Schlieren-Zurich, Switzerland).

The microplate-based immunoassay for the detection of PrPSc (TSE Version 3, Enfer Scientific®, Newhall, Naas, County Kildare, Ireland).

The sandwich immunoassay for PrPSc detection (short assay protocol) carried out following denaturation and concentration steps (TeSeE™ Purification-Detection SAP Test Kit, Bio-Rad Laboratories, Marnes-La-Coquette, France).

The microplate-based immunoassay (ELISA) which detects Proteinase K-resistant PrPSc with monoclonal antibodies (Prionics®—Check LIA BSE Antigen Test Kit, Prionics AG, Schlieren-Zurich, Switzerland).

The immunoassay using a chemical polymer for selective PrPSc capture and a monoclonal detection antibody directed against conserved regions of the PrP molecule (IDEXX® HerdChek BSE Antigen Test Kit, EIA & IDEXX® HerdChek BSE-Scrapie Antigen Test Kit, EIA, Westbrook, ME, USA).

The lateral-flow immunoassay using two different monoclonal antibodies to detect proteinase K-resistant PrP fractions (Prionics®—Check PrioSTRIP, Prionics AG, Schlieren-Zurich, Switzerland).

The two-sided immunoassay using two different monoclonal antibodies directed against two epitopes presented in a highly unfolded state of bovine PrPSc (BetaPrion® BSE EIA Test Kit, AJ Roboscreen, Leipzig, Germany).

A part from the *Prionics®* Western blotting and lateral-flow immunoassay, the remaining approved tests are based on semi-quantitative ELISA methods that produce a qualitative result relative to a cutoff value. They include a PK digestion step to unmask cryptic epitopes, except for the *IDEXX HerdChek® BSE-scrapie EIA*, which relies on conformational detection technology using a specific aggregate specific capture ligand on a dextran polymer (Seprion ligand technology, Microsens Biotechnologies, London, UK) [48]. The lateral-flow immunoassay *Prionics®—Check PrioSTRIP* produces results that can be interpreted by a computerized *PrioSCAN®* software to minimize subjectivity, although a visual interpretation by two independent readers is also validated. The *Prionics®—Check Western* is based on a Western blotting procedure. It is both a qualitative and quantitative test, as it distinguishes PrPSc in non-, mono-, and diglycoforms while expressing their respective quantitative ratio and migration positions. The diagnostic criteria for positive results are based on the exhibition of a three-band signal, the top one corresponding to a protein with an approximate molecular weight of 30 kD. Signal intensity decreases from top to bottom, but the higher band should be clearly visible immediately under the PK band.

7. Histopathological examination

The histological examination is performed on formalin-fixed, paraffin-embedded brain sections that are stained with hematoxylin and eosin (H&E). The histological C-BSE changes in the CNS, that are visible using an optical microscopy, are vacuolation of gray matter neuropil (spongiform change) and/or vacuolation of neurons, with a predilection for certain neuroanatomic locations [34, 49]; astrocytosis and neuronal degeneration may also be present [50]. The target areas at the level of the obex for the diagnosis of BSE are the solitary tract nucleus (NST) and the spinal tract nucleus of the trigeminal nerve (NSTV) (**Figures 3** and **4**). Moreover, vacuolation could be also present in central gray matter of the midbrain and mild spongiform changes of the neuropil could be observed in some cattle at the level of the thalamus. In natural cases of L-BSE (BASE), spongiosis is not consistently found in the brainstem, at the level of the obex or in more rostral areas. The frontal, parietal, and occipital cortices are apparently spared, and no vacuolation is detected in the olfactory bulb, piriform cortex, and hippocampus [4]. In experimental cases, a more severe involvement of central gray matter (periaqueductal gray) and rostral colliculus but not the vestibular nuclear complex is observed. Additional brain areas, including the olfactory areas, amygdalae, hippocampi, and dorsal horns of spinal cords, are severely involved. Ventral and dorsal roots do not show major pathological changes [51]. In experimental H-type BSE, vacuolar changes are generally observed in all the brain areas. The major vacuolation appears in the thalamic nuclei and neuropil of the central gray matter of the

http://dx.doi.org/10.5772/67332

midbrain, and mild vacuolation is found in the caudal cerebral and cerebellar cortices. In the vestibular and pontine nuclei, spongy changes are not as prominent as in the other brainstem nuclei [52].

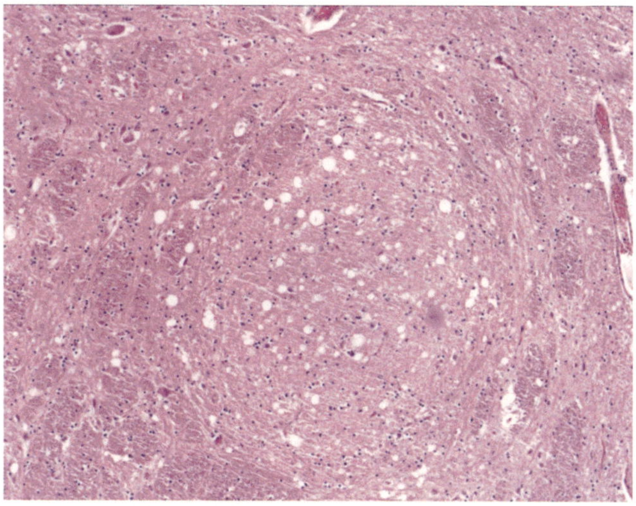

Figure 3. H&E, nucleus of the solitary tract of C-BSE: presence of spongiosis in the neuropil (20X).

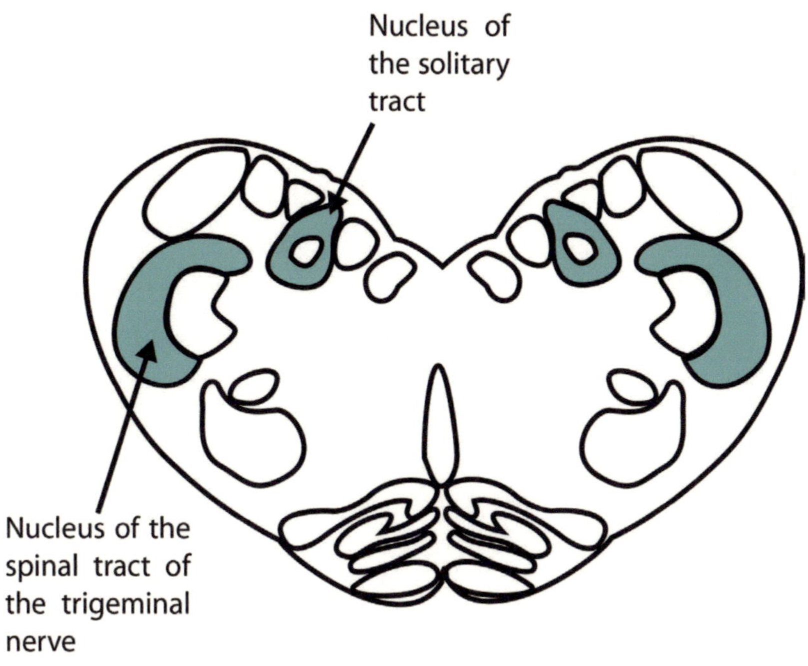

Figure 4. Section of the obex showing the target nuclei for BSE diagnosis.

8. Immunohistochemistry

Immunohistochemical analysis is performed on paraffin-embedded brain tissues in order to highlight the presence of PrPSc accumulation. The samples are deparaffinated, rehydrated, pretreated with 98% formic acid, and autoclaved at 121°C, then incubated at 4°C with monoclonal primary antibody, incubated with avidin-biotin-peroxydase, reacted with chromogen 3-3′ diaminobenzidine (DAB), and counterstained with Mayer's hemalum. Different immunohistochemical types of PrPSc deposition can be observed in the brain of C-BSE-affected cattle [53]: glial type labeling with PrPSc deposits branching out from the nucleus of glial cells on their processes conferring them a stellate appearance is predominantly in central gray matter and cerebral lamina and also within medial pontine nuclei in cerebral cortex, thalamus, and obex; a granular type that is characterized by granular PrPSc accumulations in the neuropil is commonly found in the neuropil of gray matter nuclei such as dorsal motor nucleus of vagus nerve (DMVN), NST, and in thalamic nuclei; intraneuronal type with PrPSc immunoreactivity throughout the neuronal cytoplasm is often observed in DMVN, reticular formation, olivary nuclei, vestibular complex, pontine, and thalamic nuclei and hypothalamus; perineuronal type, consisting in PrPSc deposits around individual neuronal perikarya and neuritis in caudate and putamen nuclei of basal ganglia and in DMVN; linear tract characterized by PrPSc deposits along neuronal processes in particular at the level of reticular formation of the brainstem; coalescing type seemingly arising from the merging of granular PrPSc deposits to form amorphous or mesh-like masses and intraglial type with fine punctate PrPSc adiacent to glial nuclei (**Figure 5**).

In the matter of natural cases of BASE, a distinctive feature is the presence of PrPSc deposition prevalently in the more rostral portions of the brain rather than occurs in C-BSE. At the level of the brainstem, the prevalent PrPSc deposition patterns are the punctate and granular

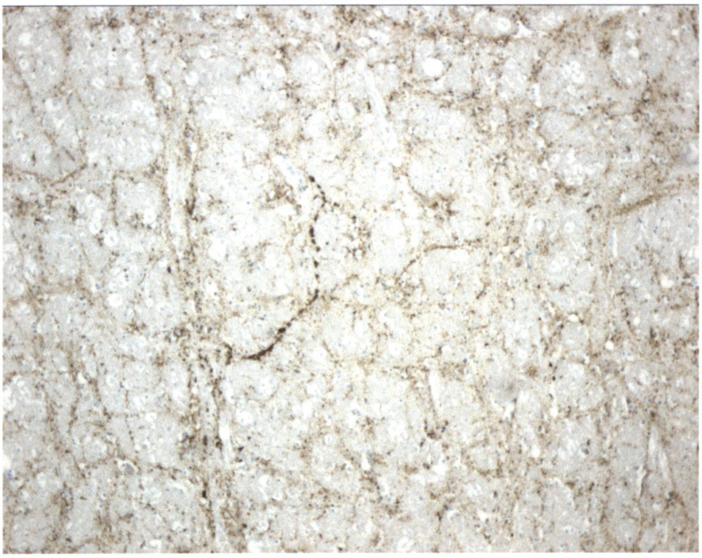

Figure 5. IHC, patterns of PrPSc of C-BSE, characterized by granular deposits and linear tracts (10X).

http://dx.doi.org/10.5772/67332

types, which are mildly present in the hypoglossal and olivary nucleus and moderately present at the level of DMVN nucleus, NST, NSTV, and reticular formation [54]. Glial, intraneuronal, perineuronal, and linear tracts are also frequent in BASE cases in different brain areas. Another characteristic of BASE cases is the presence of PrP-positive amyloid plaques; they appear as dense, unicentric, or less frequently multicentric round structures up to 25 μm in diameter with a pale core and a dark radial periphery. They are predominantly located in the thalamus, subcortical white matter, in deeper layers of cerebral cortexes and in the olfactory bulb (**Figure 6**) [4]. In experimental BASE cattle, abundant amyloid PrP-plaques are observed in subcortical white matter and in deep gray nuclei, as observed in natural BASE cases. No PrP-plaques are seen in the olfactory glomeruli, the cerebellum, or the spinal cord. Perineuronal pattern of PrPSc is also seen in ventral horn neurons of the spinal cord and in the dorsal root ganglion cells [51].

As regards natural H-type BSE, in the brainstem, granular, intraneuronal, linear, intraglial, and punctate PrPSc deposits are the most characteristic types, mainly detected at the level of the DMVN, NST, NSTV, and in the reticular formation; however, there is some variability in PrPSc distribution among different H-BSE cases [54] (**Figure 7**). Regarding experimental H-type BSE, large amounts of PrPSc are diffusely deposited in the cerebral cortex, basal ganglia, thalamus, hypothalamus, brainstem, and spinal cord. The most conspicuous type of PrPSc deposition is fine or coarse particulate-type deposition in the neuropil of the gray matter throughout the brain and spinal cord. Linear, perineuronal, and intraneuronal types of PrPSc staining are observed in the cerebral cortex, basal ganglia, thalamus, and brainstem. Glial-type PrPSc deposition is predominantly identified in the cerebral cortex, basal ganglia, thalamus, hypothalamus, and hippocampus and often in the cerebellar cortex, but is not

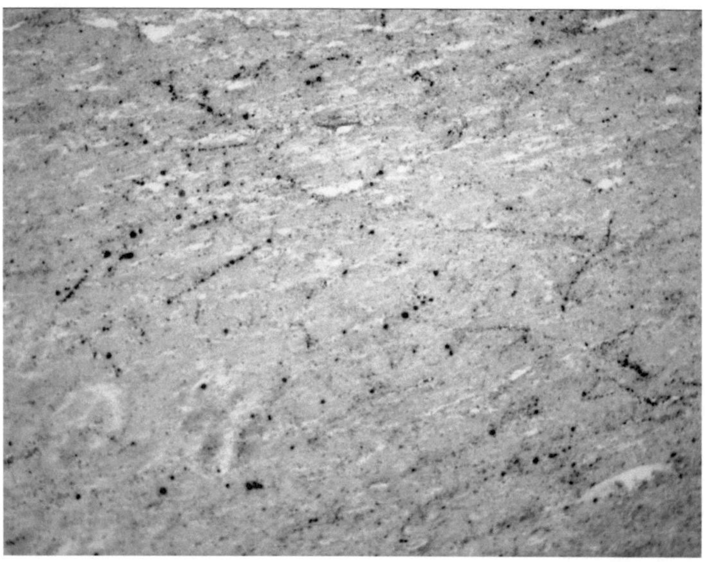

Figure 6. IHC, patterns of PrPSc of L-type BSE (BASE), characterized by amyloid plaques, granular deposits, and linear tracts (10X).

visible in the brainstem and spinal cord. Intraglial-type PrPSc deposition is very consistent throughout the white matter of the CNS and spinal cord. Some animals show the presence of PrPSc-positive plaques scattered throughout the cerebral white matter [52].

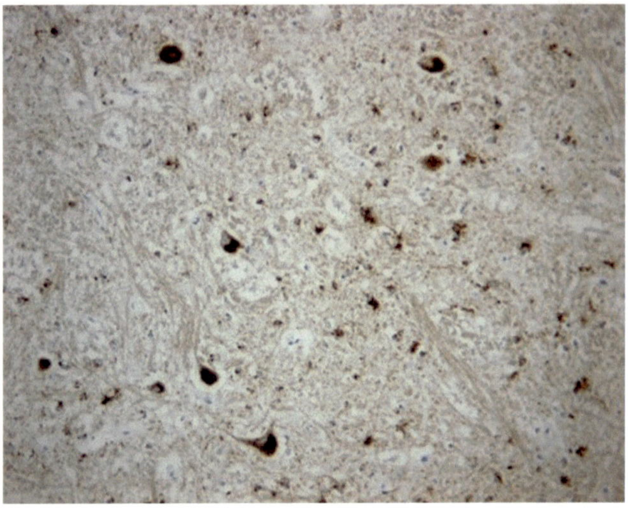

Figure 7. IHC, pattern of PrPSc of H-type BSE, characterized by intraneuronal deposits (10X).

9. Western blotting

The WB is an immunobiochemical technique widely used for the diagnosis of the prion diseases. Different WB methods have been developed since it was instituted active surveillance system in Europe, some used as screening tests and other to confirm the suspect cases identified by active but also through passive surveillance. These techniques are based on the immunodetection of the PrPSc at the level of the medulla oblongata. WB methods are very versatile since they can be applied on fresh, frozen, and autolytic tissue [55]. The SAF-immunoblot was the first such method for use in BSE diagnosis. It has similar diagnostic sensitivity to the IHC techniques, and remains the method of choice, along with IHC, for the confirmation of suspect BSE cases. It is a highly sensitive method using a large mass (2–4 g) of material and several steps to concentrate PrPSc. Alternative less time-consuming and less costly methods are now available in the different TSE Reference Laboratories in Europe to confirm the BSE cases. Unlike the published methods, in-house test applied for confirmatory purposes must be validated and their analytical sensitivity, together with the commercial tests, is continuously monitored by the TSE European Union Reference Laboratory (APHA, UK) through annual ring trial. The protocol of SAF-immunoblotting includes briefly the preparation of the homogenates from brainstem and the digestion of the samples with proteinase K. After ultracentrifugation step, the pellet is dissolved in Laemmli Buffer and an equivalent of 10 mg of wet tissue is loaded on SDS-polyacrylamide gels and, after separation, proteins are transferred onto PVDF membrane. The detection of PrPSc is performed by monoclonal antibody anti-PrP and the presence of immunosignals is revealed by a phosphatase-conjugated anti-mouse IgG, developed using a chemiluminescence system and visualized on hyperfilm ECL. In the positive cases, the confirmatory WB shows the presence of PrPSc characterized by an electrophoretic pattern consists of three bands and corresponding to the di-, mono- and nonglycosylated forms, migrating at approximately 30, 25, and 19 kDa, respectively. No PrP signals are present in the bovine cases confirmed as negative since the PrPC is completely digested by proteinase K (**Figure 8**). The application of immunoblotting methods is very important to evaluate also the molecular features of PrPSc and so to discriminate between classical and atypical BSE isolates. The H-type is characterized by a significantly higher molecular size of the nonglycosylated PrPSc form and a conventional glycopattern, while the L-type or BASE, has only a slightly lower molecular size of the nonglycosylated and a predominance of the monoglycosylated moiety (**Figure 9**).

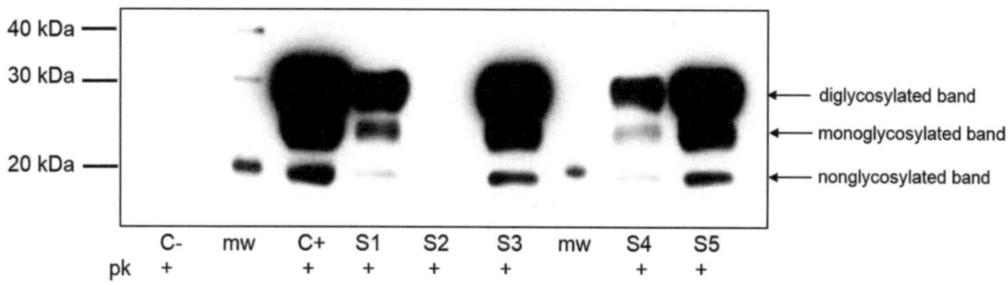

Figure 8. Western blotting analysis of positive and negative BSE cases. C−: negative BSE control; C+: positive BSE control; lanes S1, S3, S4 and S5: positive BSE samples; lane S2: negative BSE sample. Mw: molecular markers. Immunodetection was performed by monoclonal antibody 6H4.

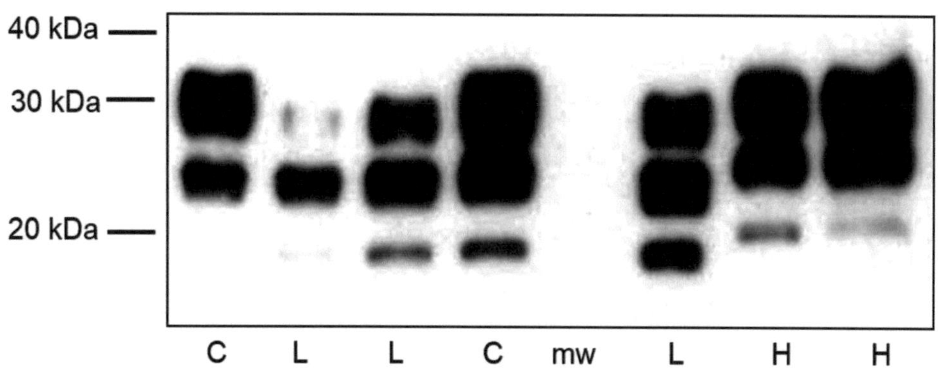

Figure 9. Western blotting analysis of PrPSc from classical and atypical BSE cases. C: classical BSE; L: low-type BSE; H: high-type BSE. Mw: molecular markers. Immunodetection was performed by monoclonal antibody 6H4.

10. Scrapie-associated fibrils

Electron microscopy highlights the BSE-associated fibrils, the bovine equivalent of SAF. The fibrils are composed of PrPSc and they are extracted from fresh, frozen, or formalin-fixed nervous tissue with the use of a homogenization treatment, differential centrifugations and digestion with proteinase K and colored with phosphotungstic acid. The observation to the electron microscopy allows us to highlight the fibrils with simple or double helix structure of 100–500 nm of length.

11. *In vitro* amplification techniques

A major problem for the effective management of animal prion diseases is the lack of rapid high-throughput assay to detect low levels of prions for the ante-mortem diagnosis of these diseases. In prion-affected animals, PrPSc is detected in a variety of peripheral tissues and body fluids, including blood, urine, saliva, cerebrospinal fluid (CSF), and nasal fluids; however, a validated diagnostic test is not available, yet. Current biochemical or immunocytochemical assays are roughly sensitive and might provide inconclusive results and consequently not reliable in a clinical or a preclinical setting of prion infected hosts in contrast to *in vitro* amplification techniques that can be used to determine whether a tissue contains any prion seeding activity. Two very efficient procedures to amplify prions in a test tube have emerged in the last decades, such as protein misfolding cyclic amplification (PMCA) or real-time quaking-induced conversion (RT-QuIC). Both depend on the detection of PrP structural conversion and polymerization upon addition of PrPSc "seeds" contained in the infected samples. These methods are usually more sensitive than the bioassay by two to three orders of magnitude, and endpoint titration can be performed in a format similar to the bioassay [56].

11.1. Protein misfolding cyclic amplification

In 2001, Soto and colleagues described a new type of *in vitro* prion conversion reaction called PMCA which greatly improved the efficiency and sensitivity compared to the initial conversion reactions of the prion protein in cell-free environment (cell-free conversion assay) [57]. The prion amplification by PMCA is based on repeated cycles of incubation and sonication during which increasing multimers of PrPSc are fragmented by sonication to induce formation and increase the effective concentration of PrPSc aggregates. In the typical reaction of PMCA, brain extracts are used as a source of PrPC. The cyclic nature of the system and the possibility to refresh the substrate at each round enables the performance of as many cycles as required to reach the amplification state needed for the detection of PrPSc in a given sample. In these conditions, the PrPSc can be amplified to detectable levels by immunoblotting. PMCA allows the detection of minute amounts of PrPSc in biological tissues or fluid samples including blood, urine, feces, or cerebrospinal fluid from many prion-infected species. This method has sufficient sensitivity for PrPSc detection in blood in the asymptomatic stages of prion diseases [58]. In recent years, this method has become very useful to study different aspects of the prion protein such as to understand the molecular mechanism of prions' replication, the cellular factors involved in the propagation of the prions, and the still unknown aspects related to the prion strains and their trans-species conversion characteristics upon passage.

Thus, PMCA has promise not only as a prion detection assay, but also as a tool to study the mechanism of prion-induced PrP conversion. Despite the progress that PMCA has facilitated in prion research, the fact that the amplification process to detect prions relies on sonication, makes it difficult to control. In addition, the limitations of PMCA include the time required to achieve optimal sensitivity and the requirement for brain-derived PrPSc as the amplification substrate. As a result, there was a need to develop an accurate, high throughput diagnostic that is automated and can be easily used in a routine diagnostic lab.

11.2. Real-time quaking-induced conversion

To avoid technical complexities associated with PMCA reactions, a new practical prion assay, quaking-induced conversion (QuIC), has been developed by Atarashi et al. [59]. The QuIC method uses recombinant prion protein (rPrPSc) produced in bacteria as a substrate for seeded polymerization and shaking instead of sonication is performed to break the generated polymers and provide new seeds for conversion in amplification rounds. As in the amyloid seeding assay, ASA, polymerization of rPrPSc into amyloid fibers can be detected by a fluorescence shift in the dye thioflavin T (ThT). The formation of these prion-seeded amyloid fibers is detected in real time by reading ThT fluorescence over time. In its real-time and multiwell plate format, the RT-QuIC has the potential to be used for the high throughput screening of samples. Since bacterially expressed rPrPSc can be produced rapidly in high purity, using the rPrP-QuIC method solves the difficulty of using the brain PrPSc as the amplification substrate. Moreover, the fact that rPrPSc can be easily mutated allows investigation into the role of specific sequences or amino acids in the conversion reaction and accelerates studies on the detection of prions. This test can be quantitative and sensitive as *in vivo* testing [56] and has been adapted to different types of TSE. The RT-QuIC assay provides rapid and highly sensitive discrimination of prion-infected and uninfected brain tissues. Furthermore, the technique has proved sensitive in detecting prions in several infected tissues and in fluids such as cerebrospinal fluid, saliva, nasal fluids and blood [59, 60]. This method does not detect prion infectivity in a given tissue, but allow detection of a seeding activity potentially associated with prion replication. Under defined conditions, this method can be used to quantitatively estimate prion concentration in fluids and tissues of interest. Indeed, based upon the quantitative correlation between prion seed concentration and the lag time to the start of the conversion reaction, qRT-QuIC allows quantification of prion infectivity in tissues, body fluids, and excreta [61]. For quantification, the amplified PrPSc signal can be compared with that seen in endpoint titrated material run in the same conditions (such as brain homogenate from animals at the terminal stage of disease) or to PrP calibration curves. By analogy with animal bioassays, RT-QuIC assay can titrate the seeding activity in endpoint diluted samples [56, 59]. Serial dilutions of a given sample are used as seeds and the seeding dose (SD) giving 50% ThT-positive replicate reactions (SD50), that is, the 50% endpoint dilution, is estimated. The SD50 is analogous to the 50% lethal dose (LD50) determined in an endpoint dilution animal bioassay. However, RT-QuIC has several major advantages over animal bioassays, including practicality, high-throughput potential, rapidity, and reduced cost. The quantitative aspect of qRT-QuIC suggests that it can provide a reliable assessment of anti-prion therapy *in vivo* in order to follow the effects of therapy on progression of prion diseases. Moreover, since qRT-QuIC provides an ultra-sensitive method for quantifying pathological amyloid aggregate seeds, this technique may also be applicable to other disease-associated proteins rich in β-pleated structures that bind T and that show seeded aggregation. Some prion strain types are known to be fairly resistant to amplification by either PMCA or RT-QuIC. However, recent studies have adapted RT-QuIC assays to the sensitive detection and discrimination of the C-BSE, L-BSE, and H-BSE (**Figure 10**) [62, 63]. Brain tissue from cattle affected by these strains were tested by the RT-QuIC assay and found that all these forms can be detected and distinguished using particular rPrPSc substrates. RT-QuIC tests have been adapted to the detection of many types of prion seeding activity; however, there are still some missing outcomes for the ante-mortem diagnosis of TSE in animals of farm interest:

- identify the most noninvasive and economic biological peripheral matrix for performing the prion test in living subjects;
- recognize classical and atypical forms of PrPSc by a unique protocol for obtaining a single diagnostic assay for TSE diseases;
- detect PrPSc from all biological fluids by removing soluble components that would inhibit the assay;
- collect pre-clinical and clinical data from subjects resulted PrPSc positive in peripheral matrices to better define the peripheral TSE infectivity distribution.

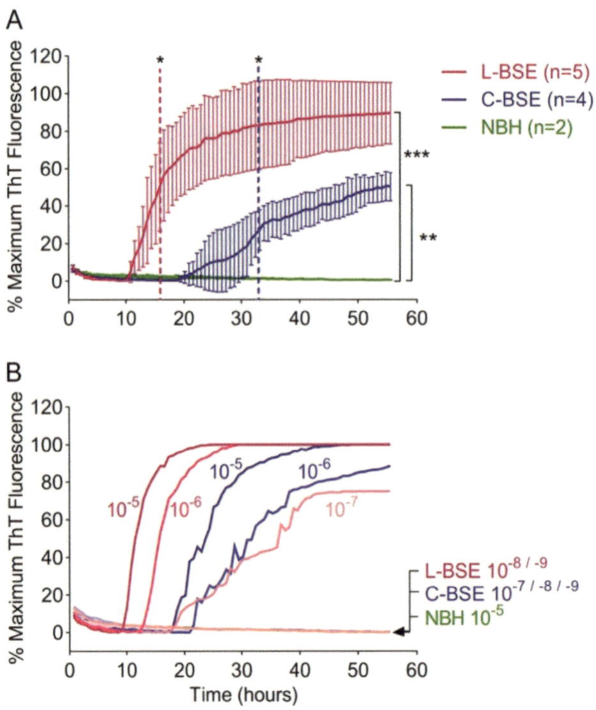

Figure 10. RT-QuIC sensitivity for C-BSE and L-BSE detection. (A) L-BSE-infected (magenta), C-BSE-infected (blue), or normal negative control (NBH, green) 10^{-5} brain tissue dilutions were used to seed quadruplicate RT-QuIC reactions using the Ha-S rPrPSen substrate. (B) Serial dilutions (10^{-5}–10^{-9}) of C-BSE-infected or L-BSE-infected brain tissue or a 10^{-5} dilution of uninfected brain tissue were used to seed quadruplicate RT-QuIC reactions with Ha-S rPrPSen as the substrate. The data show the average ThT fluorescence of four replicate wells. Each ThT reading is indicated as the percentage of the maximum value achievable by the plate readers as a function of reaction time (Orrù et al. 2015).

http://dx.doi.org/10.5772/67332

Author details

Barbara Iulini[1,2], Elena Vallino Costassa[1,2]*, Cristiano Corona[1], Daniela Meloni[1], Alessandra Favole[1], Maria Mazza[1], Maria Caramelli[1], Cristiana Maurella[1] and Cristina Casalone[1]

* Address all correspondence to: elena.vallinocostassa@izsto.it

1 Istituto Zooprofilattico Sperimentale del Piemonte, Liguria e Valle d'Aosta, Turin, Italy

2 Coauthors

References

[1] Bruce ME, Will RG, Ironside JW, McConnell I, Drummond D, Suttie A, McCardle L, Chree A, Hope J, Birkett C, Cousens S, Fraser H, Bostock CJ. Transmissions to mice indicate that 'new variant' CJD is caused by the BSE agent. Nature. 1997; 389(6650): 498–501.

[2] Collinge J, Sidle KC, Meads J, Ironside J, Hill AF. Molecular analysis of prion strain variation and the aetiology of 'new variant' CJD. Nature. 1996; 383(6602): 685–90.

[3] Scott MR, Will R, Ironside J, Nguyen HO, Tremblay P, DeArmond SJ, Prusiner SB. Compelling transgenetic evidence for transmission of bovine spongiform encephalopathy prions to humans. Proc Natl Acad Sci USA.1999; 96(26): 15137–42.

[4] Casalone C., Zanusso G., Acutis P.L., Ferrari S., Capucci L., Tagliavini F., Monaco S., Caramelli M. Identification of a second bovine amyloidotic spongiform encephalopathy: molecular similarities with sporadic Creutzfeld-Jakob disease. Proc Natl Acad Sci USA. 2004; 101: 3065–70.

[5] Biacabe AG, Laplanche JL, Ryder S, Baron T. Distinct molecular phenotypes in bovine prion diseases. EMBO Rep. 2004; 5(1): 110–15.

[6] Ducrot C, Abrial D, Calavas D, Carpenter T. A spatio-temporal analysis of BSE cases born before and after the reinforced feed ban in France. Vet Res. 2005; 36(5–6): 839–53.

[7] La Bonnardière C, Calavas D, Abrial D, Morignat E, Ducrot C. Estimating the trend of the French BSE epidemic over six birth cohorts through the analysis of abattoir screening in 2001 and 2002. Vet Res. 2004; 35(3): 299–308.

[8] Ru G, Maurella C, Ponti AM, Ingravalle F, Caramelli M. Epidemiological study of the decline of BSE in Italy. Vet Rec. 2007; 161(15): 511–14.

[9] Wilesmith JW, Ryan JB, Stevenson MA, Morris RS, Pfeiffer DU, Lin D, Jackson R, Sanson RL. Temporal aspects of the epidemic of bovine spongiform encephalopathy in Great Britain: holding-associated risk factors for the disease. Vet Rec. 2000; 147(12): 319–25.

[10] Wilesmith JW, Wells GA, Cranwell MP, Ryan JB. Bovine spongiform encephalopathy: epidemiological studies. Vet Rec. 1988; 123(25): 638–44.

[11] Salman M, Silano V, Heim D, Kreysad J. Geographical BSE risk assessment and its impact on disease detection and dissemination. Prev Vet Med. 2012; 105: 255–264.

[12] Opinion of the Scientific Panel on Biological Hazards on the revision of the Geographical BSE risk assessment (GBR) methodology. EFSA J. 2007; 463: 1–3.

[13] Donnelly CA, Ferguson NM, Ghani AC, Woolhouse MEJ, Watt CJ, Anderson RM. The epidemiology of BSE in cattle herds in Great Britain. I. Epidemiological processes, demography of cattle and approaches to control by culling. Philos Trans R Soc Lond, B, Biol Sci. 1997; 352: 781–801.

[14] Ducrot C, Arnold M, de Koeijer A, Heim D, Calavas D. Review on the epidemiology and dynamics of BSE epidemics. Vet Res. 2008; 39(4): 15. doi: 10.1051/vetres:2007053.

[15] Griffin JM. BSE and British cattle exports. Vet Rec. 1997; 141(11): 286–87.

[16] Hoinville LJ, Wilesmith JW, Richards MS. An investigation of risk factors for cases of bovine spongiform encephalopathy born after the introduction of the 'feed ban'. Vet Rec. 1995; 136(13): 312–18.

[17] Wells GA, Scott AC, Johnson CT, Gunning RF, Hancock RD, Jeffrey M, Dawson M, Bradley R. A novel progressive spongiform encephalopathy in cattle. Vet Rec. 1987; 121(18): 419–20.

[18] Wilesmith JW, Ryan JB. Bovine spongiform encephalopathy: recent observations on the age-specific incidences. Vet Rec. 1992; 130(22): 491–92.

[19] Stevenson MA, Morris RS, Lawson AB, Wilesmith JW, Ryan JBM, Jackson R. Area-level risks for BSE in British cattle before and after the July 1988 meat and bone meal feed ban. Prev Vet Med. 2005; 69(1–2): 129–44.

[20] Doherr MG, Oesch B, Moser M, Vandevelde M, Heim D. Targeted surveillance for bovine spongiform encephalopathy. Vet Rec. 1999; 145(23): 672.

[21] European Commission Regulation (EC) No. 999/2001 of the European Parliament and of the Council of 22 May 2001 laying down rules for the prevention, control and eradication of certain transmissible spongiform encephalopathies. Official Journal of the European Union. L147: 1–40 and further modifications.

[22] The TSE Roadmap COM (2005) 322 CE. Available at: https://ec.europa.eu/food/sites/food/files/safety/docs/biosafety_food-borne-disease_tse_road-map1.pdf

[23] Heppner FL, Christ AD, Klein MA, Prinz M, Fried M, Kraehenbuhl JP, Aguzzi A. Transepithelial prion transport by M cells. Nat Med. 2001; 7(9): 976–77.

[24] Terry LA, Marsh S, Ryder SJ, Hawkins SA, Wells GA, Spencer YI. Detection of disease-specific PrP in the distal ileum of cattle exposed orally to the agent of bovine spongiform encephalopathy. Vet Rec. 2003; 152(13): 387–92.

[25] Wells GA, Spiropoulos J, Hawkins SA, Ryder SJ. Pathogenesis of experimental bovine spongiform encephalopathy: preclinical infectivity in tonsil and observations on the distribution of lingual tonsil in slaughtered cattle. Vet Rec. 2005; 156(13): 401–7.

[26] Hoffmann C, Eiden M, Kaatz M, Keller M, Ziegler U, Rogers R, Hills B, Balkema-Buschmann A, van Keulen L, Jacobs JG, Groschup MH. BSE infectivity in jejunum, ileum and ileocaecal junction of incubating cattle. Vet Res. 2011; 7(42): 21. doi: 10.1186/1297-9716-42-21.

[27] Jeffrey M, González L, Espenes A, et al. Transportation of prion protein across the intestinal mucosa of scrapie-susceptible and scrapie-resistant sheep. J Pathol. 2006; 209(1): 4–14.

[28] Balkema-Buschmann A, Fast C, Kaatz M, Eiden M, Ziegler U, McIntyre L, Keller M, Hills B, Groschup MH. Pathogenesis of classical and atypical BSE in cattle. Prev Vet Med. 2011; 102(2): 112–17. doi: 10.1016/j.prevetmed.2011.04.006.

[29] Arnold ME, Ryan JB, Konold T, et al. Estimating the temporal relationship between PrPSc detection and incubation period in experimental bovine spongiform encephalopathy of cattle. J Gen Virol. 2007; 88(Pt 11): 3198–208.

[30] Espinosa JC, Morales M, Castilla J, Rogers M, Torres JM. Progression of prion infectivity in asymptomatic cattle after oral bovine spongiform encephalopathy challenge. J Gen Virol. 2007; 88(Pt 4): 1379–83.

[31] Okada H, Miyazawa K, Fukuda S, Iwamaru Y, Imamura M, Masujin K, Matsuura Y, Fujii T, Fujii K, Kageyama S, Yoshioka M, Murayama Y, Yokoyama T. The presence of disease-associated prion protein in skeletal muscle of cattle infected with classical bovine spongiform encephalopathy. J Vet Med Sci. 2014; 76(1): 103–7.

[32] Protocol for further laboratory investigations into the distribution of infectivity of Atypical BSE. EFSA J. 2014; 12(7): 3798.

[33] Iwamaru Y, Imamura M, Matsuura Y, Masujin K, Shimizu Y, Shu Y, Kurachi M, Kasai K, Murayama Y, Fukuda S, Onoe S, Hagiwara K, Yamakawa Y, Sata T, Mohri S, Okada H, Yokoyama T. Accumulation of L-type bovine prions in peripheral nerve tissues. Emerg Infect Dis. 2010; 16(7): 1151–54. doi: 10.3201/eid1607.091882.

[34] Wells GA, Hancock RD, Cooley WA, Richards MS, Higgins RJ, David GP. Bovine spongiform encephalopathy: diagnostic significance of vacuolar changes in selected nuclei of the medulla oblongata. Vet Rec. 1989; 125(21): 521–4.

[35] Merz PA, Somerville RA, Wisniewski HM, Iqbal K. Abnormal fibrils from scrapie-infected brain. Acta Neuropathol. 1981; 54(1): 63–74.

[36] Diringer H, Rahn HC, Bode L. Antibodies to protein of scrapie-associated fibrils. Lancet. 1984; 2: 345.

[37] Sampling Guidance Document v2 September 2013 TSE EURL. Available at: https://science.vla.gov.uk/tse-lab-net/documents/tse-oie-rl-samp.pdf

[38] Moynagh J, Schimmel H, Kramer GN. The evaluation of tests for the diagnosis of transmissible spongiform encephalopathy in bovines. Nature. 1999; 400: 105.

[39] Opinion of the Scientific Steering Committee on the field trial evaluation of the evaluation of two new rapid BSE post mortem tests. 2003; Available at: http://ec.europa.eu/food/fs/sc/ssc/out316_en.pdf.

[40] Wolfang P, Pavel V. The field trial of seven new rapid post mortem tests for the diagnosis of bovine spongiform encephalopathy in bovines. 2004; Available at: http://irmm.jrc.ec.europa.eu/activities/TSE_testing/Documents/globalreportphaseii.pdf.

[41] Scientific Report of the European Food Safety Authority on the evaluation of two rapid post mortem BSE tests. EFSA J. 2005; 48: 1–10.

[42] European Commission Regulation (EC) No 956/2010 of the European Parliament and of the Council amending Annex X to Regulation (EC) No. 999/2001 of the European Parliament and of the Council as regards the list of rapid tests. J European Union. L 279: 10–12.

[43] Webster K, Flowers M, Cassar C, Bayliss D. Determination of analytical sensitivity (detection limit) for currently approved TSE rapid tests. 2009; Available: http://www.efsa.europa.eu/de/scdocs/doc/1436.pdf

[44] Scientific Opinion of the European Food Safety Authority on the analytical sensitivity of approved TSE rapid tests. EFSA J. 2009; 7(12): 1436.

[45] Scientific Opinion of the European Food Safety Authority on the analytical sensitivity of approved TSE rapid tests—new data for assessment of two rapid tests. EFSA J. 2010; 8: 1591.

[46] Scientific Opinion of the European Food Safety Authority on a protocol for the evaluation of new rapid BSE post mortem tests. EFSA J. 2007; 508: 1–20.

[47] Meloni D, Davidse A, Langeveld JPM, Varello K, Casalone C, et al. EU-Approved rapid tests for bovine spongiform encephalopathy detect atypical forms: a study for their sensitivities. PLoS ONE. 2012; 7(9).

[48] Grassi J, Maillet S, Simon S, Morel N. Progress and limits of TSE diagnostic tools. Vet Res. 2008; 39: 33.

[49] Wells G.AH, Wilesmith JW. The neuropathology and epidemiology of bovine spongiform encephalopathy. Brain Pathol.1995; 5: 91–103

[50] Simmons MM, Harris P, Jeffrey M, Meek SC, Blamire IW, Wells GA. BSE in Great Britain: consistency of the neurohistopathological findings in two random annual samples of clinically suspect cases. Vet Rec. 1996; 138: 175–7.

[51] Lombardi G, Casalone C, D' Angelo A, Gelmetti D, Torcoli G, Barbieri I, Corona C, Fasoli E, Farinazzo A, Fiorini M, Gelati M, Iulini B, Tagliavini F, Ferrari S, Caramelli M, Monaco S, Capucci L, Zanusso G. Intraspecies transmission of BASE induces clinical dullness and amyotrophic changes. PLoS Pathog. 2008; 4(5):e1000075. doi: 10.1371/journal.ppat.1000075.

[52] Okada H, Iwamaru Y, Imamura M, Masujin K, Matsuura Y, Shimizu Y, Kasai K, Mohri S, Yokoyama T, Czub S. Experimental H-type bovine spongiform encephalopathy characterized by plaques and glial- and stellate-type prion protein deposits. Vet Res. 2011; 42: 79. doi: 10.1186/1297-9716-42-79.

[53] Casalone C, Caramelli M, Crescio MI, Spencer YI, Simmons MM. BSE immunohistochemical patterns in the brainstem: a comparison between UK and Italian cases. Acta Neuropathol. 2006; 111(5): 444–9.

[54] Porcario C, Hall SM, Martucci F, Corona C, Iulini B, Perazzini AZ, Acutis PL, Hamir AN, Loiacono CM, Greenlee JJ, Richt JA, Caramelli M, Casalone C. 2011. Evaluation of two sets of immunohistochemical and Western blot confirmatory methods in the detection of typical and atypical BSE cases. BMC Res Notes 4, p. 376

[55] Hayashi H, Takata M, Iwamaru Y, Ushiki Y, Kimura KM, Tagawa Y, Shinagawa M, Yokoyama T. Effect of tissue deterioration on postmortem BSE diagnosis by immunobiochemical detection of an abnormal isoform of prion protein. J Vet Med Sci. 2004; 66(5): 515–20.

[56] Wilham JM, Orrú CD, Bessen RA, Atarashi R, Sano K, Race B, Meade-White KD, Taubner LM, Timmes A, Caughey B. Rapid end-point quantitation of prion seeding activity with sensitivity comparable to bioassays. PLoS Pathog. 2010; 6:e1001217.

[57] Saborio GP, Permanne B, Soto C. Sensitive detection of pathological prion protein by cyclic amplification of protein misfolding. Nature. 2001; 411(6839): 810–3.

[58] Castilla J, Saa P, Soto C. Detection of prions in blood. Nat Med. 2005; 11(9): 982–5.

[59] Atarashi R, Satoh K, Sano K, Fuse T, Yamaguchi N, Ishibashi D, Matsubara T, Nakagaki T, Yamanaka H, Shirabe S, Yamada M, Mizusawa H, Kitamoto T, Klug G, McGlade A, Collins SJ, Nishida N. Ultrasensitive human prion detection in cerebrospinal fluid by real-time quaking-induced conversion. Nat Med. 2011; 17(2): 175–8.

[60] Orrú CD, Bongianni M, Tonoli G, Ferrari S, Hughson AG, Groveman BR, Fiorini M, Pocchiari M, Monaco S, Caughey B, Zanusso G. A test for Creutzfeldt-Jakob disease using nasal brushings. N Engl J Med 2014; 371(6): 519–29.

[61] Henderson DM, Davenport KA, Haley NJ, Denkers ND, Mathiason CK, Hoover EA. Quantitative assessment of prion infectivity in tissues and body fluids by real-time quaking-induced conversion. Gen Virol. 2015; 96(Pt 1): 210–9.

[62] Orrú CD, Favole A, Corona C, Mazza M, Manca M, Groveman BR, Hughson AG, Acutis PL, Caramelli M, Zanusso G, Casalone C, Caughey B. Detection and discrimination of classical and atypical L-type bovine spongiform encephalopathy by real-time quaking-induced conversion. J Clin Microbiol. 2015; 53(4): 1115–20.

[63] Masujin K, Orrú CD, Miyazawa K, Groveman BR, Raymond LD, Hughson AG, Caughey B. Detection of atypical H-Type bovine spongiform encephalopathy and discrimination of bovine prion strains by real-time quaking-induced conversion. J Clin Microbiol. 2016; 54(3): 676–86. doi: 10.1128/JCM.02731-15.

Chapter 2

Past, Present and Potential Future Prion Disease Treatment Strategies

Pamela J. Skinner and Davis M. Seelig

Additional information is available at the end of the chapter

http://dx.doi.org/10.5772/67193

Abstract

The prion diseases are rare and invariably fatal neurodegenerative diseases characterized by a unique, protein-only pathogenesis. Mechanistically, the prion diseases result from the coerced conversion of a protease-sensitive form of the cellular prion protein (PrP^C) into a protease-resistant infectious form (PrP^{res}). This chapter reviews the past, present, and potentially future prion disease treatment strategies. This chapter begins with an introduction to prion diseases, the misfolding of prion proteins and what is known about this process, and then proceeds to discuss approaches for treatments. Regarding approaches to treat prion diseases, we discuss (1) small molecule inhibitors, (2) antiprion protein antibodies, (3) prion gene disruption, (4) targeting of the unfolded protein response, and (5) heterologous prion proteins. We elaborate on using heterologous prion proteins to treat prion diseases, as this is an area that we are pursuing. The chapter ends with thoughts on the future direction of prion disease treatment strategies and how these strategies might be applicable to other neurodegenerative diseases involving protein misfolding. The increasing awareness of the role of protein misfolding in many neurodegenerative processes makes the development of an effective treatment strategy for prion diseases a high priority.

Keywords: prion, treatment, CJD, GSS, PrP^{res}, PrP^C, heterologous prion proteins, protein misfolding diseases, neurodegenerative disorders

1. Introduction

Prion diseases, or transmissible spongiform encephalopathies (TSEs), are unique, fatal neurodegenerative diseases with infectious, genetic, or sporadic causes. Prion diseases affect humans (e.g. Creutzfeldt-Jakob disease [CJD], Gerstmann-Straussler-Scheinker syndrome [GSS], and fatal familial insomnia [FFI]) and nonhumans (e.g. bovine spongiform encephalopathy [BSE] of cattle, chronic wasting disease [CWD] of cervids, and scrapie of sheep and goats.

Irrespective of affected species, prion diseases result in progressive neurocognitive decline following a long incubation period. No effective prion disease treatments exist and most human patients die within 14 months following diagnosis [1]. Notably, many of the fundamental characteristics of prion diseases, including the molecular and biochemical mechanisms underlying the formation, accumulation, and cell-to-cell infectivity of misfolded protein and the role of glial-mediated neuroinflammation aligns prion diseases with more common human neurodegenerative conditions, including Alzheimer's, Parkinson's, and Huntington's diseases.

In the mouse, the prion protein is encoded by the Prnp gene. The nascent 254 amino acid long peptide is then posttranslationally cleaved at its N and C terminus to produce the final 210 amino acid long protein [2–4]. Structurally, the prion protein is characterized by a disordered aminoterminal tail and a globular C-terminal domain consisting of three α-helices and two antiparallel β-sheets [5, 6]. It is anchored to the outer cell surface membrane via a glycosylphosphatidylinositol (GPI) anchor, which helps tether the protein to the outer cell surface membrane [7].

The hallmark event in the prion disorders is the misfolding of the normal cellular prion protein (denoted PrP^{C}) into a misfolded isoform (commonly denoted as PrP^{res} or PrP^{Sc}). In its normal form, PrP^{C} is a monomeric or dimeric protein with abundant alpha helical content, whereas the misfolded variant PrP^{res} is aggregated with a β-pleated sheet rich conformation [8, 9]. In addition to its structural differences, PrP^{res} is characterized by resistance to protease and chemical disinfection [10]. Although the entirety of the process has not been described, it is widely believed that PrP^{res} replication results from the induced misfolding of PrP^{C} through a nucleation-dependent polymerization mechanism [11]. This process is included in the model presented in **Figure 1**.

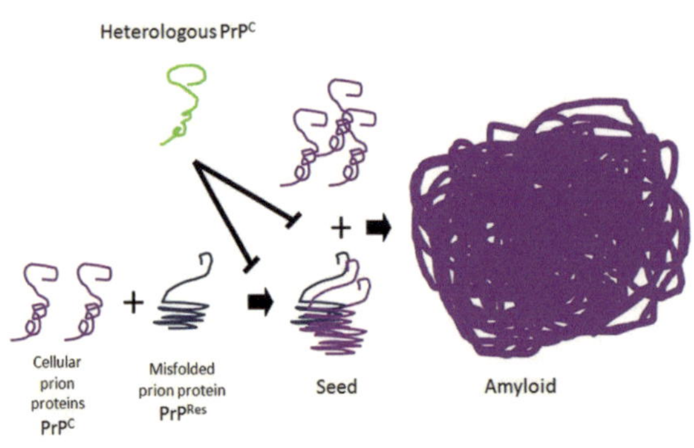

Figure 1. A proposed model of heterologous prion protein treatment in the misfolding, nucleation, and formation of amyloid. In the presence of misfolded PrP^{res}, the normal cellular prion protein (PrPc) is induced to misfold. This cycle of misfolding repeats leading to seeds of misfolded oligomers and amyloid deposits. Our studies demonstrate that heterologous prion proteins inhibit this process. We propose that heterologous prion proteins bind directly to PrP^{C} and PrP^{res} to block seed and amyloid formation.

In the pathogenesis of prion diseases, the formation of PrP^{res} is generally believed to be a key event in the disease initiation. Owing to its specificity as a marker of tissue infectivity, PrP^{res} is the most commonly used prion disease diagnostic marker. Although the inciting cause (i.e. PrP^{res} formation) and neuropathologic consequences of prion disease (i.e. gliosis, synaptic dysfunction, spongiosis, and neuronal loss) are well characterized, the mechanism(s) by which the former results in the latter remain unknown. However, it is likely that misfolded PrP^C has direct/indirect toxic properties as, as PrP^C does not appear to be detrimental [12].

The conversion of PrP^C to PrP^{res} is a highly specific process of templated conversion requiring direct interaction between the normal and abnormal forms of the protein [13]. The efficiency of this conversion is predicated upon a number of specific reaction conditions, including the secondary structure of PrP^{res}, homology of the primary and secondary structures between PrP^C and PrP^{res}, and the architecture of the PrP^C-PrP^{res} complex [14, 15]. Increased contact between PrP^C-PrP^{res} at residue 129 and the relative rigidity of the β2-α2 loops in PrP^C are two important factors in mediating the efficiency of PrP^{res} formation and TSE susceptibility [15–17]. In addition to steric factors, the formation of PrP^{res} is favored by destabilization of PrP^C as a number of destabilizing pathogenic mutations in PrP are linked with increasing misfolding rates [18–20].

The presence and primary structure of host PrP^C are major determinants in conferring susceptibility to prion disease infection. This is most expressly evident by work demonstrating that transgenic mice lacking PrP^C are conferred resistance to prion infection [21]. Beyond simple PrP^C expression, the degree of sequence homology between infecting prion and host PrP^C plays a significant role in determining the efficiency of prion infection and prion replication [22]. Moreover, differences in primary sequence between host PrP^C and infectious PrP^{res} have been proposed to underlie the species barrier that mitigates cross species prion infection as well as prion strains [23–25]. The importance of prion structure extends beyond simple amino acid homology and is also dependent upon secondary structural variations, including differences in loop/turn structures [23, 26]. In light of complementary in vitro and in vivo work, it appears as though the middle third region of the prion protein is particularly important for the autocatalytic conversion of PrP^C to PrP^{res} [27]. The potential clinical relevance of PrP^C sequence is demonstrated by work revealing that polymorphisms in this area of the protein can confer prion disease resistance, as mice expressing a variant PrP containing amino acid substitutions in the β2-α2 loop were resistant to prion infection [28].

Given studies that have revealed the pathogenic importance of a precisely formed PrP^C-PrP^{res} complex, it seems reasonable to investigate whether interference with this complex might have therapeutic potential. This approach is best described by Singh and Udgaonkar in their comprehensive review on PrP misfolding, namely to test whether or not "...any ligand, whether small or large, that binds to the native conformation of the [PrP^C] protein would stabilize that state and can therefore be expected to decrease the native-state dynamics that drive misfolding [29]." Support for such an approach has been validated by antibody-based studies, which have stabilized the α1 region of PrP^C and prevented prion disease in animals [30, 31].

In this chapter, we review past, present, and potential future strategies to treat prion diseases.

2. Small molecule inhibitors to treat prion diseases

There are a number of small molecules that have proposed as prion therapeutics, including that either inhibit the misfolding of PrP^C or promote the clearance of PrP^{res}. In general, small molecule compounds can be segregated according to their method of action into compounds that either inhibit the misfolding of PrP^C (potentially through stabilization) promote the clearance of PrP^{res}. Over the past two decades, many small molecules have been evaluated for their in vitro or in vivo antiprion efficacy.

Of the most commonly examined small molecule candidate therapies, many have not stood up to scrutiny when their in vitro efficacy was tested in vivo. This includes quinacrine, pentosan poylsufate, Congo red, amphotericin B, anthracyclines, and memantine [32–39]. Moreover, a subset of these compounds has been shown to extend the lives of prion-infected animals [40–42]. However, as noted by Caughey et al., the "clinical applicability of these compounds is severely limited by a lack of activity when administered after the onset of clinical signs of disease, poor bioavailability to the brain, and/or high toxicity [42–46]." Despite the incremental progress in the field, efforts to more efficiently identify and screen test compounds for antiprion activity are ongoing. Early work by Pruisner et al. searched the Available Chemicals Directory for molecules that inhibit prion replication based upon prior studies, identified a number of a family of compounds (pyridine dicarbonitriles) that showed in vitro efficacy in inhibiting prion replication [47, 48]. Follow-up studies by Reddy et al., who, through the design, synthesis, and screening of a series of related compounds, identified an additional compound that demonstrated efficacy at mitigating PrP^{res} formation [49]. Most recently, Ferriera et al. describe the in silico and in vitro identification and screening of new small organic antiscrapie compounds that decreased PrP^{res} accumulation and inhibit PrP aggregation [46]. Mechanistically, one of the most intriguing families of antiprion compounds is chemical chaperones. Chaperones are cellular constituents that interact with, stabilize, and assisting in the proper folding of nonfolded proteins [50]. When used pharmacologically, chaperones are small compounds that bind to proteins and either induce their refolding or stabilize their structure. Specific chaperones demonstrating in vitro and/or in vivo efficacy in prion disease systems including (along with their mechanism of action): trimethylamine N-oxide, glycerol, dimethyl sulfoxide (protein stabilization by altering solvent properties), and bile salts [51, 52].

3. Antiprion antibodies to treat prion diseases

Other treatment strategies for prion diseases have been attempted including vaccination and immunotherapy, but these strategies have had limited success [53]. Nonetheless, there have been several promising studies gaining insights into this approach and its potential. To reduce redundancies, we refer the interested reader to the chapter entitled "Immunobiology of Prion Diseases" for more information on this topic.

4. Prion gene disruption to treat prion diseases

Since the cellular prion protein is not essential for life but required for prion disease [54, 55], several groups have worked to develop and test strategies that disrupt normal cellular prion proteins, PrP^C. With this in mind, a recent treatment strategy used lentivirus vectors that expressed silencing RNAs directed against the cellular form of the prion protein [56]. These lentiviral vectors were employed to transduce mouse embryonic stem cells and the resultant transduced embryonic stem cells used to create chimeric mice expressing various levels of the silencing RNAs. After infection of these mice with scrapie, mice that were highly chimeric for the transgene and that showed reduced PrP^C expression in the brain showed increased survival times. Similarly, Mallucci et al. generated an adult-onset PrP knockout mouse model with delayed, neuron-specific deletion of PrP^C, which mitigated the clinical and neuropathologic consequences of prion disease [57, 58]. In another study, the same group used RNAi-driven gene silencing to reduce PrP^C expression. Using lenti-shRNA directed against PrP^C, treated mice experienced a significant downregulation of PrP^C expression and a delay in prion disease progression [59]. Thus, strategies that reduce or eliminate PrP^C using inhibitory RNAs show promise as a treatment for prion diseases.

An alternative approach to reducing PrP^C expression is to edit the gene using Zn-finger nucleases (ZFN), transcription activator-like effector nucleases (TALEN), or clustered regularly interspaced short palindromic repeats (CRISPR) gene editing systems. Indeed, mice, bovine and goat prion genes have been targeted using these approaches [60–62] to produce disease resistant animals, and at least one patent has been filed for gene editing of prion genes in animals [63].

5. Target the unfolded protein response to treat prion diseases

The pivotal event in prion disease pathogenesis is the formation and accumulation of misfolded PrP^{res} in the brain as it initiates a pathologic cascade of glial activation, neuronal hypometabolism, and apoptotic neuronal loss. An increasing body of work indicates that PrP^{res} triggers this pathology, in part, through the activation of the unfolded protein response (UPR) [64]. The UPR is a two-phase, cytoprotective cascade of the endoplasmic reticulum (ER) that is initiated by misfolded or aggregated protein, and it seeks to resolve cellular and ER stress. In the initial adaptive phase of the UPR, misfolded protein stimulates one (or more) of three sensing proteins: (1) PERK (protein kinase RNA-like ER kinase), (2) IRE1α (inositol-requiring protein 1), and/or (3) ATF6 (activating transcription factor-6). Subsequent homodimerization of two of these proteins (PERK and IRE1α) results in the phosphorylation and activation of intermediate messengers, including eIF2α (eukaryotic initiation factor 2 alpha), ATF4 (activating transcription factor), and XBP1 (X-box folding protein). The end result of the adaptive phase of the UPR is an attenuation of protein synthesis, an increased synthesis of ER chaperones, and a mitigation of ER protein processing [65, 66]. However, if these initial adaptive efforts fail, the UPR transitions to a second, apoptotic phase involving the activation of caspases 3, 6, 7, and 8.

Previous work has demonstrated involvement of both phases of the UPR in human and rodent prion disease [67, 68]. In addition to triggering apoptosis, it is increasing clear that the UPR is able to induce the deleterious, glial-mediated inflammatory response that is characteristic of both prion and other neurodegenerative diseases [69]. Specifically, Moreno et al. have shown that prion replications results in unchecked eIF2α activation that contributes to synaptic failure, neuronal loss, and clinical deficits in prion-infected mice [70]. However, the role of the UPR in human prion disease is less clear. Although Hetz et al. demonstrated increased levels of ER stress associated with misfolded protein in the brains of human patients with sporadic or variant CJD [71], subsequent immunohistochemical studies examining the brains of human patients with CJD for activated forms of PERK and eIF2α have failed confirm consistent involvement of the UPR [72].

Despite the inconclusive mechanistic data linking the UPR with prion disease pathogenesis, a small number of groups have examined the efficacy of therapeutic strategies directed at mitigating its activation. The therapeutic potential of targeting the UPR pathway is best demonstrated by work performed by Mallucci and Moreno. In their initial studies, they report that genetic mitigation of eIF2α activation decreases synaptic loss and neuronal loss in prion-infected mice [70]. Moreover, in follow-up work they demonstrate that upstream blockade of UPR activation through pharmacological inhibition of the activation of PERK reverses cognitive deficits and prevents clinical disease in prion-infected mice [67]. A smaller body of work has revealed that pharmacologic inhibition of the UPR using the neuroprotective, antiapoptotic bile acids tauroursodeoxycholic acid (TUDCA) and ursodeoxycholic acid (UDCA), results in decreased levels of activated eIP2α in organotypic cerebellar slices as well as decreased neuroinflammation and prolonged survival in mice. The reported benefits of bile acids result, in part, from their ability to inhibit the UPR activation across all three sensing pathways as reflected by lower levels of phosphorylated eIF2α, ATF4, PERK, ATF6, and IRE1α [73–76].

6. Heterologous prion proteins to treat prion diseases

The concept of heterologous prion proteins (HetPrP) as potential therapeutics is based on a body of research, including studies performed in cell free, cell culture, and animal models, in which prion proteins from different species were allowed to interact. Horiuchi et al. demonstrate that inclusion of a heterologous species PrP^{c} in a cell-free conversion system was capable of interfering with the formation of PrP^{res} between two homologous species [24]. When they divide the process of PrP^{res} formation into two steps, namely initial binding between PrP^{C} and PrP^{res} followed by acquisition of protease resistance, the interfering effect of HetPrP appears to occur during the latter [24]. Further, the expression of hamster prion protein (HaPrP) in scrapie-infected mouse cells in vitro lead to near complete elimination of PrP^{res} [77] supporting a role for heterologous HaPrP in either inhibiting PrP^{res} production or enhancing its clearance. Moreover, the induced expression rabbit prion proteins in scrapie-infected mouse cells led to substantially less PrP^{res} as compared to mouse cells that do not express rabbit prion proteins, supporting a role for rabbit prion proteins interfering with mouse PrP^{res} formation [23].

In our work, we extended these in vitro observations into the mouse using the rocky mountain laboratories (RML)-Chandler strain of scrapie and HetPrP therapy using bacterially expressed and purified recombinant HaPrP amino acids 23-231 [78]. For this study, mice were intracerebrally inoculated with an RML-Chandler strain brain homogenate combined with either recombinant HaPrP or vehicle control. The following day, mice were treated with HaPrP orally. We assessed the effect of HaPrP dosage using two treatment groups, including a high dose of recombinant protein (0.7 mg/ml, high dose) and a low dose (0.35 mg/ml). Lastly, two control groups were included, those being a mock treatment group comprised of mice that were infected and treated with vehicle only, and mice that were not infected and not treated. We assessed the impact of treatment on clinical disease by evaluating mice daily following infection, weekly during the first months and then daily in later months for signs of scrapie-related symptoms including decreased motility, flattened stature, ataxic gait, hind limb paresis, dull eyes, weight loss, and kyphosis.

Treatment with the high dose HaPrP effectively and significantly delayed the onset of clinical symptoms, and prolonged survival compared to the vehicle-treated animals [78]. Moreover, when the study was terminated at 452 days postinfection, half of the high-dose-treated animals were still free of scrapie symptoms. **Figure 2** shows the survival times.

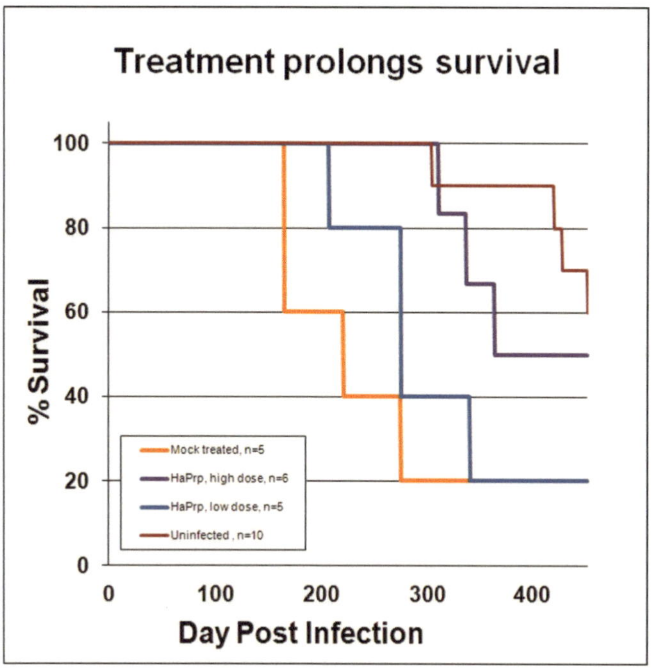

Figure 2. Treatment with heterologous recombinant HaPrP prolonged survival. Kaplan-Meier plots showing the survival times of mock-treated (orange, $n = 5$), low-dose-treated (blue, $n = 5$), high-dose-treated mice (purple, $n = 6$) and uninfected (red, $n = 10$). We tested for differences between groups using a modified version of the Gehan-Wilcoxon test and found a statistically significant difference between the mock infected group and the high-dose group ($p = 0.0348$).

In addition to abrogating the clinical signs of prion disease, mice receiving the high-dose of HaPrP, compared to mice treated with a low dose of HaPrP or with vehicle only, accumulated significantly less PrP^{res} in both brain and spleen. Furthermore, HaPrP partially mitigated the neuropathologic consequences of prion infection as high-dose-treated animals showed a trend towards fewer activated astrocytes as revealed by immunohistochemistry for glial fibrillary acidic protein and less severe neuropil spongiosis in total brain and highly significant reductions in the thalamus.

Although we demonstrated that treatment with $HetPrP^C$ inhibits both the formation of PrP^{res} and the clinical consequences of prion infection, the mechanism underlying this phenomenon is not known. We think that HetPrP binds to both PrP^{res} and PrP^C and blocks the production and elongation of PrP^{res} chains and amyloid formation. This is modeled in **Figure 1**.

The work of Horiuchi et al. offers two possible mechanistic models for this interference, based upon number and type of binding sites for PrP^C on PrP^{res} [24]. They posit in a "one binding system," that the binding of HetPrP to a growing PrP^{res} oligomer creates an aggregate that is incapable of generating the steric interactions necessary for the continued production of PrP^{res}. Alternately, they propose in a "two binding system" that the growing PrP^{res} oligomer contains two binding sites, namely a conversion-inducing site and a nonconverting site. In this two-site system, HetPrP interferes with the formation of PrP^{res} by binding and blockading conversion site without blocking the nonconverting site.

In addition to biochemical mechanisms described, it is possible that the protective effect of HetPrP in our study resulted from an evoked immune response that impacted PrP^{res} formations. However, our data do not support this hypothesis. By western blot analysis of serum from study mice, we did not detect the presence of antihamster PrP antibodies in treated compared to control animals. Lastly, it is important to note that because mice were simultaneously intracerebrally inoculated with both scrapie prions and HaPrP, it is quite likely that the HaPrP in the inoculum served to inactivate the scrapie prion by binding to PrP^{res} and forming an inactive complex due to sequence incongruence.

It is increasingly apparent that HetPrP treatment safely inhibits the PrP^C to PrP^{res} conversion process. In vitro and in vivo studies render feasible the prospect of treating human prion diseases with HetPrP. While demonstrating efficacy, in our study the treatment regime used (intracerebral instillation of HetPrP at the time of infection followed by oral ingestion of heterologous PrP^C) which is not ideal for treating patients with existing prion disease. Delivery via intracerebral injection is certainly not anticipated to allow HetPrP to make contact with and inactivate all PrP^{res} in the system. As such, future studies are needed to develop more practical HetPrP delivery modalities as well as to evaluate potentially more effective HetPrP sequences.

While a wide range of mammal species are susceptible to prion infection, the efficiency of interspecies transmission is varied and governed by a "species barrier," the integrity of which is inversely proportional to the strength of the interaction between host PrP^C and incoming PrP^{res}. Interestingly, rabbits have been shown to be unusually resistant to prion disease inoculation, as attempts to transmit CJD, Kuru, sheep scrapie, TME, and mouse-adapted scrapie to rabbits failed [79, 80]. While subsequent groups have confirmed that the rabbit is not absolutely resistant or prion infection, there is general agreement that they are only minimally susceptible [81, 82]. The degree of primary sequence homology is important in determining the robustness of the species barrier. The rabbit prion protein shows relatively low sequence homology to other species prion proteins. Based upon this work, we propose that a rabbit PrP-based HetPrP treatment strategy may be more effective than HaPrP at inhibiting prion disease.

While we used IC injection of HetPrP in our study, the clinical evolution of this approach necessitates a more effective and simpler means of delivery. One such approach could be delivery via the bloodstream and use blood vessels to efficiently deliver HetPrP to all areas of the brain. In addition, it may be possible to use peptides derived from HetPrP rather than whole proteins. Indeed Chabry et al. showed in vitro inhibition of PrP conversation with synthetic peptides derived from mouse and hamster PrP [83, 84]. Another such possibility for HetPrP treatment is the adoption of a gene therapy-based approach using lentiviral vectors. Thus, further studies are warranted to optimize both the form of HetPrP as well as its mode of delivery.

In related studies, other groups have found promising therapeutic results as well. Meier et al. engineered PrP^{C} fused to immunoglobulin Fcgamma, termed PrP-Fc(2) [85]. Wild-type mice expressing PrP-Fc(2) and subsequently infected with scrapie prions showed delayed PrP^{res} accumulation and onset of disease [85]. In follow-up studies, they further showed that expression of PrP-Fc(2) transduced by a lentiviral vector at 170 days postinfection was able to reduce prion infectivity by 3–4 logs [86]. Toupet et al. created a recombinant lentiviral vector that transduces expression of a dominant negative mouse prion protein that recapitulates sheep PrPQ171R and human PrPE219K polymorphisms associated with prion disease resistance [87]. They showed that chronic injection of this vector directly into the brains of prion disease infected mice led to reduced astrocytic gliosis and extended survival [87]. Moreover, Soto et al. designed beta sheet breaker peptides corresponding to the conserved region of PrP 115-122 that is thought to play a central role in conversion of PrP^{C} to PrP^{res} [88–91]. These beta sheet peptides partly reversed PrP^{res} to PrP^{c} in vitro, and when mixed with scrapie prions and injected into mice, decreased infectivity by 90–95% [88]. Thus, multiple strategies have been developed and tested in mice that use prion proteins or related peptides to target and reduce prion infectivity and have demonstrated efficacy.

7. Potential future strategies to treat prion diseases

Understanding pathogenesis is key to developing new therapies for prion diseases. For example, we [92, 93] and others have gained insights into prion disease pathogenesis by studying in changes in gene expression that occur during the disease process. These expression alterations provide insights to underlying pathological processes, and key mediators of these processes might be targeted in future prion treatment strategies. Another example comes from Hetz et al., who determined in a scrapie infected cell culture system that PrP^{sc} toxicity and apoptosis induction was associated in an increase in an endoplasmic reticulum resident enzyme caspase-12, and a corresponding increase in caspase-12 was also seen in humans affected by CJD [94]. With this knowledge of a key process in pathogenesis, they were able to inhibit apoptosis by overexpression of a catalytic mutant of caspase-12 [94]. In another set of studies, the 37 kDa/67 kDa laminin receptor LPR/LR was targeted based on knowledge that LPR/LR is a cell surface receptor for PrP^{c} [95] and required for PrP^{res} propagation in scrapie-infected cells [96]. Zuber et al. created and infused single-chain Fv antibodies directed against LPR/LR into mice just prior to inoculation with scrapie prions and weekly afterwards, and found an ~40% reduction in PrPres in spleen [97]. In similar experiments, Pflanz et al. injected lentiviral vectors that transduce small interfering RNAs directed against LPR/LR precursor mRNA into the brains of mice, then infected them with scrapie, and found a 41% reduction in PrP^{res} and prolongation of the preclinical phase [98]. Thus, gaining understanding of the molecular event underlying prion disease pathogenesis can identify potential targets for future prion disease therapeutics.

Moving forward to a viable treatment and cure for prion diseases in humans will likely involve a combination of therapies. For example, this might involve a combination of approaches such as gene editing to create disease resistant prion gene alleles, a drug that inhibits apoptosis, a small molecule that stabilizes PrP^{c} and regular injections of heterologous prion proteins that bind and clear nascent PrP^{res}.

Importantly, strategies that work for treating prion diseases may also be effective when applied to other neurodegenerative diseases that involve protein misfolding, such as Alzheimer's disease and Huntington's chorea. There is increasing evidence of underlying similarities in the pathogenesis of protein misfolding neurodegenerative diseases. Hence, similar cure strategies may be feasible.

8. Conclusion

In conclusion, an ever-expanding understanding of basic prion pathogenesis, combined with the rapidly ever-expanding development of new biotechnologies, combined with existing strategies to treat prion diseases, will likely to lead to a feasible and effective treatment for prion diseases in the near future. Already, innovations such as genome editing, inhibitory RNAs, and improved gene therapy vectors are being applied to and advancing treatment strategies to create improved treatments. In addition, strategies that show efficacy that target separate components of disease pathogenesis can be combined. Thus, in the coming years, the outlook is very promising for the development of an effective treatment and potential cure for individuals with prion diseases. Furthermore, strategies used to treat prion diseases might be broadly applicable and effective when applied to other protein misfolding diseases. The increasing awareness of the role of protein misfolding in many neurodegenerative processes makes the development of an effective treatment strategy for prion diseases a high priority.

http://dx.doi.org/10.5772/67193

Abbreviations and acronyms

TSEs	Transmissible spongiform encephalopathies
CJD	Creutzfeldt-Jakob disease
GSS	Gerstmann-Straussler-Scheinker syndrome
FFI	Fatal familial insomnia
BSE	Bovine spongiform encephalopathy
CWD	Chronic wasting disease
Denoted PrPC	Cellular prion protein
Commonly denoted as PrP^{res} or PrP^{Sc}	Misfolded isoform
HetPrP	Heterologous prion proteins
HaPrP	Hamster prion protein

Author details

Pamela J. Skinner[1]* and Davis M. Seelig[2]

*Address all correspondence to: skinn002@umn.edu

1 University of Minnesota, Department of Veterinary and Biomedical Sciences, Saint Paul, MN, USA

2 University of Minnesota, Department of Veterinary Clinical Sciences, Saint Paul, MN, USA

References

[1] Valleron AJ, Boelle PY, Will R, Cesbron JY. Estimation of epidemic size and incubation time based on age characteristics of vCJD in the United Kingdom. *Science.* 2001;294(5547):1726–1728. doi: 10.1126/science.1066838.

[2] Basler K, Oesch B, Scott M, et al. Scrapie and cellular PrP isoforms are encoded by the same chromosomal gene. *Cell.* 1986;46(386272089):417–428.

[3] Mange A, Beranger F, Peoc'h K, Onodera T, Frobert Y, Lehmann S. Alpha- and beta-cleavages of the amino-terminus of the cellular prion protein. *Biol Cell.* 2004;96(2):125–132. doi: 10.1016/j.biolcel.2003.11.007.

[4] Westaway D, Prusiner SB. Conservation of the cellular gene encoding the scrapie prion protein. *Nucleic Acids Res.* 1986;14(586176712):2035–2044.

[5] Riek R, Hornemann S, Wider G, Glockshuber R, Wuthrich K. NMR characterization of the full-length recombinant murine prion protein, mPrP(23-231). *FEBS Lett.* 1997;413(297424376):282–288.

[6] Riek R, Hornemann S, Wider G, Billeter M, Glockshuber R, Wuthrich K. NMR structure of the mouse prion protein domain PrP(121-321). *Nature*. 1996;382(658796317593):180–182.

[7] Stahl N, Borchelt DR, Hsiao K, Prusiner SB. Scrapie prion protein contains a phosphatidylinositol glycolipid. *Cell*. 1987;51(288027007):229–240.

[8] Pan KM, Baldwin M, Nguyen J, et al. Conversion of alpha-helices into beta-sheets features in the formation of the scrapie prion proteins. *Proc Natl Acad Sci U S A*. 1993;90(2394068524):10962–10966.

[9] Gasset M, Baldwin MA, Fletterick RJ, Prusiner SB. Perturbation of the secondary structure of the scrapie prion protein under conditions that alter infectivity. *Proc Natl Acad Sci U S A*. 1993;90(193126320):1–5.

[10] Taylor DM. Inactivation of BSE agent. *Dev Biol Stand*. 1991;7592175414:97–102.

[11] Jarrett JT, Lansbury PT, Jr. Seeding "one-dimensional crystallization" of amyloid: a pathogenic mechanism in Alzheimer's disease and scrapie? *Cell*. 1993;73(693292067):1055–1058.

[12] Hetz C, Maundrell K, Soto C. Is loss of function of the prion protein the cause of prion disorders? *Trends Mol Med*. 2003;9(6):237–243. doi: S1471491403000698 [pii].

[13] Caughey B, Chesebro B. Transmissible spongiform encephalopathies and prion protein interconversions. *Adv Virus Res*. 2001;56:277–311.

[14] Prusiner SB, Scott M, Foster D, et al. Transgenetic studies implicate interactions between homologous PrP isoforms in scrapie prion replication. *Cell*. 1990;63(491029499):673–686.

[15] Mallik S, Yang W, Norstrom EM, Mastrianni JA. Live cell fluorescence resonance energy transfer predicts an altered molecular association of heterologous PrPSc with PrPC. *J Biol Chem*. 2010;285(12):8967–8975. doi: 10.1074/jbc.M109.058107 [doi].

[16] Bett C, Fernandez-Borges N, Kurt TD, et al. Structure of the beta2-alpha2 loop and interspecies prion transmission. *FASEB J*. 2012;26(7):2868–2876. doi: 10.1096/fj.11-200923.

[17] Giachin G, Biljan I, Ilc G, Plavec J, Legname G. Probing early misfolding events in prion protein mutants by NMR spectroscopy. *Molecules*. 2013;18(8):9451–9476. doi: 10.3390/molecules18089451.

[18] Singh J, Udgaonkar JB. Structural effects of multiple pathogenic mutations suggest a model for the initiation of misfolding of the prion protein. *Angew Chem Int Ed Engl*. 2015;54(26):7529–7533. doi: 10.1002/anie.201501011.

[19] Liemann S, Glockshuber R. Influence of amino acid substitutions related to inherited human prion diseases on the thermodynamic stability of the cellular prion protein. *Biochemistry (N Y)*. 1999;38(1199178830):3258–3267.

[20] Apetri AC, Surewicz K, Surewicz WK. The effect of disease-associated mutations on the folding pathway of human prion protein. *J Biol Chem*. 2004;279(17):18008–18014. doi: 10.1074/jbc.M313581200.

[21] Bueler H, Aguzzi A, Sailer A, et al. Mice devoid of PrP are resistant to scrapie. *Cell*. 1993;73(793313963):1339–1347.

[22] Rigter A, Bossers A. Sheep scrapie susceptibility-linked polymorphisms do not modulate the initial binding of cellular to disease-associated prion protein prior to conversion. *J Gen Virol*. 2005;86(Pt 9):2627–2634. doi: 86/9/2627.

[23] Vorberg I, Groschup MH, Pfaff E, Priola SA. Multiple amino acid residues within the rabbit prion protein inhibit formation of its abnormal isoform. *J Virol*. 2003;77(3):2003–2009.

[24] Horiuchi M, Priola SA, Chabry J, Caughey B. Interactions between heterologous forms of prion protein: Binding, inhibition of conversion, and species barriers. *Proc Natl Acad Sci U S A*. 2000;97(1120283912):5836–5841.

[25] Priola SA, Vorberg I. Molecular aspects of disease pathogenesis in the transmissible spongiform encephalopathies. *Mol Biotechnol*. 2006;33(1):71–88.

[26] Moore RA, Taubner LM, Priola SA. Prion protein misfolding and disease. *Curr Opin Struct Biol*. 2009;19(1):14–22. doi: 10.1016/j.sbi.2008.12.007.

[27] Priola SA. Prion protein and species barriers in the transmissible spongiform encephalopathies. *Biomed Pharmacother*. 1999;53(1):27–33. doi: S0753332299800572.

[28] Kurt TD, Jiang L, Bett C, Eisenberg D, Sigurdson CJ. A proposed mechanism for the promotion of prion conversion involving a strictly conserved tyrosine residue in the beta2-alpha2 loop of PrPC. *J Biol Chem*. 2014;289(15):10660–10667. doi: 10.1074/jbc.M114.549030.

[29] Singh J, Udgaonkar JB. Molecular mechanism of the misfolding and oligomerization of the prion protein: Current understanding and its implications. *Biochemistry*. 2015;54(29):4431–4442. doi: 10.1021/acs.biochem.5b00605.

[30] Heppner FL, Musahl C, Arrighi I, et al. Prevention of scrapie pathogenesis by transgenic expression of anti-prion protein antibodies. *Science*. 2001;294(5540):178–182.

[31] White AR, Enever P, Tayebi M, et al. Monoclonal antibodies inhibit prion replication and delay the development of prion disease. *Nature*. 2003;422(6927):80–83. doi: 10.1038/nature01457.

[32] Haik S, Brandel JP, Salomon D, et al. Compassionate use of quinacrine in Creutzfeldt-Jakob disease fails to show significant effects. *Neurology*. 2004;63(12):2413–2415. doi: 63/12/2413.

[33] Whittle IR, Knight RS, Will RG. Unsuccessful intraventricular pentosan polysulphate treatment of variant creutzfeldt-jakob disease. *Acta Neurochir (Wien)*. 2006;148(6):677–9; discussion 679. doi: 10.1007/s00701-006-0772-y.

[34] Farquhar C, Dickinson A, Bruce M. Prophylactic potential of pentosan polysulphate in transmissible spongiform encephalopathies. *Lancet*. 1999;353(9147):117. doi: S0140-6736(98)05395-1.

[35] Caughey B, Ernst D, Race RE. Congo red inhibition of scrapie agent replication. *J Virol.* 1993;67(1093381832):6270–6272.

[36] Demaimay R, Adjou KT, Beringue V, et al. Late treatment with polyene antibiotics can prolong the survival time of scrapie-infected animals. *J Virol.* 1997;71(1298037685):9685–9689.

[37] Tagliavini F, McArthur RA, Canciani B, et al. Effectiveness of anthracycline against experimental prion disease in syrian hamsters. *Science.* 1997;276(531597293259):1119–1122.

[38] Muller WE, Ushijima H, Schroder HC, et al. Cytoprotective effect of NMDA receptor antagonists on prion protein (PrionSc)-induced toxicity in rat cortical cell cultures. *Eur J Pharmacol.* 1993;246(394039507):261–267.

[39] Muller WE, Laplanche JL, Ushijima H, Schroder HC. Novel approaches in diagnosis and therapy of Creutzfeldt-Jakob disease. *Mech Ageing Dev.* 2000;116(2-3):193–218. doi: S0047637400001123.

[40] Cashman NR, Caughey B. Prion diseases—close to effective therapy? *Nat Rev Drug Discov.* 2004;3(10):874–884.

[41] Trevitt CR, Collinge J. A systematic review of prion therapeutics in experimental models. *Brain.* 2006;129(Pt 9):2241–2265. doi: awl150.

[42] Sim VL. Prion disease: Chemotherapeutic strategies. *Infect Disord Drug Targets.* 2012; 12(2):144–160. doi: IDDT-EPUP-20120314-001.

[43] Collins SJ, Lewis V, Brazier M, Hill AF, Fletcher A, Masters CL. Quinacrine does not prolong survival in a murine Creutzfeldt-Jakob disease model. *Ann Neurol.* 2002;52(4):503–506. doi: 10.1002/ana.10336.

[44] Caughey B, Caughey WS, Kocisko DA, Lee KS, Silveira JR, Morrey JD. Prions and transmissible spongiform encephalopathy (TSE) chemotherapeutics: a common mechanism for anti-TSE compounds? *Acc Chem Res.* 2006;39(9):646–653. doi: 10.1021/ar050068p.

[45] Kocisko DA, Caughey B. Mefloquine, an antimalaria drug with antiprion activity in vitro, lacks activity in vivo. *J Virol.* 2006;80(2):1044–1046. doi: 80/2/1044.

[46] Ferreira NC, Marques IA, Conceicao WA, et al. Anti-prion activity of a panel of aromatic chemical compounds: In vitro and in silico approaches. *PLoS One.* 2014;9(1):e84531. doi: 10.1371/journal.pone.0084531.

[47] Perrier V, Wallace AC, Kaneko K, Safar J, Prusiner SB, Cohen FE. Mimicking dominant negative inhibition of prion replication through structure-based drug design. *Proc Natl Acad Sci U S A.* 2000;97(1120283952):6073–6078.

[48] Kaneko K, Wille H, Mehlhorn I, et al. Molecular properties of complexes formed between the prion protein and synthetic peptides. *J Mol Biol.* 1997;270(4):574–586. doi: S0022–2836(97)91135-9.

[49] Reddy TR, Mutter R, Heal W, et al. Library design, synthesis, and screening: pyridine dicarbonitriles as potential prion disease therapeutics. *J Med Chem.* 2006;49(2):607–615. doi: 10.1021/jm050610f.

[50] Hartl FU, Hayer-Hartl M. Molecular chaperones in the cytosol: from nascent chain to folded protein. *Science*. 2002;295(5561):1852–1858. doi: 10.1126/science.1068408.

[51] Tatzelt J, Prusiner SB, Welch WJ. Chemical chaperones interfere with the formation of scrapie prion protein. *EMBO J*. 1996;15(2397133266):6363–6373.

[52] Cortez LM, Campeau J, Norman G, et al. Bile acids reduce prion conversion, reduce neuronal loss, and prolong male survival in models of prion disease. *J Virol*. 2015;89(15):7660–7672. doi: JVI.01165-15.

[53] Li L, Napper S, Cashman NR. Immunotherapy for prion diseases: Opportunities and obstacles. *Immunotherapy*. 2010;2(2):269–282. doi: 10.2217/imt.10.3.

[54] Brandner S, Isenmann S, Raeber A, et al. Normal host prion protein necessary for scrapie-induced neurotoxicity. *Nature*. 1996;379(656396149246):339–343.

[55] Brandner S, Raeber A, Sailer A, et al. Normal host prion protein (PrPC) is required for scrapie spread within the central nervous system. *Proc Natl Acad Sci U S A*. 1996;93(2397075133):13148–13151.

[56] Pfeifer A, Eigenbrod S, Al-Khadra S, et al. Lentivector-mediated RNAi efficiently suppresses prion protein and prolongs survival of scrapie-infected mice. *J Clin Invest*. 2006;116(12):3204–3210. doi: 10.1172/JCI29236.

[57] Mallucci GR, Ratte S, Asante EA, et al. Post-natal knockout of prion protein alters hippocampal CA1 properties, but does not result in neurodegeneration. *EMBO J*. 2002;21(3):202–210. doi: 10.1093/emboj/21.3.202.

[58] Mallucci G, Dickinson A, Linehan J, Klohn PC, Brandner S, Collinge J. Depleting neuronal PrP in prion infection prevents disease and reverses spongiosis. *Science*. 2003;302(5646):871–874. doi: 10.1126/science.1090187.

[59] White MD, Farmer M, Mirabile I, Brandner S, Collinge J, Mallucci GR. Single treatment with RNAi against prion protein rescues early neuronal dysfunction and prolongs survival in mice with prion disease. *Proc Natl Acad Sci U S A*. 2008;105(29):10238–10243. doi: 10.1073/pnas.0802759105.

[60] Bevacqua RJ, Fernandez-Martin R, Savy V, et al. Efficient edition of the bovine PRNP prion gene in somatic cells and IVF embryos using the CRISPR/Cas9 system. *Theriogenology*. 2016;86(8):1886–1896.e1. doi: 10.1016/j.theriogenology.2016.06.010.

[61] Kaczmarczyk L, Mende Y, Zevnik B, Jackson WS. Manipulating the prion protein gene sequence and expression levels with CRISPR/Cas9. *PLoS One*. 2016;11(4):e0154604. doi: 10.1371/journal.pone.0154604.

[62] Ni W, Qiao J, Hu S, et al. Efficient gene knockout in goats using CRISPR/Cas9 system. *PLoS One*. 2014;9(9):e106718. doi: 10.1371/journal.pone.0106718.

[63] Weinstein E, Simmons P, Cui X, inventors. Genomic editing of prion disorder-related genes in animals. Patent US20110023147 A1. 2011.

[64] Ferreiro E, Costa R, Marques S, Cardoso SM, Oliveira CR, Pereira CM. Involvement of mitochondria in endoplasmic reticulum stress-induced apoptotic cell death pathway triggered by the prion peptide PrP(106–126). *J Neurochem*. 2008;104(3):766–776. doi: JNC5048.

[65] Maly DJ, Papa FR. Druggable sensors of the unfolded protein response. *Nat Chem Biol*. 2014;10(11):892–901. doi: 10.1038/nchembio.1664.

[66] Ron D, Walter P. Signal integration in the endoplasmic reticulum unfolded protein response. *Nat Rev Mol Cell Biol*. 2007;8(7):519–529. doi: nrm2199.

[67] Moreno JA, Halliday M, Molloy C, et al. Oral treatment targeting the unfolded protein response prevents neurodegeneration and clinical disease in prion-infected mice. *Sci Transl Med*. 2013;5(206):206ra138. doi: 10.1126/scitranslmed.3006767; 10.1126/scitranslmed.3006767.

[68] Hetz C, Maundrell K, Soto C. Is loss of function of the prion protein the cause of prion disorders? *Trends Mol Med*. 2003;9(6):237–243. doi: S1471491403000698.

[69] Salminen A, Kauppinen A, Suuronen T, Kaarniranta K, Ojala J. ER stress in Alzheimer's disease: A novel neuronal trigger for inflammation and Alzheimer's pathology. *J Neuroinflammation*. 2009;6:41-2094-6-41. doi: 10.1186/1742-2094-6-41.

[70] Moreno JA, Radford H, Peretti D, et al. Sustained translational repression by eIF2alpha-P mediates prion neurodegeneration. *Nature*. 2012;485(7399):507–511. doi: 10.1038/nature11058.

[71] Hetz CA, Soto C. Stressing out the ER: a role of the unfolded protein response in prion-related disorders. *Curr Mol Med*. 2006;6(1):37–43.

[72] Unterberger U, Hoftberger R, Gelpi E, Flicker H, Budka H, Voigtlander T. Endoplasmic reticulum stress features are prominent in Alzheimer disease but not in prion diseases in vivo. *J Neuropathol Exp Neurol*. 2006;65(4):348–357. doi: 10.1097/01.jnen.0000218445.30535.6f.

[73] Lo AC, Callaerts-Vegh Z, Nunes AF, Rodrigues CM, D'Hooge R. Tauroursodeoxycholic acid (TUDCA) supplementation prevents cognitive impairment and amyloid deposition in APP/PS1 mice. *Neurobiol Dis*. 2013;50:21–29. doi: 10.1016/j.nbd.2012.09.003.

[74] Castro-Caldas M, Carvalho AN, Rodrigues E, et al. Tauroursodeoxycholic acid prevents MPTP-induced dopaminergic cell death in a mouse model of Parkinson's disease. *Mol Neurobiol*. 2012;46(2):475–486. doi: 10.1007/s12035-012-8295-4.

[75] Keene CD, Rodrigues CM, Eich T, Chhabra MS, Steer CJ, Low WC. Tauroursodeoxycholic acid, a bile acid, is neuroprotective in a transgenic animal model of Huntington's disease. *Proc Natl Acad Sci U S A*. 2002;99(16):10671–10676. doi: 10.1073/pnas.162362299.

[76] Dromparis P, Paulin R, Stenson TH, Haromy A, Sutendra G, Michelakis ED. Attenuating endoplasmic reticulum stress as a novel therapeutic strategy in pulmonary hypertension. *Circulation*. 2013;127(1):115–125. doi: 10.1161/CIRCULATIONAHA.112.133413.

[77] Priola SA, Caughey B, Race RE, Chesebro B. Heterologous PrP molecules interfere with accumulation of protease-resistant PrP in scrapie-infected murine neuroblastoma cells. *J Virol*. 1994;68(8):4873–4878.

[78] Skinner PJ, Kim HO, Bryant D, et al. Treatment of prion disease with heterologous prion proteins. *PLoS One*. 2015;10(7):e0131993. doi: 10.1371/journal.pone.0131993.

[79] Gibbs CJ,Jr., Gajdusek DC. Experimental subacute spongiform virus encephalopathies in primates and other laboratory animals. *Science*. 1973;182(10773250694):67–68.

[80] Barlow RM, Rennie JC. The fate of ME7 scrapie infection in rats, guinea-pigs and rabbits. *Res Vet Sci*. 1976;21(176245654):110–111.

[81] Chianini F, Fernandez-Borges N, Vidal E, et al. Rabbits are not resistant to prion infection. *Proc Natl Acad Sci U S A*. 2012;109(13):5080–5085. doi: 10.1073/pnas.1120076109.

[82] Vidal E, Fernandez-Borges N, Pintado B, et al. Bovine spongiform encephalopathy induces misfolding of alleged prion-resistant species cellular prion protein without altering its pathobiological features. *J Neurosci*. 2013;33(18):7778–7786. doi: 10.1523/JNEUROSCI.0244-13.2013.

[83] Begley DJ. Transport of prion proteins across the blood-brain barrier. *Exp Neurol*. 2009;220(2):217–218. doi: 10.1016/j.expneurol.2009.08.006.

[84] Chabry J, Caughey B, Chesebro B. Specific inhibition of in vitro formation of protease-resistant prion protein by synthetic peptides. *J Biol Chem*. 1998;273(2198250777):13203–13207.

[85] Meier P, Genoud N, Prinz M, et al. Soluble dimeric prion protein binds PrP(sc) in vivo and antagonizes prion disease. *Cell*. 2003;113(1):49–60.

[86] Genoud N, Ott D, Braun N, et al. Antiprion prophylaxis by gene transfer of a soluble prion antagonist. *Am J Pathol*. 2008;172(5):1287–1296. doi: 10.2353/ajpath.2008.070836.

[87] Toupet K, Compan V, Crozet C, et al. Effective gene therapy in a mouse model of prion diseases. *PLoS One*. 2008;3(7):e2773. doi: 10.1371/journal.pone.0002773.

[88] Soto C, Kascsak RJ, Saborio GP, et al. Reversion of prion protein conformational changes by synthetic beta- sheet breaker peptides. *Lancet*. 2000;355(919920137584):192–197.

[89] De Gioia L, Selvaggini C, Ghibaudi E, et al. Conformational polymorphism of the amyloidogenic and neurotoxic peptide homologous to residues 106-126 of the prion protein. *J Biol Chem*. 1994;269(1194179145):7859–7862.

[90] Zhang H, Kaneko K, Nguyen JT, et al. Conformational transitions in peptides containing two putative alpha- helices of the prion protein. *J Mol Biol*. 1995;250(495341684):514–526.

[91] Chabry J, Caughey B, Chesebro B. Specific inhibition of in vitro formation of protease-resistant prion protein by synthetic peptides. *J Biol Chem*. 1998;273(21):13203–13207.

[92] Kim HO, Snyder GP, Blazey TM, Race RE, Chesebro B, Skinner PJ. Prion disease induced alterations in gene expression in spleen and brain prior to clinical symptoms. *Adv Appl Bioinform Chem*. 2008;1:29–50.

[93] Skinner PJ, Abbassi H, Chesebro B, Race RE, Reilly C, Haase AT. Gene expression alterations in brains of mice infected with three strains of scrapie. *BMC Genomics*. 2006;7:114.

[94] Hetz C, Russelakis-Carneiro M, Maundrell K, Castilla J, Soto C. Caspase-12 and endoplasmic reticulum stress mediate neurotoxicity of pathological prion protein. *EMBO J*. 2003;22(20):5435–5445. doi: 10.1093/emboj/cdg537.

[95] Gauczynski S, Peyrin JM, Haik S, et al. The 37-kDa/67-kDa laminin receptor acts as the cell-surface receptor for the cellular prion protein. *EMBO J*. 2001;20(21):5863–5875. doi: 10.1093/emboj/20.21.5863.

[96] Leucht C, Simoneau S, Rey C, et al. The 37 kDa/67 kDa laminin receptor is required for PrP(sc) propagation in scrapie-infected neuronal cells. *EMBO Rep*. 2003;4(3):290–295. doi: 10.1038/sj.embor.embor768.

[97] Zuber C, Knackmuss S, Rey C, et al. Single chain fv antibodies directed against the 37 kDa/67 kDa laminin receptor as therapeutic tools in prion diseases. *Mol Immunol*. 2008;45(1):144–151. doi: S0161-5890(07)00197-6.

[98] Pflanz H, Vana K, Mitteregger G, et al. Microinjection of lentiviral vectors expressing small interfering RNAs directed against laminin receptor precursor mRNA prolongs the pre-clinical phase in scrapie-infected mice. *J Gen Virol*. 2009;90(Pt 1):269–274. doi: 10.1099/vir.0.004168-0.

Section 2

Molecular Mechanism of Prion Disease

Chapter 3

Structure-Property Relationship of Amyloidogenic Prion Nanofibrils

Myeongsang Lee, Hyunsung Choi, Jae In Kim,
Gwonchan Yoon and Sungsoo Na

Additional information is available at the end of the chapter

http://dx.doi.org/10.5772/66448

Abstract

The structure and its property for the prion nanofibrils, which exhibit self-assembled steric zipper, amyloid fibrils, are described in this chapter. There is the belief of origin for the infectiousness of the prion can be its molecular structure. It is due to the amyloid toxicity, which is related to its beta sheet rich molecular structure and self-aggregated long fibrils. There is evidence that the difference between PrP^{c} and PrP^{sc} is transitioned beta sheet from alpha helix to self-assemble and then to the amyloidogenic fibrils. Therefore, the scope of this chapter is the amyloidogenic structural characteristics of prion fibrils and its relationship to the property. The molecular structural characteristics can be changed by properties such as affinity, toxicity, infectivity, and so on, so this is a key factor to understand the origin of prion disease and develop the therapeutic strategy. One of the main properties of amyloid fibrils that we want to describe here is mechanical property such as dynamic property and material property for prion nanofibrils. This chapter can shed light on understanding the infectious characteristics of prion and the relationship of its molecular structures.

Keywords: prion, amyloid fibrils, physiological conditions, heterogeneity interaction, cross seeding, HET-s, singlet, triplet, mechanical characterization, molecular dynamics, coarse-grained model

1. Introduction

The molecular structure and properties of prion nanofibrils, which exhibit self-assembled steric zipper and amyloid fibrils, result in fatal prion diseases such as transmissible spongiform encephalopathies and neurodegenerative diseases such as Alzheimer's disease. Various origins for the infectious nature of prions have been suggested, including the molecular structure; amyloid diseases exert their toxicity by forming self-aggregated β-sheets and self-assembled long fibrils. For example, hIAPP fibrils induce apoptosis of insulin-secreting β-cells in the pancreas for its hardness and self-propagation characteristics. For the prion, PrP^{C} and PrP^{Sc} differ because of the transition from an α-helix to a β-sheet, respectively, to self-assemble into amyloidogenic fibrils. This chapter describes the amyloidogenic structural characteristics of prion fibrils and their relationship with their functions. The molecular structural characteristics can be quantified based on affinity, toxicity, and infectivity, among others, which are key factors for understanding the origin of prion diseases and developing therapeutic strategies. We focus on the mechanical properties of amyloid fibrils such as the dynamic and material properties of the HET-s prion.

Prion proteins exist in forms such as fibrils, oligomers, and lattice-like plate structures under different physiological conditions. A common structural feature of prion and amyloid proteins is that prions disrupt normal cell function and exhibit toxic behavior; thus, it is necessary to understand the different conformations of prion proteins under various physiological conditions. Different conformations of prion proteins have been reported under various pH conditions determined using various experimental techniques. Furthermore, some computational groups investigated the development of secondary prion structures as well as protonation status of specific prion residues, which enable secondary structures of prions to form oligomer conformation and grow into fibrillar or plaque structures. Similarly, toxic and nontoxic characteristics of prion proteins for β-helices in the presence of physiological agents were determined through the structural stability and mechanical property analyses.

Various experimental and computational studies have provided insight into the amyloid fibril-forming mechanism. Recently, computational studies were performed to overcome the limitation of experimental methods, which are unable to reveal the detailed molecular structures. For several decades, many studies evaluated the mechanical properties (such as bending and torsional rigidities) and mechanical behaviors of amyloid fibrils. These studies increased the understanding of the mechanism of fibril formation. Most studies evaluated homogeneous amyloid fibrils. However, other experiments revealed that heterogenetic interactions are possible for different amyloid monomers. Alpha-synuclein Aβ, Aβ-amylin, and Aβ-tau are well-known heterogenetic interactions.

Previous experimental and computational studies reported that depending on the conformation of amyloids or prion proteins, 2D material-based amyloids including fibrillar and plaque were deposited, which disrupted normal cell functions. Additionally, 1D materials, based on amyloids such as monomers and oligomers, showed toxic characteristics. These various forms of amyloid and prion proteins are affected by physiological conditions such as thermal fluctuation, internal flow, pH, and ionic strength. For instance, Aβ amyloid proteins exhibit various conformations such as cross-β zipper structures and β-turn-β motif structures. Based on their structural conformation features, the generation and development

http://dx.doi.org/10.5772/66448

of oligomeric and fibrillar Aβ amyloids are different. Specifically, the existence of metal ions including copper, zinc, and aluminum affects the development of oligomeric or fibrillar Aβ amyloids. Therefore, understanding the various conformations of Aβ amyloid and their characteristics under different physiological conditions is necessary for revealing their toxic behaviors.

In this chapter, we introduce the mechanism of formation of amyloid fibrils and diverse molecular structures of prion fibrils. Moreover, the structure-property relationships and mechanical characterization *in silico* are described using HET-s amyloidogenic prion fibrils as an example.

2. Seeding and aggregation mechanisms of prion nanofibrils

In this section, the seeding mechanism and characteristics of prions are introduced with homogeneous/heterogenetic amyloidogenic prion fibrils.

2.1. Prion, amyloid folding, and amyloid fibrils

Prion proteins, known as proteinaceous infectious agents, constitute a subclass of amyloids. Prion infection involves the conversion of proteins from their normal functional conformations, via an unfolded intermediate state, into amyloids. The conversion of the α-helical, isoform of the prion protein (PrP^{c}) into the insoluble, β-sheet-rich, and infectious form (PrP^{sc}) induces the accumulation of β-sheets and formation of fibrils and bundle structures [1]. After seeding, self-propagation is induced by providing templates for further assemblies [2–4]. This is known as the initial event in prion-inducing disease [5–9]. It is important to understand the propagation and amyloid fibril-forming mechanism for the development of therapeutic agents [10–12]. To understand amyloid fibril formation, numerous experimental and computational studies have been conducted. The molecular and atomic structure of mammalian and fungal prion fibrils should be determined to understand the propensity for polypeptides to form amyloid fibrils. In many cases, mammalian amyloid fibrils, which are known to induce amyloid disease, such as Aβ, α-synuclein, and amylin, do not form structures determined by their amino acid sequences. It is known that for self-propagation, molecular polymorphisms lead to different structures, and various polymorphic structures have been observed under diverse laboratory conditions, as depicted in **Figure 1**. For example, Tycko et al. showed that $A\beta_{1-40}$ has two main polymorphic structures that form fibrils [13]. One is a twofold, and the other is a threefold β-sheet array. According to the interaction directions of the β-sheet layers, templates for fibril structures were determined. Furthermore, self-propagation of HET-s fungal amyloid fibril was studied previously using high-resolution techniques, offering insight into structural changes induced by pH variations [4].

Advanced experimental techniques such as X-ray crystallography, transmission electron microscopy, scanning electron microscopy, and cryo-electron microscopy have revealed high-resolution amyloid conformations and the self-propagation and fibril formation mechanisms [14–20]. Amyloid fibrils were suggested to aggregate via a dense inherent hydrogen-bond-network and steric-zipper-like interactions between β-sheet layers, resulting in fiber formation along the fibril axis. Amyloid fibrils showed good structural complementarity and highly ordered conformations. However, although the physiochemical characteristics of amyloid proteins have been revealed, the structures and seeding processes remain unclear, and determining the molecular motion of amyloid proteins is challenging.

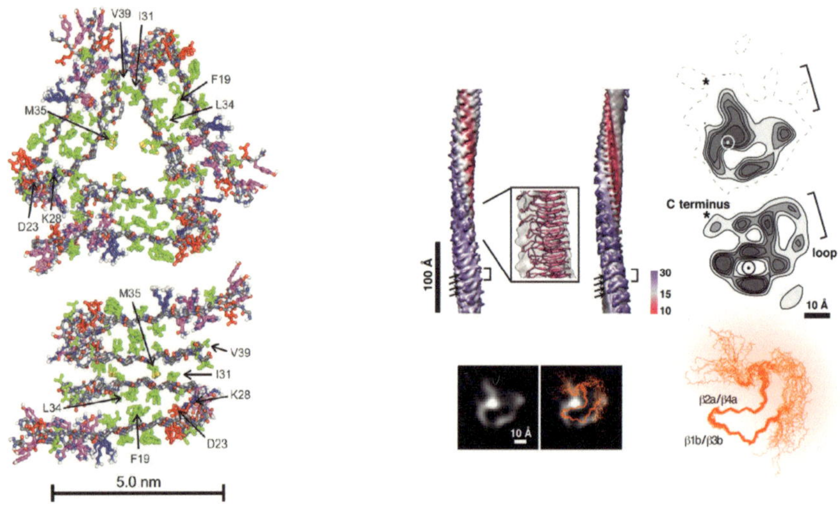

Figure 1. Various conformations for amyloid fibrils along to different cross-sectional area [13] and pH conditions [4].

2.2. Self-seeding and cross-seeding of amyloids

Diseases related to the toxicity of amyloid proteins are induced by the accumulation of amyloids, which consists of fibrillar forms and tangles. Experimental studies revealed that amyloid fibrils extracted from patients with amyloid disease brain had a fibrillar form and residual nonfibrillar materials [3]. The extracted fibrils showed widths and morphologies similar to those of synthetic amyloid fibrils *in vitro*, but the precise morphologies of the extracted amyloid fibrils are difficult to assess because of the self-association of fibrils and adhesive particles. Aβ amyloid fibrils from amyloid disease brains presumably contained chain length variations and chemical modifications. Previously, experimental and computational studies evaluated the kinetics of amyloid fibril formation. For both extracted and synthetic amyloid fibrils, the growth rate of amyloid fibrils was accelerated and amplified by seeding. However, nonfibrillar particles were not accelerated, and they did not show seeding behavior. Typically, amyloid fibrils are constructed by adding amyloid protein blocks composed of 4 or 5 parallel- or anti-parallel-layered β-sheets. These structures may also be 'tetramers' or 'pentamers', depending on the number of layers present. Monomers referred to as seeds act as "Lego blocks," and single amyloid fibrils are constructed in a specific elongation direction when seed monomers are added. Particularly, single monomers can be regarded as templates for fibril formation. Previous studies evaluated the elongation processes of uniformly composed monomers to understand the self-propagation process [2, 3, 21]. The process is referred to as "self-seeding" and homogeneous amyloid block monomers form fibrillar conformations. Previous studies also provided insight into the structural and physiochemical characteristics of diverse amyloid fibrils. However, accumulated amyloid agents, which are present in neurodegenerative disease, are not uniform. Thus, better models are needed to understand the polymorphic features of the fibril formation mechanism. Recent studies have evaluated the different types of amyloid block monomers that can bind to each other to form fibrils and tangles through a specific mechanism known as "cross-seeding". The key point of this mechanism is that one block monomer of amyloid proteins can be regarded as a template for other block monomers, even if the blocks have different physiochemical characteristics and are constructed with different conformations and compositions [22–25]. The cross-seeding mechanism can explain the formation of heterogeneous-composed amyloid fibrils and polymorphic fibrils, and these models offered better insight into amyloid accumulation processes. Experimental studies showed that seeding with amyloid-like fibrils made from short synthetic peptides from other amyloid proteins or fibrils of a completely different nature; for example, bacterial curli or Sup35 from *Saccharomyces* may function through other interactions [26]. It appears likely that the β-sheet structure of the seed has a general effect on the seeded material, inducing misfolding, and production of a new seed that can proceed to an amyloid fibril. In addition, Yan et al. examined the effect of coinjection of murine senile apolipoprotein A-II amyloid and reactive protein A amyloid amyloidosis to determine the heterologous transmissible seeding mechanism [22] shown in **Figure 2**.

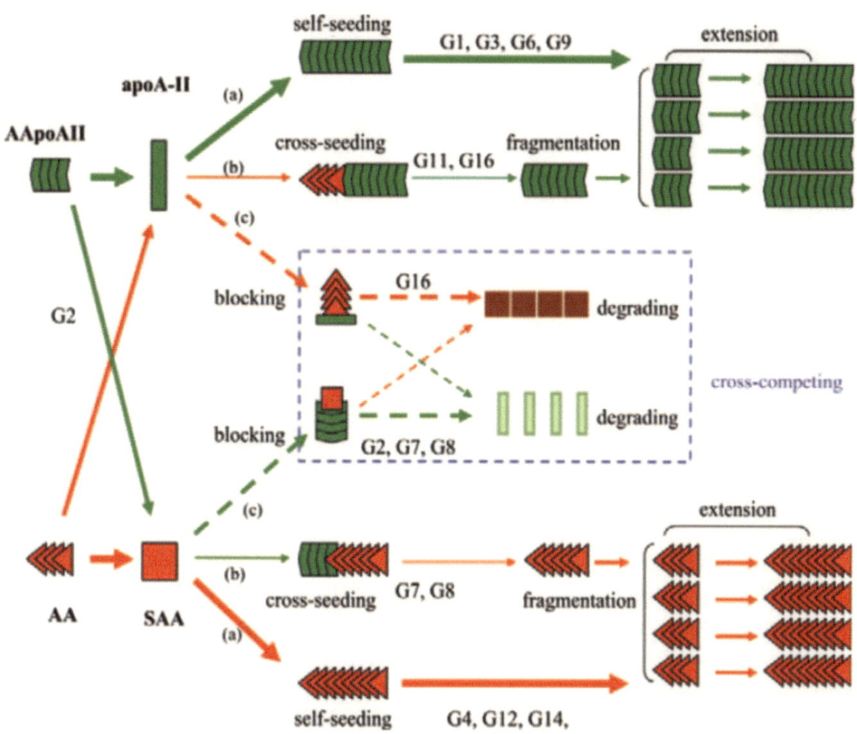

Figure 2. Cross-seeding mechanism of heterogeneous amyloid fibrils [22].

2.3. Cross-seeded fibrils

Recently, computational studies were performed to overcome the limitation of experimental studies, which are unable to determine molecular structures in detail. For several decades, many studies have evaluated the mechanical properties and behaviors of amyloid fibrils [27–32], providing insight into the amyloid fibril formation mechanism. Most studies examined homologous amyloid fibrils. Experimentally, it was revealed that heterogeneous interactions enabled different amyloid monomers to aggregate with each other. Alpha synuclein-Aβ, Aβ-amylin, and Aβ-tau, which are well-known heterologous amyloid fibrils, have been used to understand the effect of structural affinity on amyloid fibril formation [33–38]. Recent studies revealed the structural and interaction features of cross-seeded amyloid oligomers and proto-fibrils. Oligomeric Aβ-tau heterologous amyloid is one example of a cross-seeded amyloid protein. Aβ and U-shaped tau monomers are structural similar in that both have a common U-shaped β-turn-β structure. In addition, Miller et al. determined the structural stabilities of possible compositions of Aβ-tau heterologous oligomers using experimental and computational methods [38], as shown in **Figure 3**. They studied the interactions between heterologous monomers. Furthermore, Choi et al. studied the mechanical and physicochemical features of heterologous oligomers with diverse-mutated Tau monomers [37]. They found that different binding directions showed different structural stabilities. It was observed that amyloid beta monomers and other monomers could act as templates for seeding processes.

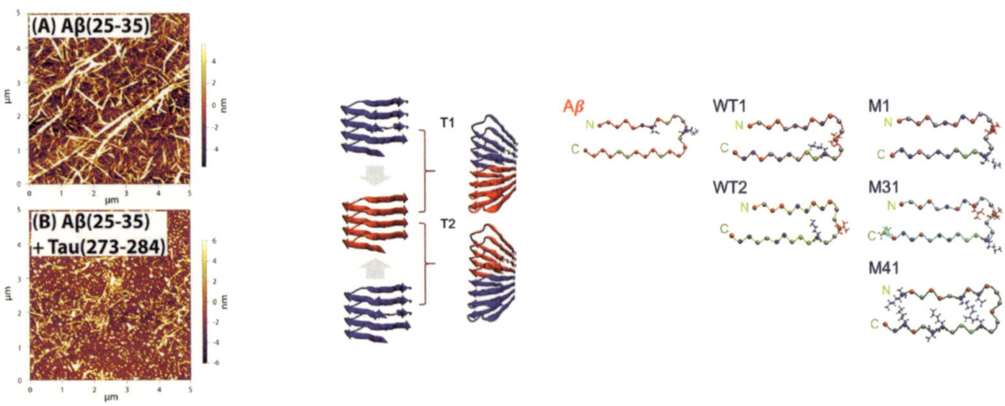

Figure 3. Experimental result for heterogeneous amyloid fibrils (*left panel*) [36] and schematic constraint for simulation of heterogeneous amyloid fibrils (*right panel*) [37].

Many computational studies showed that not only structural similarity but also specific interactions between residues of amyloid proteins play a major role in seeding processes. Elongation of amyloid fibrils along the fibril axis is related to the binding features of the seed amyloids and their structural stabilities. The binding sites on monomers enable the attachment of other monomers [39]. The specific interactions can be classified as intra-layer interactions and inter-layer interactions, which confer structural stability, as depicted in **Figure 4**.

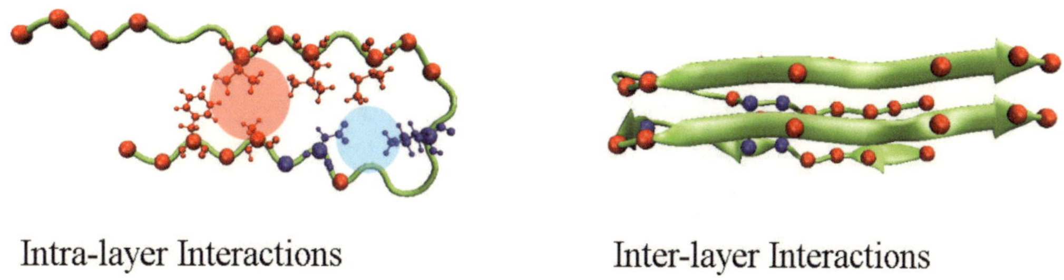

Figure 4. Intra-layer interaction and inter-layer of heterogeneous mixture of amyloid proteins [37].

It was revealed that the structural stabilities of intra-layers were affected by steric-zipper-like interactions [40–42] and salt-bridge interactions [37]. Intra-structural stabilities are dominantly affected by specific interactions. Hydrophobic residues in interior regions of amyloid fibrils form steric-zipper-like structures and help maintain cross-sectional structures. Although heterologous monomers contain different residues, hydrophobic residues commonly construct dry-regions and affect structural stabilities. In addition, charged residues such as lysine (K) and aspartic acid (D) form salt-bridge regions and affect intra-stabilities.

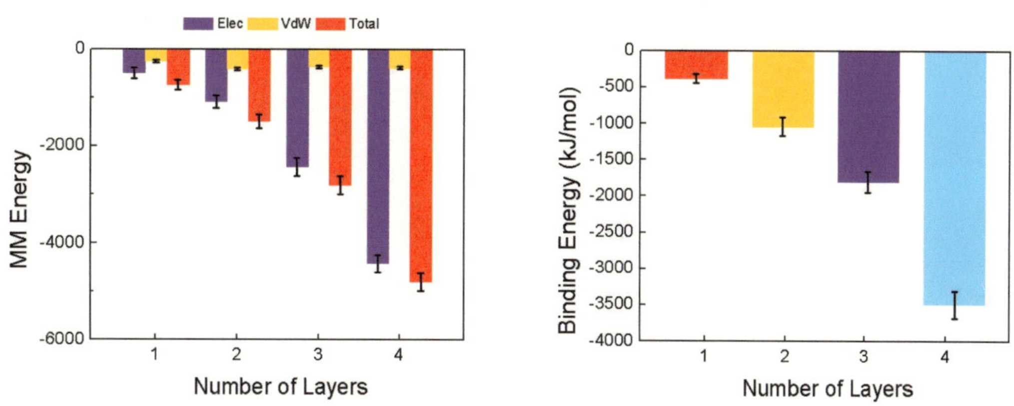

Figure 5. MM and binding energies of Aβ-tau mixtures after 20-ns equilibrium MD simulations [37].

The stabilities of inter-layers are also affected by hydrogen-bonding networks and nonbonding interaction energies, such as Van der Waals and electrostatic energy induced by interactions between residues of layers that face each other. Interactions between single layers are dominantly affected by electrostatic and Van der Waals energies. However, as the number of layers is increased, the effect of electrostatic energies becomes dominant. In the fibril formation processes of heterologous amyloids, binding between monomers is affected by electrostatic energies (**Figure 5**).

3. Molecular structure of prions in various physiological environments

In the previous section, we described the general aggregation and seeding mechanism of amyloid-like prion fibrils based on homogeneous and heterogeneous structures. During the aggregation of prion fibrils in the seeding mechanism, the external environment affects growth of prion-like amyloid fibrils. Here, the effect of the external environment is referred to as the physiological conditions, which have been shown to affect molecular conformational variation in the fibrillary growth of PrP^{C}, HET-s, and Sup35, in detail.

First, the development of prion proteins is caused by the conversion of native prion protein monomeric PrP^{C} as misfolded and denatured PrP^{Sc} because of external conditions such as partial mutation, internal flow, pH, ionic strength, and temperature variations. This PrP^{C} protein is glycosylated and functions similar to components of the extracellular surface of neurons, which play a significant role in signal transduction. This native PrP^{C} is converted to monomeric PrP^{Sc}, which gradually aggregates to form oligomeric, fibrillar, and plaque structures. These converted monomeric PrP^{Sc} act as seeds at specific concentrations with a lag phase, which induce the aggregation of fibrillar and plaque prions. This conversion is frequently observed in amyloidosis including Alzheimer's disease by Aβ from amyloid precursor protein and cardiovascular diseases by transthyretin (105–115) from native functional transthyretin monomers [6, 43, 44]. As shown in **Figure 6**, aggregation of converted PrP^{Sc} from PrP^{C} monomer deposited near the brains of human and mouse represents the hallmark of neuropathological features [45].

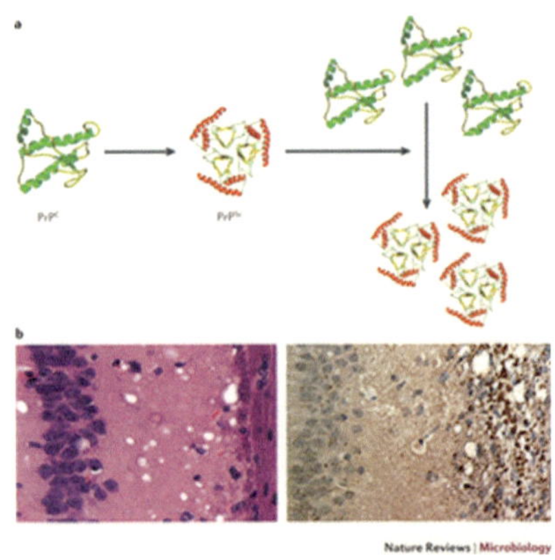

Figure 6. Prion proteins. (a) Conversion mechanism from PrP^{C} to PrP^{Sc} and (b) experimental result of PrP prion proteins [45].

The other type of prion proteins is the HET-s prion protein. According to Govaerts et al., the left-handed β-rich helical structures containing α-helices are located outside of the β-helical structures of prion fibers and are responsible for their toxicity (refer **Figure 6(a)**) [46]. In contrast, right-handed prion proteins are not toxic based on combined experimental and computational studies. HET-s prion amyloid proteins were also reported to have β-solenoid conformations and triangular hydrophobic cores [47]. In 2008, Wasmer et al. determined detailed structural information of HET-s (219–289) via solid-state nuclear magnetic resonance techniques as shown in **Figure 7**.

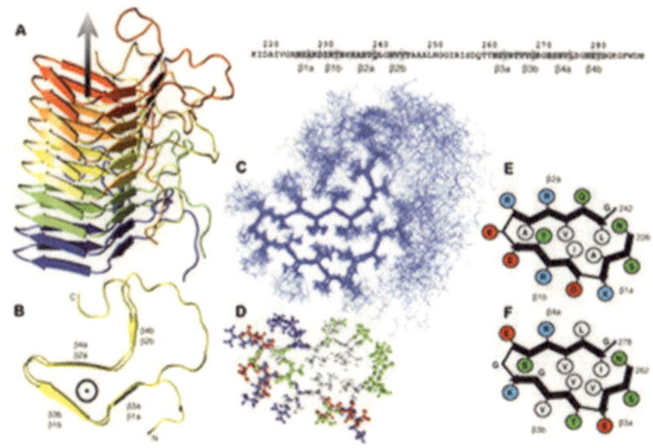

Figure 7. (A) Side view of HET-s prion fibrils (B) Top view (C) NMR structure (D) Type of amino acid for single layer of HET-s (E) Side chain interaction of first layer (F) Side chains for second layer [47].

A third type of prion proteins is known as the Sup35 prion proteins, which exhibit cross-β characteristics with steric zipper structures as shown in **Figure 3** [48, 49] and are similar to other proteins that cause several degenerative diseases such as Alzheimer's diseases, type II diabetes, and dialysis-related amyloidosis by Aβ, human islet polypeptide, and β_2-microglobulin [41]. Specifically, partial prion proteins fragment from the Sup35 prion protein and show polymorphic features including lateral thickness increases (**Figures 8** and **9**) with changes in physiological conditions such as pH, thermal variation, internal flow, and ionic strength [50].

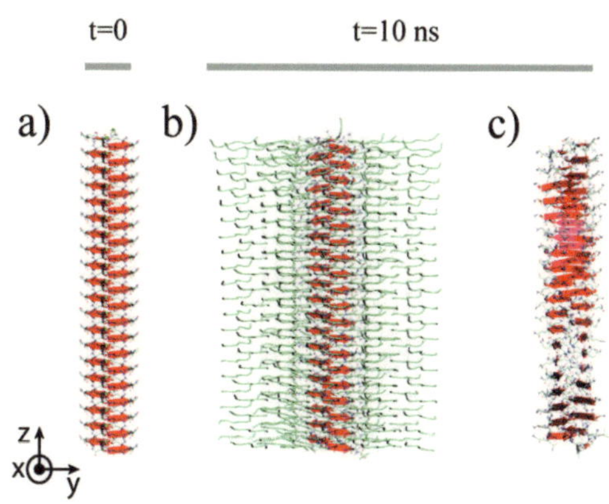

Figure 8. Lateral thickness composition of Sup 35 prion proteins. (a) Unit protofilament crystalline structures, (b) lateral thickness composition of Sup 35 prion fibrils, and (c) equilibrium result of unit protofilament prion protein [51].

Fibrillar and plaque forms of PrP^{Sc} prion proteins are frequently observed because of their considerable infectivity ability. These fibrillar and plaque types of prion proteins can be generated through repetitive fragmentation and elongation mechanisms. The prion proteins grow by adding monomers or attracting other fragmented prion segments. A previous study showed that fragmented and denatured prion proteins add PrP^{C} to grow PrP^{Sc} based on protein-misfolding cycling amplification techniques [45] (refer to **Figure 10**).

Colby et al. investigated the prion propagation mechanism via repetitive fragmentation and elongation by adding additional prion monomers and evaluated the kinetics study and conducted imaging analysis [15]. Through the repetitive process of fragmentation and elongation mechanism, neuro-toxic prion oligomers could be generated. In this aggregation, after conversion from PrP^{C} to PrP^{Sc}, prion proteins showed toxic characteristics and affected intercellular processes. Similarly, for the fragmentation and elongation mechanisms of HET-s prion proteins, Mizuno et al. investigated similar fibrillar and plaque proteins such as prion, particularly HET-s, under various pH conditions [4]. Fragmentation and addition of prion seeds generated different types of fibrillar HET-s near pH 2 and 3, while lattice-like HET-s was observed under neutral physiological conditions. Between pH 2 and 3, a tight fibrillar HET-s structure was observed, while fibrillar HET-s exhibited a cavity at pH 3 [4, 37]

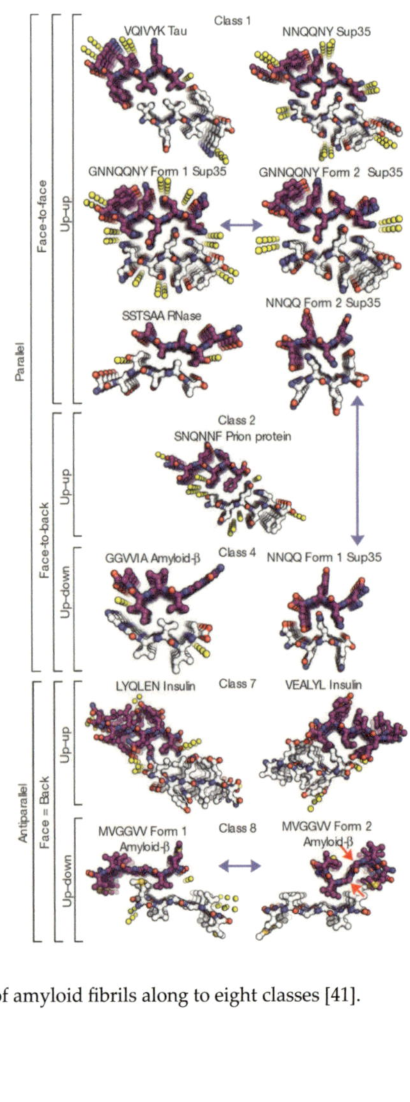

Figure 9. Polymorphic schematic of amyloid fibrils along to eight classes [41].

http://dx.doi.org/10.5772/66448

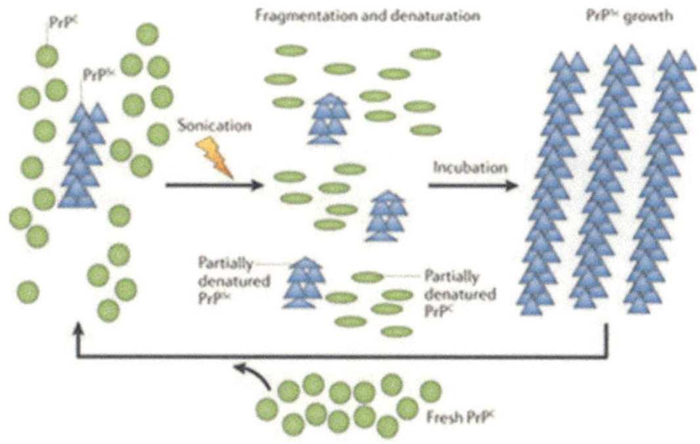

Figure 10. Schematic for protein-misfolding cyclic amplification [45].

To discuss the structural characteristics of plaque and fibrillar prions from converted PrP^{Sc}, in this section, we described the conversion mechanism of PrP^C from PrP^{Sc} prion proteins at the atomic scale based on computational results. As described previously, native PrP^C proteins varied from misfolded PrP^C to PrP^{Sc} based on the physiological conditions [52–56]. In 2001, Daggett et al. reported computational results for the conversion of PrP^C when pH conditions were varied from neutral to low pH conditions [56]. They observed that the core region of PrP^C was stabilized, while the N-terminus exhibited considerable structural fluctuations compared to the core and C-terminal regions. In addition, they reported the conversion process from PrP^C to PrP^{Sc} over time.

As shown in **Figure 11**, additional β-strands were generated at the N-terminal regions with lengthening of the β-strands after 2 ns. Furthermore, they found that Met-129 at the N-terminal region triggered the conversion of the turn-rich N-terminal region into β-strands. Therefore, external physiological factors such as ionic strength and pH altered the native PrP^C resulting in misfolding into PrP^{Sc} structures with the additional generation of β-strands, which may be related to the aggregation of PrP^{Sc} structures.

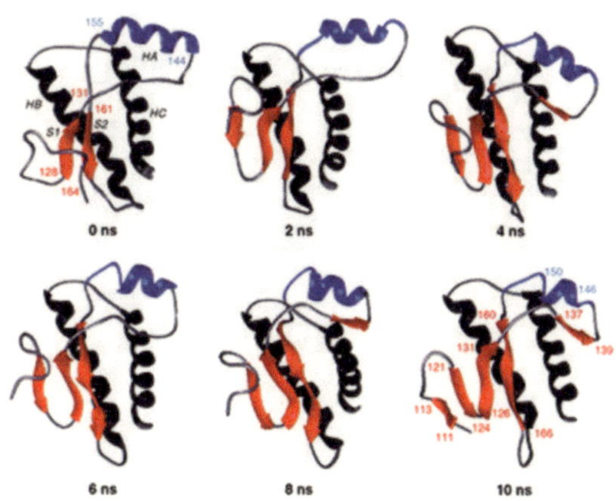

Figure 11. Trajectory variation of PrP^C at low pH with respect to time trajectories [56].

Another study observed protofibril formation of scrapie prion protein, which contained numerous β-strand conformation variations [55]. They computationally found that the conversion from monomeric syrian PrP^{C} segments to PrP^{Sc} occurred because of a point asparagine mutation at the 147th aspartate residue (D147N) under neutral and low pH conditions. Subsequently, they observed that the prion protofibril was stabilized and compared their computational results to the experimental results of DeMarco et al. [55]. The monomeric conversion from D147N PrP^{C} to PrP^{Sc} occurred near β-strands at the 1st and 2nd β-sheet regions of the original structures. In this procedure, they determined the critical role of additionally generated β-strands in the conversion of PrP^{C} structures through computational analysis. The salt bridge region between the 147th aspartate and 151st arginine residue was disrupted; this event did not critically alter the structural stability of D147N PrP^{C} structures, but the D147 mutation affected expansion of the N-terminal region, generating additional β-strands regions. These results support their previous computational results for the role of the Met-129 residue.

Based on the converted PrP^{Sc} unit monomers, they constructed the basic protofibril unit of the converted PrP^{Sc} monomer by connecting adjacent β-strand regions of the monomer. As shown in **Figure 12(a)**, basic trimer structures of prion protofibril units using converted PrP^{Sc} monomer under acidic conditions were constructed and stabilized based on molecular dynamics simulations. By superimposing the trimer structures along the fibril axis as shown in **Figure 12(b)** with a 60° rotation, they replicated the sixfold symmetry of prion fibril structures. Using this computationally constructed prion protofibril model, they compared the results with the previously reported experimental results of Cauhey et al. Electron microscopy images were consistent with the constructed computational model of the prion protofibril.

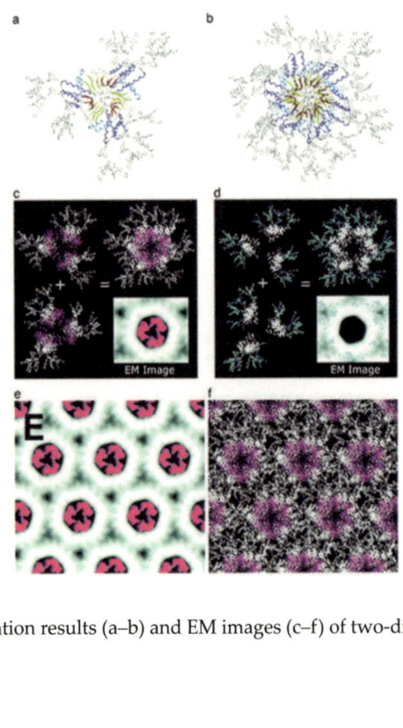

Figure 12. Comparison with simulation results (a–b) and EM images (c–f) of two-dimensional PrP structures [55].

Additionally, they observed conformational variation in the full-length bovine PrP prion at low pH using molecular dynamics [53]. The conformational variation of native full-length bovine PrP prion structures was found to be PrP^{Sc} with additional generation of β-strands; the role of the Met-129 residue was determined by conformational and secondary structure analysis, as shown in **Figure 13**.

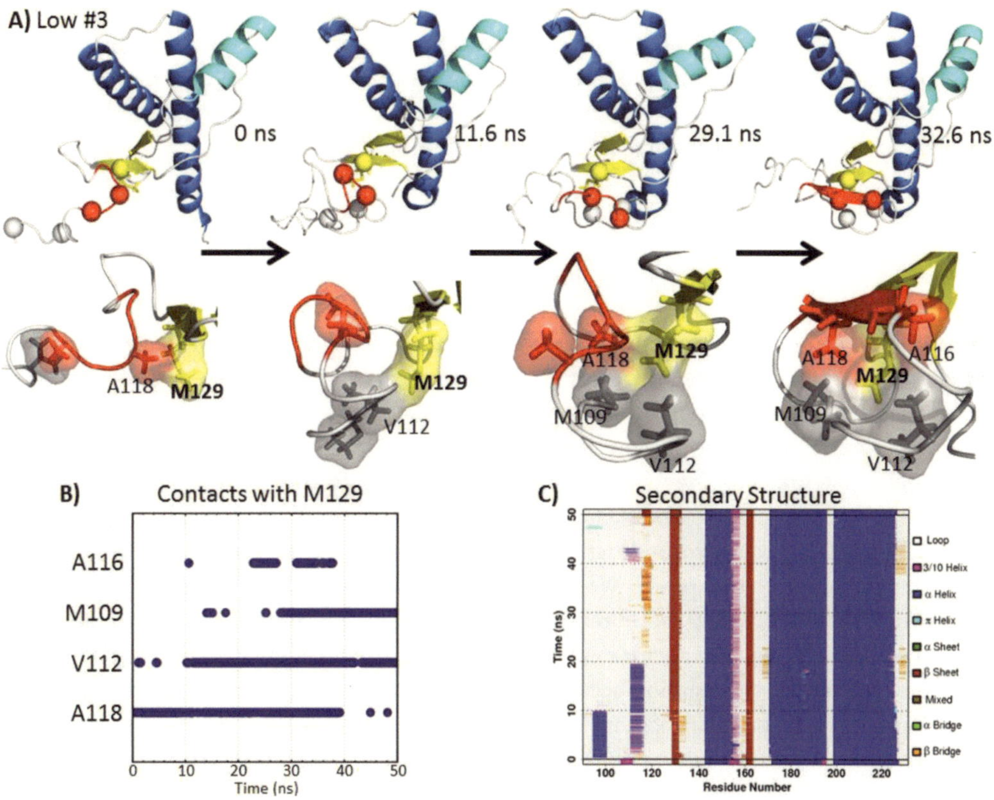

Figure 13. Representation of β-strands formation at the N-terminal region due to the N-terminal hydrophobic contacts with M129 in low pH. (a) Top panel describes the bovine PrP with crucial hydrophobic residue described as sphere, (b) hydrophobic contact with M129 respect whole time trajectories, and (c) secondary structure analysis of PrP [54].

Based on computational studies of prion proteins, physiological conditions such as pH, ionic strength, point mutation, and temperature variation have a considerable effect on structural variations in HET-s and native PrP^{C} structures as PrP^{Sc} structures; some conditions enlarge the N-terminal region and cause formation of additional β-strands, which are similar to reported experimental results. Converted PrP^{Sc} with additional β-strands can connect to protofibril structures. Therefore, understanding prion proteins under external physiological conditions may be useful for preventing the generation of fibril structures and their toxic behaviors.

4. Characterization of amyloid molecular structure by mechanical testing

Above, we introduced the generation of amyloid-like prion fibrils via self-aggregation and seeding mechanisms based on previously reported experimental and computational studies. Specifically, we described the aggregation mechanism from native PrP^{C} segments to denatured PrP^{Sc} segments under physiological conditions, where pH variation caused partially disordered N-terminal regions of PrP^{C} to convert to β-strands at the N-terminal region of PrP^{Sc}. These denatured PrP^{Sc} segments aggregated as fibrillar prion amyloids, which are toxic to cell function and delete the lipid bilayer of membranes. In this section, we explain the role of the β-sheet-rich prion fibrils and their toxic characteristics from a mechanical perspective determined through experimental and computational studies.

4.1. Importance of mechanical properties of amyloid fibrils

4.1.1. Disease—breakage and infections

Amyloid fibrils are disease-related proteins found in various types of neurodegenerative and degenerative diseases. Aggregated fibrils were detected in diseased cells. Understanding the mechanical behavior of amyloid fibrils is important because it is related to fibril breakage. Misfolded amyloids do not initially form long fibrils. Single amyloid monomers inside the body begin to aggregate. They stack into small oligomers, forming aggregates, which grow into the fibrillar form. These fibers may be up to 100-nm long [5]. In humans, amyloid fibrils eventually break. In our surroundings, breakage of an item is not a good thing. For example, if a ruler is broken into two pieces, we do not use it anymore. Because we cannot measure the length which it was made to measure. However, Long amyloid fibrils breakage creates small oligomers, which become seeds for new fibrils. Additionally, in environments containing both fibrils and oligomers, aggregation occurs more rapidly than in environments containing only oligomers [5]. Thus, breakage of amyloid fibrils generates additional fibrils. Understanding when the fibril will break may be determined by measuring mechanical properties of amyloid fibrils.

4.1.2. Bio-materials

Several studies have compared the mechanical properties (e.g., Young's modulus) of amyloid fibrils with those of other bio-materials. Amyloid fibrils exhibit a Young's modulus comparable to those of wood and silk, and its strength is comparable to those of metals such as aluminum or steel (**Figure 14**) [57]. Comparable mechanical properties of amyloid fibrils with these materials indicate that amyloid fibril is a potentially useful bio-material. Compared to proteinaceous biomaterials such as actin filaments, amyloid fibrils exhibit longer persistence length [19]. Persistence length is a basic mechanical property quantifying the stiffness of a polymer. Materials with shorter lengths than its persistence length behave as elastic materials and form longer polymers. The mechanical properties and behaviors of elastic materials and polymers are very different. Polymers are materials that act as soft chains, making them unsuitable for use as support materials. Proteins are composed of poly-peptide chains and are polymers. The poly-peptide chain folds as a globular protein (or misfolds as an amyloid), and the structure is maintained by noncovalent interactions between amino-acids. Amyloid fibrils or actin filaments are large structures constructed by large numbers of proteins composed of polypeptide chains.

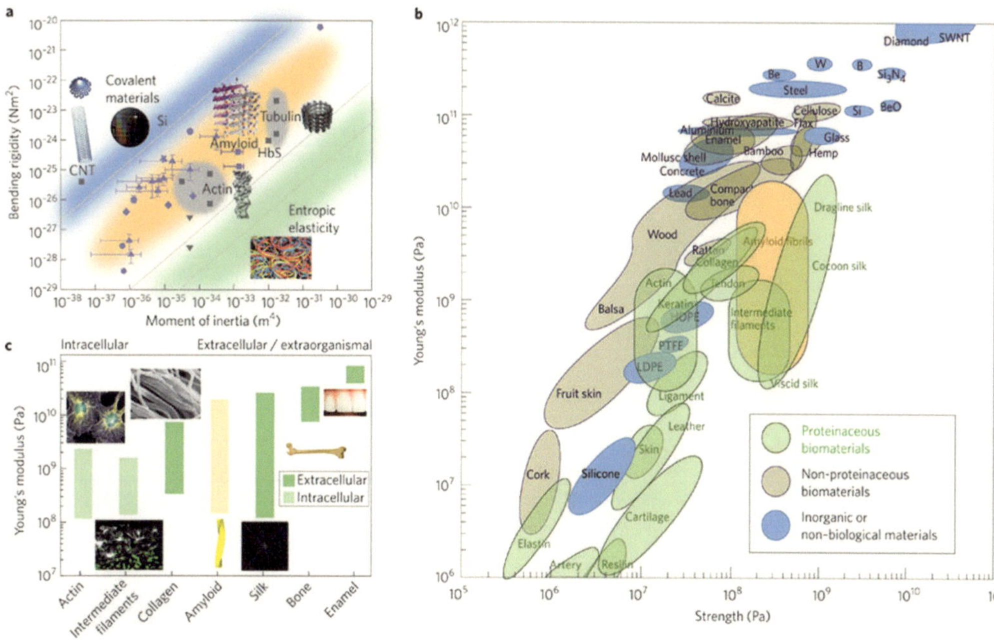

Figure 14. (a) Bending rigidity of amyloid fibrils compared to other materials (b) Young's modulus of amyloid fibrils (c) Young's modulus of biomaterials [57].

4.2. Determination of mechanical properties

4.2.1. Experiments

Studies have focused on the relationship between amyloid fibril mechanical properties and behaviors in biology. One of the pioneer studies of mechanical property measurement of amyloid fibril was conducted by Smith et al. in 2006 [58]. In their study, the mechanical properties of insulin fibrils (not prions) were measured using atomic fore microscopy to determine ultimate strength, Young's modulus, persistence length, bending rigidity, shear modulus, and torsional rigidity (**Figure 15**). Young's modulus and persistence length were measured to be 3.3 ± 0.4 GPa and 22 ± 3 μm, respectively. Several studies revealed that amyloid fibril's mechanical properties are comparable to those of silk, a well-known and broadly used biomaterial [57–59]. Interestingly, amyloid fibrils share some structural characteristics with silk: (1) frequently repetitive primary sequences; (2) stable and irreversible β-sheet-enriched state; (3) structural similarity with β-sheet rich structure; (4) self-assembling behavior to fibrillary structures in solution; and (5) hydrogen bonding between β-sheets. Comparable mechanical properties and structural features indicate that amyloid fibrils can also be used in various applications [59]. The Young's modulus of various amyloid fibrils ranged from 10^9 to 10^{10} Pa, which is similar to that of silk [57].

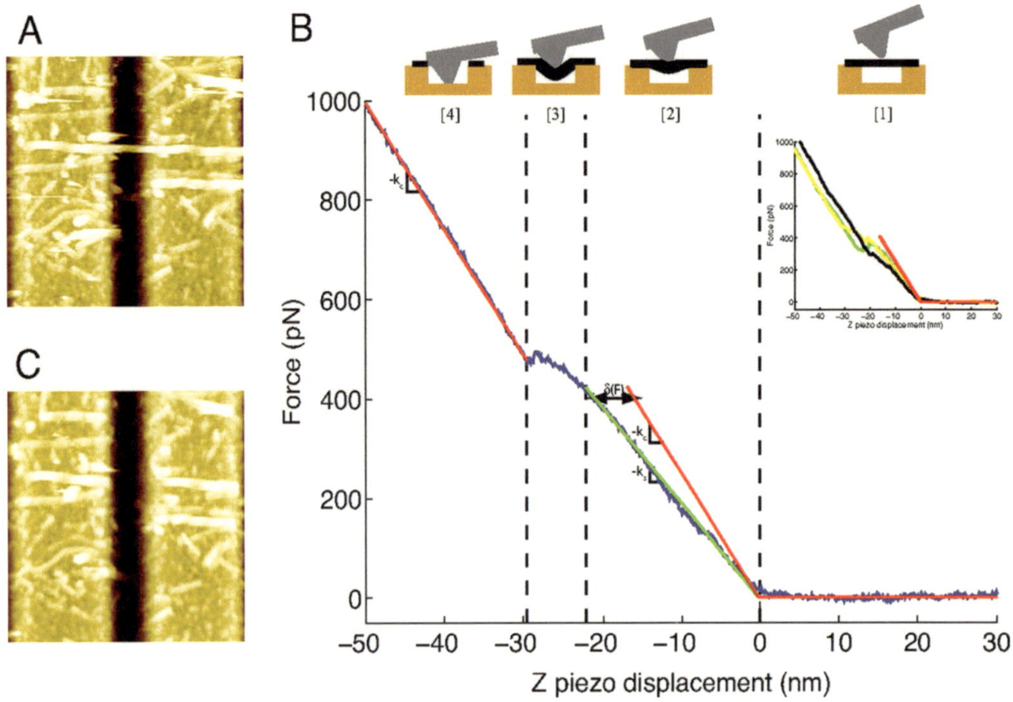

Figure 15. (A) Image of insulin amyloid fibrils before breakage (B) Force displacement curve for bending with atomic force microscope (C) Image after breakage [58].

The mechanical properties of amyloid fibrils are not affected by covalent bonds constructing the β-sheets, but rather by noncovalent bonds between β-sheets. Hydrogen bonds are important for maintaining amyloid fibrils and their mechanical properties; other non-covalent bonds (e.g., electrostatic interactions, π-π interactions, etc.) can also affect strength depending on the amyloid fibril structures.

4.2.2. Simulations

Experimental studies have revealed that various types of amyloid fibrils exist. Not only disease-related fibril types such as Alzheimer's disease, Jakob-Cruetzfeld disease, type 2 diabetes, and Parkinson's disease, among others but also those that form amyloid fibrils in same phenotypes of amyloids are important. For example, human islet amyloid polypeptide (hIAPP), which is found in cells of type 2 diabetes patients, forms eight different fibril types by stacking in different directions [17, 41]. Differences in the composition of amyloid fibrils lead to different mechanical behaviors and fractions in the body. Small fraction structures are more difficult to form than large fraction structures. Simulation methods constitute an easier approach for evaluating these variations in amyloid fibrils. A common structural characteristic of the amyloid fibril is its repetitive structure of β-sheets. Structural information determined experimentally may differ from that determined computationally.

Detailed structural information (distance between β-sheets, twist angle between layers, etc.) of amyloid fibrils is clearly needed to rapidly and effectively build the fibrils [17]. An important simulation study evaluated the size-dependent mechanical properties of $A\beta_{1-40}$ [60]. In this study, two different types of Aβ amyloid fibrils were constructed: a twofold symmetric structure and threefold symmetric structure. A computational model was prepared using an elastic network model (ENM), and normal mode analysis (NMA) was applied to calculate eigenvalue eigenvectors of the structure. Torsional modulus, bending rigidity, and Young's modulus were calculated for different types of amyloid fibrils, with the twofold symmetric structure showing better mechanical properties. Yoon et al. analyzed four configurations of hIAPP amyloid fibrils. They also applied ENM to calculate the mechanical properties of hIAPP amyloid fibrils. Despite this detailed chemical interaction information, each structure exhibited different mechanical properties related to differences in H-bond interactions [61]. Additionally, the effects of mutations on the mechanical properties of amyloid fibrils [62] or multi-strand effects can be calculated [63].

4.3. Structural effect of prion

4.3.1. Structural variation depending on environment and its properties

Proteins functioning in living bodies interact with various surroundings such as water, ion, proteins, ligands, and DNA. Protein conformation, which is determined by sequence and length of the polypeptide chain, is important in the interactions with the surroundings of a protein. Some environmental conditions may favor amyloid formation (which may lead to an unhealthy condition). Studies of prions revealed that prions form a certain shape or structure under specific conditions, indicating that amyloid structure depends on the surroundings [4]. In this study, prions were exposed to different pH conditions, including pH 2, 3, 4, and 7. In each state, prions formed triplets, singlets and triplets, an angled-layer aggregate, and bundles at pH 2, 3, 4, and 7, respectively. The stability of each conformation changed when the pH was changed (surroundings). For example, a triplet structure formed at pH 2 and 3 but with different conformations. Additionally, a singlet was detected at pH 3. When the pH was changed to 4, the triplet fibril disappeared while the angled-layer structure remained. These structures may be related to the mechanical properties or interactions between fibrils. Triplet prion fibrils are stable and noninfectious (pH 2). However, when pH is increased, the triplet fibril structure is broken into singlets (pH 3) and become infectious. These singlet fibrils can easily break and form new fibrils from new seeds, forming an angled-layered structure (pH 4) as shown in **Figure 16**.

4.3.2. Simulation methods

Changes in pH affect the chemical interactions of prion amyloid fibrils. Although simulation researches do not reveal chemical interaction, they provide other useful information.

A study conducted in 2013 compared the mechanical properties of prion amyloid fibrils (left-handed turn) and nonprion fibrils (right-handed turn) using ENM and NMA [27]. Basic structural units were very similar β-sheets, but mechanical properties such as elastic modulus and bending rigidity differed for both fibrils as shown in **Figure 17**. In fact, a toxic prion fibril exhibited higher mechanical properties. Additionally, left-handed prion fibrils had more local contacts than non-prion fibrils, which are consistent with the results of a previous study analyzing hydrogen bonds.

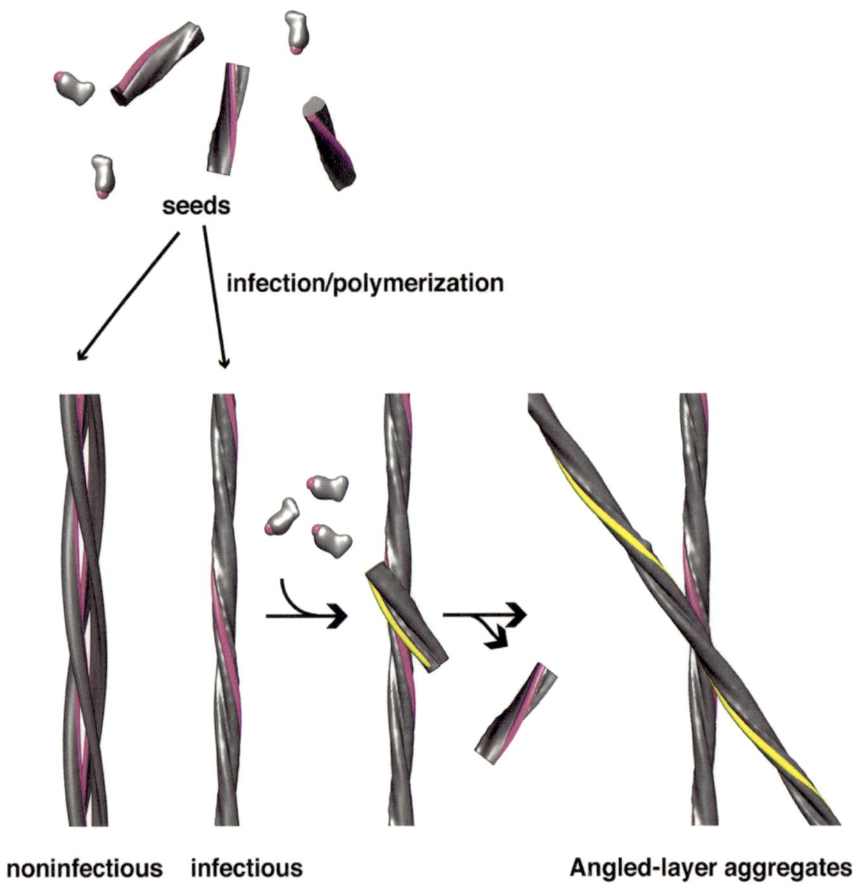

Figure 16. Surface seeding model for assembly of HET-s prion disease fibrils [4].

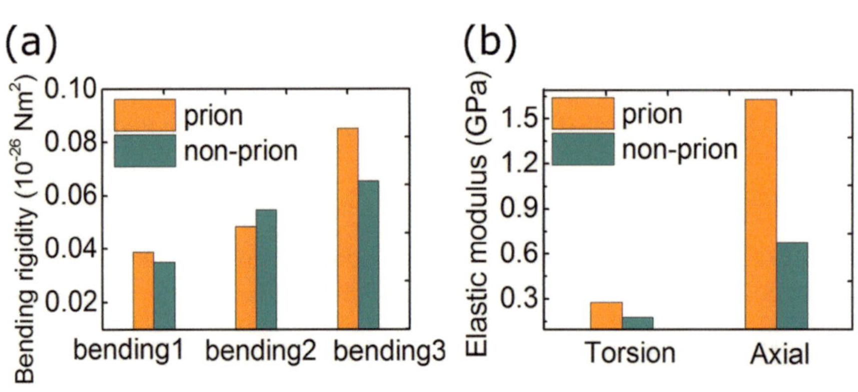

Figure 17. Difference of mechanical properties between prion fibril (orange) and non-prion fibril (a) Bending rigidities (b) Torsional and axial elastic modulus [27].

Triplet fibrils were also examined by ENM and NMA [64]. In this study, prion triplet fibrils were compared at pH 2 and 3. Mechanical properties such as bending rigidity and torsional modulus were calculated for both models; fibrils for the pH 2 model showed better values for both parameters. This indicates that the pH 2 model was more stable than the pH 3 model, which is known to be noninfectious [4]. However, the pH 3 triplet showed a bending rigidity of 0.6×10^{-26} Nm^2, which is much larger than the value of 0.3×10^{-26} Nm^2 determined for a singlet fibril in a previous study [27]. The structure and mechanical properties of prion fibrils are related, explaining their toxicities. Moreover, in the previous study, the potential for conformational changes between the pH 2 and 3 models was observed. NMA provides results in eigenvalues and eigenvectors, which are connected to natural frequencies and normal modes. A normal mode corresponds to a single natural frequency, and the low frequency normal mode describes large motions of structures (i.e., for amyloid fibril, bending, twisting, and extension). Comparison of the normal mode calculated from the pH 2 model and direction vector between the pH 2 and 3 model showed that low-frequency normal modes up to the 23rd mode described conformational changes in triplet fibril caused by pH change. These results indicate that conformational changes are caused by pH changes, but the conformational change direction can reveal structure information (**Figure 18**).

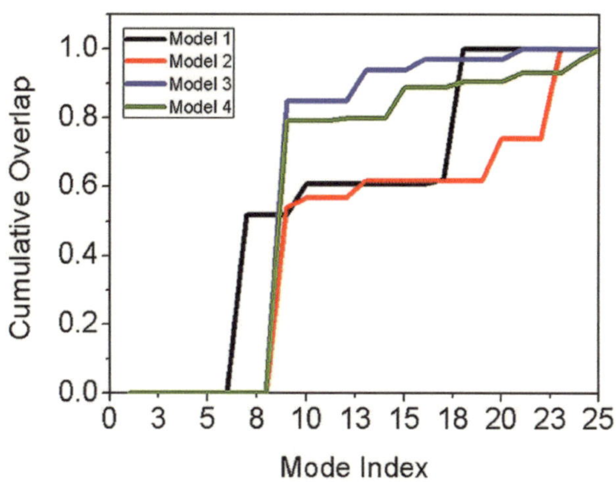

Figure 18. Cumulative overlap between normal modes calculated from pH 2 model and direction vector between pH 2 and pH 3 model [64].

5. Summary

In this chapter, the formation of amyloidogenic prion nanofibrils and the relationship between molecular structure and its properties are presented. In the first section, the seeding mechanisms of prions for the homogenous and heterogeneous fibrils are introduced, and the molecular structure differences in the assembly process of amyloid fibrils under environmental conditions are described in the second section. Finally, the mechanical characterization of amyloid fibrils *in vitro* and *in silico* is explained. It remains challenging to determine the infectiousness and toxicity of prions and amyloids. Therefore, additional studies are needed to determine the molecular structure, aggregation kinetics, and properties of prions and amyloids. Increasing the understanding of these molecules will aid in the development of therapeutic strategies for prion diseases.

Author details

Myeongsang Lee[1], Hyunsung Choi[1], Jae In Kim[1], Gwonchan Yoon[1,2*] and Sungsoo Na[1]

*Address all correspondence to: gwonchanyoon@gmail.com and nass@korea.ac.kr

1 Department of Mechanical Engineering, Korea University, Seoul, Republic of Korea

2 Department of Electrical and Computer Engineering, Texas Tech University, Lubbock, Texas, USA

References

[1] Stöhr J, Weinmann N, Wille H, Kaimann T, Nagel-Steger L, Birkmann E, et al. Mechanisms of prion protein assembly into amyloid. Proceedings of the National Academy of Sciences. 2008;105:2409–2414.

[2] Kihara M, Chatani E, Sakai M, Hasegawa K, Naiki H, Goto Y. Seeding-dependent maturation of β2-microglobulin amyloid fibrils at neutral pH. Journal of Biological Chemistry. 2005;280:12012–12018.

[3] Paravastu AK, Qahwash I, Leapman RD, Meredith SC, Tycko R. Seeded growth of β-amyloid fibrils from Alzheimer's brain-derived fibrils produces a distinct fibril structure. Proceedings of the National Academy of Sciences. 2009;106:7443–7448.

[4] Mizuno N, Baxa U, Steven AC. Structural dependence of HET-s amyloid fibril infectivity assessed by cryoelectron microscopy. Proceedings of the National Academy of Sciences. 2011;108:3252–3257.

[5] Merlini G, Bellotti V. Molecular mechanisms of amyloidosis. New England Journal of Medicine. 2003;349:583–596.

[6] Soto C. Unfolding the role of protein misfolding in neurodegenerative diseases. Nature Reviews Neuroscience. 2003;4:49–60.

[7] Chiti F, Dobson CM. Protein misfolding, functional amyloid, and human disease. Annual Review of Biochemistry. 2006;75:333–366.

[8] Pepys MB. Amyloidosis. Annual Review of Medicine. 2006;57:223–241.

[9] Eisenberg D, Jucker M. The amyloid state of proteins in human diseases. Cell. 2012;148: 1188–1203.

[10] Merlini G, Seldin DC, Gertz MA. Amyloidosis: pathogenesis and new therapeutic options. Journal of Clinical Oncology. 2011;29:1924–1933.

[11] Wang C, Yang A, Li X, Li D, Zhang M, Du H, et al. Observation of molecular inhibition and binding structures of amyloid peptides. Nanoscale. 2012;4:1895–1909.

[12] Baral Pravas K, Swayampakula M, Rout Manoj K, Kav Nat NV, Spyracopoulos L, Aguzzi A, et al. Structural basis of prion inhibition by phenothiazine compounds. Structure. 2014;22:291–303.

[13] Tycko R, Wickner RB. Molecular structures of amyloid and prion fibrils: consensus versus controversy. Accounts of Chemical Research. 2013;46:1487–1496.

[14] Kad NM, Myers SL, Smith DP, Alastair Smith D, Radford SE, Thomson NH. Hierarchical assembly of β2-microglobulin amyloid *in vitro* revealed by atomic force microscopy. Journal of Molecular Biology. 2003;330:785–797.

[15] Madine J, Jack E, Stockley PG, Radford SE, Serpell LC, Middleton DA. Structural Insights into the polymorphism of amyloid-like fibrils formed by region 20–29 of amylin revealed by solid-state NMR and X-ray fiber diffraction. Journal of the American Chemical Society. 2008;130:14990–15001.

[16] Mylonas E, Hascher A, Bernadó P, Blackledge M, Mandelkow E, Svergun DI. Domain conformation of tau protein studied by solution small-angle X-ray scattering. Biochemistry. 2008;47:10345–10353.

[17] Nielsen JT, Bjerring M, Jeppesen MD, Pedersen RO, Pedersen JM, Hein KL, et al. Unique identification of supramolecular structures in amyloid fibrils by solid-state NMR spectroscopy. Angewandte Chemie. 2009;121:2152–2155.

[18] Adamcik J, Jung J, Flakowski J, Rios De Los P, Dietler G, Mezzenger R. Understanding amyloid aggregation by statistical analysis of atomic force microscopy images. Nature Nanotechnology. 2010;5:423–428.

[19] Sachse C, Grigorieff N, Fändrich M. Nanoscale flexibility parameters of alzheimer amyloid fibrils determined by electron cryo-microscopy. Angewandte Chemie International Edition. 2010;49:1321–1323.

[20] Xu LP, Liu Y, Zhang X. Interfacial self-assembly of amino acids and peptides: scanning tunneling microscopy investigation. Nanoscale. 2011;3:4901–4915.

[21] Yamaguchi KI, Takahashi S, Kawai T, Naiki H, Goto Y. Seeding-dependent propagation and maturation of amyloid fibril conformation. Journal of Molecular Biology. 2005;352:952–960.

[22] Yan J, Fu X, Ge F, Zhang B, Yao J, Zhang H, et al. Cross-seeding and cross-competition in mouse apolipoprotein A-II amyloid fibrils and protein A amyloid fibrils. The American Journal of Pathology. 2007;171:172–180.

[23] Ono K, Takahashi R, Ikeda T, Yamada M. Cross-seeding effects of amyloid β-protein and α-synuclein. Journal of Neurochemistry. 2012;122:883–890.

[24] Seeliger J, Evers F, Jeworrek C, Kapoor S, Weise K, Andreetto E, et al. Cross-amyloid interaction of Aβ and IAPP at lipid membranes. Angewandte Chemie International Edition. 2012;51:679–683.

[25] Morales R, Moreno-Gonzalez I, Soto C. Cross-seeding of misfolded proteins: implications for etiology and pathogenesis of protein misfolding diseases. PLoS Pathogens. 2013;9:e1003537.

[26] Lundmark K, Westermark GT, Olsén A, Westermark P. Protein fibrils in nature can enhance amyloid protein A amyloidosis in mice: cross-seeding as a disease mechanism. Proceedings of the National Academy of Sciences. 2005;102:6098–6102.

[27] Yoon G, Kab Kim Y, Eom K, Na S. Relationship between disease-specific structures of amyloid fibrils and their mechanical properties. Applied Physics Letters. 2013;102:011914.

[28] Kim JI, Lee M, Baek I, Yoon G, Na S. The mechanical response of hIAPP nanowires based on different bending direction simulations. Physical Chemistry Chemical Physics. 2014;16:18493–18500.

[29] Lee M, Baek I, Chang HJ, Yoon G, Na S. The bond survival time variation of polymorphic amyloid fibrils in the mechanical insight. Chemical Physics Letters. 2014;600:68–72.

[30] Choi B, Yoon G, Lee SW, Eom K. Mechanical deformation mechanisms and properties of amyloid fibrils. Physical Chemistry Chemical Physics. 2015;17:1379–1389.

[31] Lee M, Chang HJ, Kim D, Lee Y, Suh H, Ahn N, et al. Relationship between structural composition and material properties of polymorphic hIAPP fibrils. Biophysical Chemistry. 2015;199:1–8.

[32] Lee M, Kwon J, Na S. Mechanical behavior comparison of spider and silkworm silks using molecular dynamics at atomic scale. Physical Chemistry Chemical Physics. 2016;18:4814–4821.

[33] Guo JP, Arai T, Miklossy J, McGeer PL. Aβ and tau form soluble complexes that may promote self aggregation of both into the insoluble forms observed in Alzheimer's disease. Proceedings of the National Academy of Sciences of the United States of America. 2006;103:1953–1958.

[34] Li DW, Mohanty S, Irbäck A, Huo S. Formation and growth of oligomers: a monte carlo study of an amyloid tau fragment. PLoS Computational Biology. 2008;4:e1000238.

[35] Raz Y, Miller Y. Interactions between Aβ and mutated tau lead to polymorphism and induce aggregation of Aβ-mutated tau oligomeric complexes. PLoS One. 2013; 8:e73303.

[36] Do TD, Economou NJ, Chamas A, Buratto SK, Shea JE, Bowers MT. Interactions between Amyloid-β and tau fragments promote aberrant aggregates: implications for amyloid toxicity. The Journal of Physical Chemistry B. 2014;118:11220–11230.

[37] Choi H, Lee M, Park HS, Na S. The effect of structural heterogeneity on the conformation and stability of A[small beta]-tau mixtures. RSC Advances. 2016;6:52236–52247.

[38] Miller Y, Ma B, Nussinov R. Synergistic Interactions between repeats in tau protein and Aβ amyloids may be responsible for accelerated aggregation via polymorphic states. Biochemistry. 2011;50:5172–5181.

[39] Peralta MDR, Karsai A, Ngo A, Sierra C, Fong KT, Hayre NR, et al. Engineering amyloid fibrils from β-solenoid proteins for biomaterials applications. ACS Nano. 2015;9:449–463.

[40] Jie Z, Buyong M, Ruth N. Consensus features in amyloid fibrils: sheet–sheet recognition via a (polar or nonpolar) zipper structure. Physical Biology. 2006;3:P1.

[41] Sawaya MR, Sambashivan S, Nelson R, Ivanova MI, Sievers SA, Apostol MI, et al. Atomic structures of amyloid cross-[bgr] spines reveal varied steric zippers. Nature. 2007;447:453–457.

[42] Matthes D, Gapsys V, Daebel V, de Groot BL. Mapping the conformational dynamics and pathways of spontaneous steric zipper peptide oligomerization. PLoS One. 2011;6:e19129.

[43] Haass C, Selkoe DJ. Soluble protein oligomers in neurodegeneration: lessons from the Alzheimer's amyloid [beta]-peptide. Nature Reviews Molecular Cell Biology. 2007;8:101–112.

[44] Xue Q, Zheng QC, Zhang JL, Cui YL, Chu WT, Zhang HX. Mutation and low pH effect on the stability as well as unfolding kinetics of transthyretin dimer. Biophysical Chemistry. 2014;189:8–15.

[45] Colby DW, Prusiner SB. De novo generation of prion strains. Nature Reviews Microbiology. 2011;9:771–777.

[46] Govaerts C, Wille H, Prusiner SB, Cohen FE. Evidence for assembly of prions with left-handed β-helices into trimers. Proceedings of the National Academy of Sciences of the United States of America. 2004;101:8342–8347.

[47] Wasmer C, Lange A, Van Melckebeke H, Siemer AB, Riek R, Meier BH. Amyloid fibrils of the HET-s(218–289) prion form a β solenoid with a triangular hydrophobic core. Science. 2008;319:1523–1526.

[48] Schmidt A, Annamalai K, Schmidt M, Grigorieff N, Fändrich M. Cryo-EM reveals the steric zipper structure of a light chain-derived amyloid fibril. Proceedings of the National Academy of Sciences. 2016;113:6200–6205.

[49] Esposito L, Pedone C, Vitagliano L. Molecular dynamics analyses of cross-β-spine steric zipper models: β-sheet twisting and aggregation. Proceedings of the National Academy of Sciences. 2006;103:11533–11538.

[50] Krone MG, Hua L, Soto P, Zhou R, Berne BJ, Shea JE. Role of water in mediating the assembly of Alzheimer amyloid-β Aβ16–22 protofilaments. Journal of the American Chemical Society. 2008;130:11066–11072.

[51] Periole X, Rampioni A, Vendruscolo M, Mark AE. Factors that affect the degree of twist in β-sheet structures: a molecular dynamics simulation study of a cross-β filament of the GNNQQNY peptide. The Journal of Physical Chemistry B. 2009;113:1728–1737.

[52] Chen W, van der Kamp Marc W, Daggett V. Structural and dynamic properties of the human prion protein. Biophysical Journal. 2014;106:1152–1163.

[53] Cheng C, Daggett V. Molecular dynamics simulations capture the misfolding of the bovine prion protein at acidic pH. Biomolecules. 2014;4:181.

[54] van der Kamp MW, Daggett V. Pathogenic mutations in the hydrophobic core of the human prion protein can promote structural instability and misfolding. Journal of Molecular Biology. 2010;404:732–748.

[55] DeMarco ML, Daggett V. From conversion to aggregation: Protofibril formation of the prion protein. Proceedings of the National Academy of Sciences of the United States of America. 2004;101:2293–2298.

[56] Alonso DOV, DeArmond SJ, Cohen FE, Daggett V. Mapping the early steps in the pH-induced conformational conversion of the prion protein. Proceedings of the National Academy of Sciences. 2001;98:2985–2989.

[57] Knowles TPJ, Buehler MJ. Nanomechanics of functional and pathological amyloid materials. Nature Nanotechnology. 2011;6:469–479.

[58] Smith J, Knowles T, Dobson C, MacPhee C, Welland M. Characterization of the nanoscale properties of individual amyloid fibrils. Proceedings of the National Academy of Sciences. 2006;103:15806–15811.

[59] Cherny I, Gazit E. Amyloids: not only pathological agents but also ordered nanomaterials. Angewandte Chemie International Edition. 2008;47:4062–4069.

[60] Xu Z, Paparcone R, Buehler MJ. Alzheimer's Aβ(1–40) amyloid fibrils feature size-dependent mechanical properties. Biophysical Journal. 2010;98:2053–2062.

[61] Yoon G, Kwak J, Kim JI, Na S, Eom K. Mechanical characterization of amyloid fibrils using coarse-grained normal mode analysis. Advanced Functional Materials. 2011;21:3454–3463.

[62] Yoon G, Lee M, Kim JI, Na S, Eom K. Role of sequence and structural polymorphism on the mechanical properties of amyloid fibrils. PLoS One. 2014;9:e88502.

[63] Gwonchan Y, Myeongsang L, Kyungwoo K, Jae In K, Hyun Joon C, Inchul B, et al. Morphology and mechanical properties of multi-stranded amyloid fibrils probed by atomistic and coarse-grained simulations. Physical Biology. 2015;12:066021.

[64] Choi H, Chang HJ, Shin Y, Kim JI, Park HS, Yoon G, et al. The molecular mechanism of conformational changes of the triplet prion fibrils for pH. RSC Advances. 2015;5:49263–49269.

Chapter 4

The Role of the Hsp40 Chaperone Sis1 in Yeast Prion Propagation

Michael Reidy

Additional information is available at the end of the chapter

http://dx.doi.org/10.5772/66449

Abstract

Yeast prions are self-templating amyloid aggregates composed of misfolded cellular proteins. In order to propagate, yeast prions must be broken into heritable seeds that are passed to subsequent generations. The replication step of the prion propagation cycle is accomplished by the actions of molecular chaperones, which bind to and serve the fibers through a process called disaggregation. Prions can be thought of as molecular diseases that have hijacked the chaperones for their continued existence. When viewed in this way, the study of yeast prions has been very informative about the interactions among of the molecular chaperones. This chapter focuses on the role of a single Hsp40 or J-protein, Sis1, in the propagation of yeast prions. While Sis1 seems to be required for the maintenance of many different prions, various prions depend on Sis1 in different ways, perhaps due to differences in underlying amyloid structure. New evidence is emerging that Sis1 is important for processes that may not involve prion replication activity, providing an intriguing alternative explanation for the observed differences in the prions' reliance on Sis1.

Keywords: Sis1, yeast prion, [*PSI*$^+$], [URE3], [*RNQ*$^+$], Hsp40, J-protein, prion propagation, amyloid

1. Introduction

In 1994, Reed Wickner solved a puzzle that had beguiled *Saccharomyces cerevisiae* (budding yeast) geneticists for decades [1–4]. He showed that certain genetic elements that did not follow the classical rules of DNA-based inheritance were due to alternative structures that an otherwise normal protein could adopt [5, 6]. These cytoplasmic genetic elements, some examples being [*PSI*$^+$] or [URE3] (the brackets denote the non-Mendelian character of the phenotype), were dominant in crosses but were present in all meiotic progeny, a clear violation of Mendelian inheritance. Inspired by contemporary work in human health that suggested the agent of long-known livestock diseases such as scrapie and its human counterparts kuru and Creutzfeldt-Jakob disease (CJD) was a misfolded variant of a protein found in all mammals (and coining a new term "prion"—for proteinaceous infectious virion-like particle [7]), Wickner's group demonstrated that [*PSI*⁺] and [URE3] propagated as misfolded versions of the yeast Sup35 or Ure2 protein, respectively [8, 9]. Soon, a new field emerged and several other yeast prions have been discovered and characterized (the story of the discovery of yeast prions is reviewed in Ref. [10]). **Table 1** lists the yeast prions known to date and the protein determinant that adopts the alternative fold. It was quickly discovered that the prions' continued propagation in the cytosol of yeast cells was highly dependent upon the molecular chaperones [11, 12], a strictly conserved suite of diverse proteins that evolved to protect the other proteins in the cell from the harshness of the environment.

The molecular chaperones were first identified in *Drosophila melanogaster* in the late 1970s as proteins that appeared or greatly increased in abundance after exposure to stress, such as heat [19]. These heat shock proteins (HSPs) are characterized by their apparent molecular weight in poly-acrylamide gels, for example, Hsp90, Hsp70, Hsp60 and Hsp40. Each class of HSP usually contains multiple isoforms that have overlapping and specific roles in various processes. **Table 2** lists the major chaperone families and their general activities. The molecular chaperones protect cells from stress and to varying extents are able to overcome the effects of stress. Importantly, molecular chaperones are also involved in myriad processes that are not related to stress, but are crucial to the overall proper function of the cell. Such processes include transport of proteins across membranes, assisting in the proper folding of newly syn-

Name	Determinant	Phenotype	Notes	Reference
[*PSI*$^+$]	Sup35	Nonsense suppression	Weak and strong variants	[1]
[URE3]	Ure2	Derepression of nitrogen utilization pathways		[3]
[*RNQ*$^+$]	Rnq1	Rnq1 aggregation; decrease in de novo [*PSI*$^+$] appearance	Also known as [*PIN*$^+$], for [*PSI*$^+$] inducibility, has several variants	[13]
[*ISP*$^+$]	Sfp1	Antisuppression (reverse of [*PSI*$^+$] phenotype)	Not dependent on Hsp104	[14]
[*SWI*$^+$]	Swi1	Poor growth on alternative carbon sources		[15]
[*OCT*$^+$]	Cyc8	Cyc8 deletion		[16]
[*MOT3*$^+$]	Mot3	Pseudohyphal growth and biofilm formation		[17]
[*MOD*$^+$]	Mod5	Fluconazole resistance	Prion-forming domain is not Q/N rich	[18]

Table 1. Amyloid-based yeast prions identified to date.

Class	Structure and function	Yeast	*E. coli*
Hsp100	Hexameric AAA+ ATPase disaggregase	Hsp104	ClpB
Hsp90	Dimeric posttranslational modifier of client activity	Hsc82, Hsp82	HtpG
Hsp70	Holdase; binds and releases unfolded polypeptides	Ssa1 through Ssa4; Ssb1, Ssb2	DnaK
Hsp60	Tetradecameric mitochondrial chaperonin	Hsp60	GroEL
Hsp40	Also called J-protein; dimeric stimulator of Hsp70 ATPase; substrate specificity	Sis1, Ydj1, Jjj1; 23 others (reviewed in Ref. [20])	DnaJ, CbpA, DjlA
Small HSPs	Crystallins, promoters of aggregation	Hsp42, Hsp26	

Table 2. The classes and names of cytosolic molecular chaperones and their general functions.

thesized proteins, protein turnover and cell division. Indeed, several entire classes of chaperones, such as Hsp70 and Hsp90, are essential to eukaryotic viability.

The first findings that molecular chaperones played a role in yeast prions were the discovery that overexpression of the AAA+ ATPase disaggregase Hsp104 "cured" cells of the [*PSI*$^+$] prion [11, 21]. While curing mediated by Hsp104 overexpression is a phenomenon unique to the [*PSI*$^+$] prion, (reviewed in Ref. [22]), the unexpected subsequent finding that deletion of the *HSP104* gene also resulted in inability to propagate [*PSI*$^+$] is a hallmark of most yeast prions, such as [URE3] and [*RNQ*$^+$] [11, 23, 24]. Yeast prions are highly ordered fibrous aggregates called amyloid, composed of a misfolded version of a normal yeast cytosolic protein. These amyloid fibers undergo a continual cycle of determinant protein addition and breakage that allows for sustained growth and transmission to new generations. Indeed, it is the action of the Hsp104 disaggregase, in concert with its Hsp70 and Hsp40 partners, that causes breakage and thus creation of new prion "seeds." These seeds are then passed to daughter cells where amyloid growth, breakage by chaperones and transmission to daughters continue unabated until the system is perturbed. Such perturbations include inhibition of Hsp104 activity by millimolar quantities of guanidine HCl or mutations in any of the chaperones involved. Thus, yeast prions are a valuable tool for studying molecular chaperones in vivo (reviewed in Ref. [25]).

This chapter focuses on the role of the Hsp40 Sis1 in yeast prion biology. **Figure 1** shows a cartoon of Sis1 domain structure. In addition to playing a central role in yeast prion propagation, Sis1 is essential for cell viability [26]. While the exact nature of Sis1's essential function remains unknown, it is clear that its regulation of Hsp70 function (via stimulation of Hsp70 ATPase, reviewed in Ref. [27]) is important, since the minimal Sis1 fragment required for growth is the Hsp70-interacting J-domain and the adjacent glycine/phenylalanine region [28]. Likewise, a single point mutation in any of the three universally conserved residues of the HPD (histidine, proline and aspartate) motif abolishes stimulation of Hsp70 ATPase in vitro [29] and is lethal in vivo [28]. Whether the essential function of Sis1 is also required for prion propagation is unclear, as will be discussed. The nonessential functions of Sis1 can easily

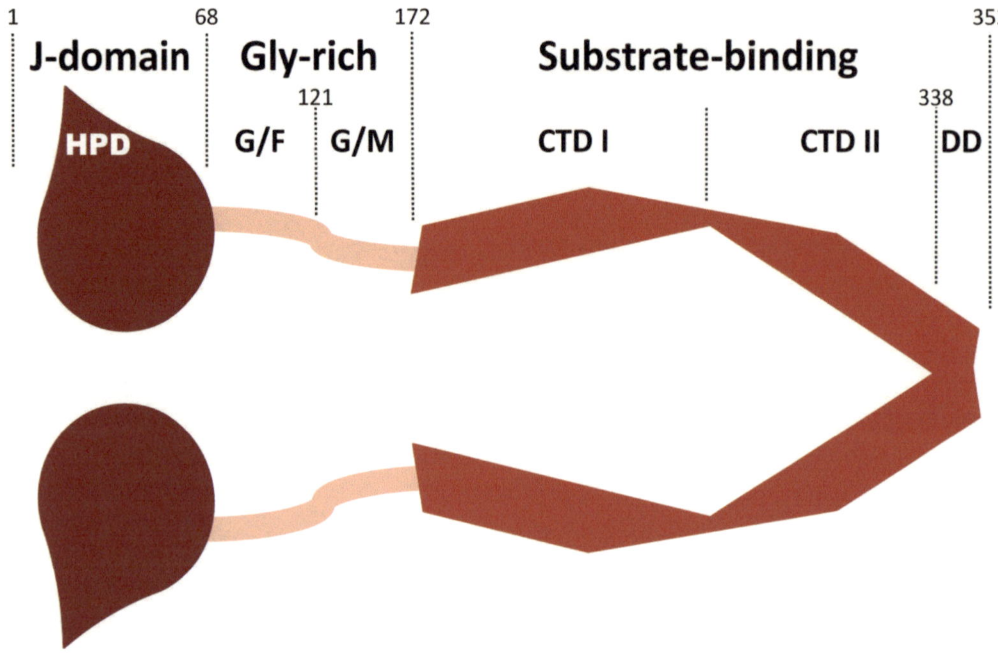

Figure 1. Cartoon of Sis1 domain structure. The J-domain is highly conserved and interacts with Hsp70 to stimulate ATPase and thus substrate transfer to Hsp70. The glycine-rich and substrate-binding domains are the areas of the most divergence between J-proteins and are thought to play a role in substrate selectivity. HPD: conserved Hsp70-interacting motif; Gly-rich: glycine-rich domain; G/F: glycine- and phenylalanine-rich region; G/M: glycine- and methionine-rich region; CTD I and CTD II are subdomains of the Sis1 substrate binding domain [34]; and DD: dimerization domain. The numbers above indicate amino acid position.

be studied using yeast prions, because the different yeast prions all seem to have differing requirements of Sis1 [30–33]. It is these nonessential Sis1 functions that are the focus of this chapter.

2. Yeast prion biology

Most yeast prions share a similar in-register parallel beta-sheet amyloid core composed of a prion-forming domain that is rich in asparagine and glutamine residues [35–37]. In the prion minus state, these domains are mostly unstructured and the protein is soluble and active. In the prion plus state, the prion-forming domains of newly synthesized prion protein molecules are recruited to the ends of an amyloid fiber. The in-register character of the beta-sheet core serves as a template for the incoming soluble molecule [38]. In addition to the different prions shown in **Table 1**, some prions such as [*PSI*$^+$] exhibit a range of distinct phenotypes called prion "variants" [39, 40]. In the case of [*PSI*$^+$], these variants roughly fall into two categories: strong and weak. It is known that phenotypically "strong" [*PSI*$^+$] variants are composed of thermodynamically unstable amyloid fibers, while "weak" [*PSI*$^+$] variants are composed of much sturdier amyloids [41]. Thus, the Sup35 protein can adopt multiple amyloid structures

http://dx.doi.org/10.5772/66449

that give rise to different phenotypes. It is likely that the locations of the turns between the beta-strands within the beta-sheet amyloid core govern amyloid thermostability and thus prion phenotype [42].

Most prion proteins also have globular domains that do not misfold to participate in the amyloid core [43, 44]. However, because the amyloid fiber as a whole is insoluble, these globular domains are essentially depleted from the cytosol. For two of the most studied prions, [*PSI*$^+$] and [URE3], depletion of the protein's function as a result of being in the prion plus state has been genetically coupled to the adenine biosynthetic pathway. Sup35, the determinant protein of the [*PSI*$^+$] prion, is the yeast eRF3 homolog, a GTPase that facilitates translation termination [45, 46]. When Sup35 is in the [*PSI*$^+$] state, there is read-through of stop codons [1, 2]. The presence of a nonsense mutation in certain genes of the adenine biosynthetic pathway, such as *ADE1* or *ADE2*, allows [*PSI*$^+$] to be monitored readily as growth on media-lacking adenine, due to suppression of the nonsense mutation. Likewise, [*psi*$^-$] cells are adenine auxotrophs. Using the adenine biosynthetic pathway to monitor prions has an added benefit. The substrates of the *ADE1* and *ADE2* gene products form pigments that are red in color and the accumulation of them within cells not expressing functional Ade1 or Ade2 proteins causes yeast colonies growing on limiting adenine media to appear red. Thus, [*PSI*$^+$] colonies are white and [*psi*$^-$] colonies are red. In the case of [*PSI*$^+$] prion variants, white colonies are categorized as phenotypically strong and weak variants appear pink on the same media. This variation in colony color is due to the relative amount of soluble, active Sup35 protein in the cell. The less soluble Sup35, the more read-through of the nonsense mutation and thus more Ade2 protein is made and less red pigment accumulates. The amount of soluble protein is directly related to the thermodynamic stability of the amyloid core of the prion. Strong phenotypes arise from thermodynamically unstable amyloids because they break more readily, exposing more ends and therefore effecting a more rapid depletion of the soluble prion protein pool. Conversely, weak variants have amyloids that are more thermostable, which break less and therefore have fewer sites of soluble protein recruitment, resulting in relatively more soluble, active protein [41]. This increase in Sup35 solubility leads to less read-through of the nonsense mutation and more accumulation of red pigment, resulting in pink colony color.

Ure2, the determinant of the [URE3] prion, is a regulator of yeast nitrogen catabolism [47, 48]. In the presence of certain nitrogen sources, soluble Ure2 binds to and sequesters transcription factors such as Gln3 in the cytoplasm [49]. When Ure2 is depleted, the transcription factors are free to move into the nucleus, where they activate genes such as *DAL5* that are essential for catabolism of poor nitrogen sources. By replacing the *ADE2* promoter with that from the *DAL5* gene, a similar red/white system for [URE3] was developed [50]. So, [URE3] cells are white and Ade$^+$ and cells lacking the prion, designated [ure-o], are red and ade$^-$. Rnq1, the determinant of the [*RNQ*$^+$] prion, has an unknown function [51]. Thus, it has not been linked to the adenine pathway without fusion to Sup35, which may complicate interpretations. The presence of the [*RNQ*$^+$] prion is most easily observed by visualization of prion aggregates in cells expressing green fluorescent protein (GFP)-tagged Rnq1 [52, 53].

Spontaneous breakage of amyloid fibers, even thermodynamically unstable ones, does not occur often enough to maintain the prion phenotype in an expanding yeast population. This inefficient breakage is evident in the reliance of all amyloid-based yeast prions, except one (see **Table 1**) [54], on the activity of the Hsp104 molecular disaggregase. The absence of the *HSP104* gene is incompatible with amyloid-based prion propagation, as are inhibition of Hsp104 by millimolar amounts of guanidine HCl in the growth media [55, 56] or by expression of dominant negative alleles that poison the functional hexamer [57]. Hsp104 hexamers adopt an open barrel-like structure into which denatured and aggregated proteins are fed [58, 59]. Upon exit of the substrate through the central pore, it is then allowed to refold either spontaneously or assisted by other chaperones. While Hsp104 plays a pivotal role in yeast prion propagation, Hsp104 does not work alone. In fact, under normal conditions Hsp100 disaggregases, such as Hsp104 and its *Escherichia coli* ortholog ClpB, are inactive without the cooperation of Hsp70 and the obligate Hsp70 cochaperone J-protein (also known as Hsp40), both in vivo and in vitro [60, 61].

3. Generalized role of Sis1 in prion propagation

The first report that the essential yeast J-protein Sis1 was involved in prion propagation was in 2001 by a collaborative effort between Elizabeth Craig and Susan Lindquist [62]. Following up on earlier reports and communications that Sis1 co-immunoprecipitated with Rnq1 [26], the determinant of the [*RNQ*$^+$] prion [51], Sondheimer and colleagues first showed that Sis1 (and the Hsp70 Ssa1) interacted with Rnq1, but only in strains that were [*RNQ*$^+$]. Thus, Sis1 only interacted with Rnq1 when it was in its amyloid conformation. Furthermore, they identified the glycine/phenylalanine (G/F)-rich region of Sis1 as being crucial for the interaction with the amyloid form of Rnq1. This finding agreed with earlier findings from the Craig lab that the G/F region somehow functioned in substrate selectivity [28]. Using strains expressing GFP-labeled Rnq1, they then observed effects of Sis1 mutations on the size and distribution of Rnq1 aggregates (that result from being in the [*RNQ*$^+$] prion state), suggesting that certain Sis1 functions were important for prion maintenance. This idea was strengthened by the results of Sis1 mutational analysis on the propagation of a hybrid Rnq1-Sup35 prion (that allowed for assay of the prion state using the adenine-requiring system described above), which showed that Sis1 lacking any nonessential region was unable to support the hybrid prion. Thus, Sis1 was identified as playing a major role in the propagation of yeast prions. However, the nature of this role remained unknown, as important questions remained as to what step in the prion cycle Sis1 was involved.

A major step toward answering these questions came from the Craig lab in 2007 [63]. Aron and colleagues introduced into their strains a tetracycline-repressible system that shuts off transcription of target genes, which they called "TET-Off" [64], in this case *SIS1*. While the *SIS1* gene is essential, either the amount of expression is leaky enough or the turnover of the preexisting protein is slow enough, or some combination of these two factors that cells were able to grow up to 80 generations after initial treatment with the repressor. By expressing Rnq1-GFP in these cells, the authors showed that [*RNQ*$^+$] aggregates initially grew in size and then were accompanied by increase in diffuse fluorescence followed by appearance of cells that were completely diffuse and thus "cured" of the prion. They also demonstrated that the diffuse fluorescence observed during the Sis1 depletion time course was from newly synthesized Rnq1, suggesting that the in the absence of Sis1 the amyloid had stopped recruiting new soluble molecules. This observation was consistent with the notion that amyloid growth is dependent upon continuous generation of new ends through fiber breakage. Importantly, the authors went on to show that Sis1 acted through Hsp70 in the propagation process, since mutations in the Hsp70-interacting HPD motif resulted in prion loss. Finally, a correlation of the effects of Hsp104 inactivation and Sis1 depletion on [*RNQ*+] aggregates was demonstrated, suggesting that the two chaperones worked together in the same process. The authors concluded that Sis1 works together with Hsp104 and Hsp70 to break prion aggregates that are then transmitted to daughter cells. However, the exact role of Sis1 in the process was still unclear, for example, whether it worked upstream or downstream of Hsp104.

Having established that the [*RNQ*+] prion relied on the activity of Sis1, the Craig lab subsequently showed the reliance on Sis1 of two other yeast prions, a strong variant of [*PSI*+] and [URE3] [30]. In doing so, Higurashi and colleagues discovered that the three prions seemed to have differential dependence on Sis1. In this study, the authors first showed that any other nonessential yeast Hsp40 can be deleted and not affect either [*RNQ*+] or [*PSI*+] propagation, suggesting a unique role for Sis1. They then monitored loss of the prions after depleting Sis1 levels through the TET-Off system. While cells completely lost [*RNQ*+] by the 20th generation after depletion of Sis1, [*PSI*+] was not completely lost until the 80th generation. They next found that the [URE3] prion was most sensitive to Sis1 depletion, with all cells having become [ure-o] by the 10th generation of growth in doxycycline. These findings opened new paths of investigation that are discussed below. While this report was important for the discoveries therein, a robust understanding of the exact nature of Sis1's role in prion propagation was still lacking, but not for long.

In 2008 Jonathan Weissman's laboratory answered one of the most important remaining questions: What does Sis1 do in prion propagation [65]? By creating chimeric domain-swapped constructs between Hsp104 and the *E. coli* ortholog ClpB, which the authors showed is unable to rescue deletion of the *HSP104* gene when expressed exogenously in yeast, Tipton and colleagues determined that the "upper ring" of the Hsp104 barrel, composed of the N-terminal, first AAA ATPase domain and the coiled coil region, worked together to support prion propagation and thermotolerance. Thermotolerance is defined as survival to a lethal heat shock (~50°C) after a short, slightly elevated temperature pretreatment (37°C) and is a non-prion-related function of Hsp104 [66]. To maintain function, all three of these regions must be from the yeast version. However, the C-terminal AAA domain, which is thought to mainly play a role in hexamerization [67], could be swapped with the *E. coli* version without loss of Hsp104 activities. Next, the authors took advantage of the activity of this chimera and introduced a system previously used to monitor ClpB substrates in *E. coli*. A single point mutation in the C-terminal AAA ATPase domain of ClpB allows interaction with the chamber-like peptidase ClpP. By combining this mutant ClpB with a catalytically inactive version of ClpP called TRAP, which trapped substrates but did not destroy them, the identity of ClpB substrates were identified via co-immunoprecipitation with TRAP [68, 69]. Tipton and colleagues engineered their active Hsp104-ClpB chimera to feed substrates into co-expressed TRAP in yeast cells propagating various prions. They found Sup35 or Rnq1 co-immunoprecipitated with

TRAP in prion plus, but not prion minus versions of their cells. This finding showed that Sup35 and Rnq1 are Hsp104 substrates only when they exist in their amyloid form, reinforcing the findings from the Sondheimer and Aron studies. This conclusion in turn implied that Sis1 or some other factor was involved in the selection of the amyloid form of Sup35 or Rnq1 over the soluble form. When Tipton and colleagues combined their TRAP system with the Sis1 TET-Off system borrowed from the Craig lab, they discovered that with reduced levels of Sis1, Sup35 and Rnq1 were no longer bound to TRAP. These results suggested that Sis1 worked upstream of Hsp104, delivering substrates to it, most likely in cooperation with Hsp70.

The investigations into the collaborative barrier that exists between prokaryotic and eukaryotic Hsp100s and Hsp70s ended up reinforcing the notion that Sis1 provides the disaggregation machinery's specificity for amyloid substrates. In 2010 and 2011, two studies revealed the underlying reason of why ClpB cannot function in yeast and Hsp104 cannot function in *E. coli*, even though the two proteins are 43% identical and share very similar structure [70, 71]. In one, Miot and coauthors created chimeras between Hsp104 and ClpB similar to those in the Tipton study, but using slightly different junction points and with more domain-swapped combinations. Through in vitro refolding reactions, where purified chaperones work together to reactivate denatured enzymes such as luciferase and in vivo thermotolerance experiments in yeast, the authors showed that the coiled-coil domain conferred a species-specific collaboration. Thus, a chimeric construct that contained only the coiled-coil domain of Hsp104, with the rest of the molecule being ClpB sequence, could rescue loss of Hsp104 activity in vivo or could effectively work with yeast Hsp70 and Hsp40 chaperones in vitro [71]. Both papers showed that it was the Hsp70 component of the machinery that interacted at the coiled-coil domain of Hsp104 or ClpB [70, 71]. Thus, Hsp104 could only work with yeast Hsp70 (Ssa1) and ClpB could only work with *E. coli* Hsp70 (DnaK). These findings implied that ClpB could not function properly in yeast because its preferred Hsp70 partner was absent, not because it was unable to disentangle yeast protein substrates. These findings were further substantiated in 2016 by the Bukau lab. Kummer and colleagues showed that ClpB and Hsp104 disaggregases use the same conserved mechanism [61]. The authors reported that Hsp70 interaction with the coiled-coil domain of the Hsp100, along with substrate binding, was an essential requirement for disaggregation activity in both the prokaryotic and eukaryotic systems. Furthermore, the authors went on to show that certain mutations in the Hsp104 coiled-coil domain, which were previously reported to activate Hsp104 in the absence of cofactors [72], also required Hsp70 to work properly [61]. This study highlighted the central role of Hsp70 and its essential cofactor Hsp40 plays in the disaggregation process.

In a follow-up to the Miot study, the Masison lab extended these findings to the prions [*PSI*$^+$], [URE3] and [*RNQ*$^+$] [60]. Reidy and colleagues tested the Hsp104-ClpB chimeras used in the Miot study for prion propagation and showed that the coiled-coil domain of Hsp104 was crucial for the maintenance of prions. Since a chimera that was mostly ClpB could propagate yeast prions as long as it contained the Hsp70-interacting domain from the yeast molecule, the authors reasoned that if other *E. coli* chaperones were co-expressed, perhaps wild-type ClpB could propagate prions and support thermotolerance in yeast. Thus, the authors used *hsp104Δ* yeast cells as living test tubes to find combinations of *E. coli* chaper-

http://dx.doi.org/10.5772/66449

ones that could rescue loss of Hsp104 functions. Remarkably, they found that in addition to the prokaryotic Hsp70 DnaK, which was expected, the Hsp70 nucleotide exchange factor GrpE was also required in order for ClpB to function properly in both thermotolerance and propagation of [*PSI*+]. These findings conflicted with earlier reports that suggested that Hsp104 could work alone in luciferase reactivation and amyloid remodeling [73] but agreed with other reports that found Hsp104 required additional factors to process aggregates [74]. Furthermore, the results of the Reidy study showed that ClpB was able to work on amyloid substrates, as long as the cognate Hsp70 and nucleotide exchange factors were present, strong evidence against the notion that Hsp104 had coevolved with yeast prions [65, 73, 75, 76]. Regardless, the finding that the *E. coli* Hsp40, DnaJ, was not required in order for the prokaryotic system to function in yeast was intriguing and strongly suggested that a yeast J-protein was involved. This idea was not controversial since it was already known that the Hsp40s did not display the same species-specific barrier that the Hsp100s and Hsp70s exhibited. The collaboration of a yeast J-protein with the bacterial chaperones was demonstrated via a single point mutation in DnaK that was shown earlier to block interaction with Hsp40 [77]. Together with normal ClpB and GrpE, this mutant DnaK failed to function in yeast, indicating that a yeast J-protein was involved [60]. Finally, Reidy and colleagues took advantage of a known compensatory mutation in Hsp40's HPD motif that restored interaction with the defective DnaK [77]. They introduced this mutation into Sis1 or Ydj1, the two major yeast Hsp40s and after introduction into the system expressing ClpB, GrpE and the mutant DnaK, they discovered that, remarkably, Sis1 is the Hsp40 that the system collaborated with propagate prions, but the same system worked with Ydj1 in thermotolerance [60]. Thus, the Hsp40 component of the system specified the substrate type, with Sis1 required for amyloid substrates (prions) and Ydj1 required for heat-induced non-structured aggregates.

4. Specialized roles of Sis1 in propagation of the different prions

Amyloid fiber breakage is a process that is fundamental for the propagation of yeast prions. Left alone, intracellular amyloid fibers would be a fleeting phenomenon. This failure to propagate is due simply to the fact that without breakage, upon mitosis there are two cells but only one amyloid fiber. While it is easy to imagine an unstable amyloid fiber able to generate enough seeds for propagation spontaneously, prions that do not require Hsp104 have been rarely observed [54] and this does not necessarily mean that propagation occurs by spontaneous breakage. Rather, amyloid-based yeast prions require molecular chaperones and specifically they require Sis1, as we have seen. At the same time, not all amyloids are the same in terms of their thermodynamic and structural properties [41]. It makes sense that a thermodynamically sturdy amyloid fiber would need an increased capability to resolve complex structures compared to an amyloid composed of the same protein but in less stable conformation. The emerging view is that Sis1 plays a major role in meeting the different demands imposed by various amyloids. The discovery and characterization of distinct prion variants have proven to be a valuable tool in shaping the field's understanding of the redundancy and variability of chaperone functions [27].

As noted previously, Higurashi showed that while the three most-studied prions, strong [*PSI*+], [*RNQ*+] and [URE3], all required Sis1 for their existence, each of the three prions displayed different sensitivities to Sis1 depletion [30]. In 2011 the Masison laboratory showed that loss or impairment of any nonessential functions of Sis1, that is, mutations outside of the Hsp70-interacting J-domain, had no deleterious effect on the propagation of strong [*PSI*+] [31]. Kirkland and coauthors reported that a minimal Sis1 construct consisting of the J-domain and the adjacent G/F region supported both growth and strong [*PSI*+]. Mutations in any other region of Sis1 did not affect the prion. It remained unclear whether the Sis1 function required for strong [*PSI*+] was the same function, in a different context, as the essential function of Sis1, or if Sis1 was not actually required by strong [*PSI*+]. This latter possibility conflicted with reports from other groups, notably the Craig lab and the issue was further muddied by differences in prion variant and yeast genetic background. A report by the Masison lab discussed above that involved expression of bacterial chaperones in yeast showed unequivocally that Sis1 was required for the same strong [*PSI*+] variant and genetic background as that used in the Kirkland study [31, 60]. The major findings of the Kirkland paper were not in doubt, however and were reinforced by a study from the laboratory of Justin Hines [32]. In complete agreement with Kirkland, Harris and colleagues observed multiple strong [*PSI*+] variants were efficiently propagated by the minimal Sis1 construct. In contrast, Harris showed that these same constructs could not propagate any of three different weak [*PSI*+] variants they tested. When Harris and coauthors compared the effects of various Sis1 domain truncations on the propagation of strong and weak [*PSI*+] to [*RNQ*+], they uncovered mutually exclusive requirements on the G/F region by weak [*PSI*+] and [*RNQ*+]. In other words, the G/F region of Sis1 was dispensable for weak [*PSI*+] propagation, in contrast to [*RNQ*+], for which the G/F is absolutely required [62]. Additionally, weak [*PSI*+] required activities of the C-terminal domain of Sis1 that were not required by either strong [*PSI*+] or [*RNQ*+]. Thus, each prion tested had distinct requirements for Sis1. The underlying reason for these distinct Sis1 functional requirements is probably related to structure, since different amyloids composed of the identical polypeptide, for example, strong [*PSI*+] and weak [*PSI*+], had unique dependencies on Sis1.

Higurashi showed that [URE3] was lost much more rapidly than strong [*PSI*+] and [*RNQ*+] upon depletion of Sis1, suggesting that [URE3] is more dependent upon Sis1 [30]. These findings were confirmed and expanded upon in 2014 [33]. Reidy and coauthors first expanded upon their earlier findings that Sis1 was the Hsp40 working with the *E. coli* Hsp100, Hsp70 and nucleotide exchange factor (ClpB, DnaK and GrpE, respectively) in prion propagation and Ydj1 directed the same disaggregation machinery to heat stress-induced aggregates. By creating domain-swapped chimeras between Sis1 and Ydj1 and combining them with the prokaryotic chaperone compensatory system described above that forced the target Hsp40 to interact only with a mutant DnaK, the authors showed that the C-terminal domains of the Hsp40 molecule determined whether the chimera behaved like Sis1, able to propagate prions, or like Ydj1, able to provide thermotolerance. The authors then investigated the ability of their chimeras to complement Sis1 or Ydj1 function in normal yeast cells not expressing the prokaryotic chaperones. They found only the chimeras with the Sis1 C-terminal domain were able to support viability and propagation of strong [*PSI*+] in strains carrying a deletion of the chromosomal *SIS1* gene. Likewise, only those chimeras that had the C-terminal domain of Ydj1 supported thermotolerance and Hsp90-related processes in cells lacking the *YDJ1* gene. Additionally, in vitro reactivation reactions using substrates that exclusively required either Sis1 or Ydj1 as the J-protein component of the disaggregation machinery in order to be resolved supported the in vivo results. The chimera that contained the Sis1 C-terminal domain could reactivate substrates that required Sis1 and the chimera that contained the Ydj1 C-terminal domain could reactivate substrates that required Ydj1.

When Reidy and colleagues investigated whether their Sis1-Ydj1 chimeras could propagate [URE3], they discovered that in addition to the C-terminal domain of Sis1, the glycine-rich domain (consisting of both the G/F region and the glycine/methionine (G/M) region) was also required. They then employed the suite of Sis1 domain truncations used in the Yan, Kirkland and Harris papers to determine the specific requirements for Sis1 on [URE3] propagation, information that was lacking. Remarkably, [URE3] was lost or greatly destabilized by any of the mutations in Sis1 that were tested [33]. In some cases, the prion could be selected for and maintained in the presence of a particular Sis1 truncation, such as deletion of the dimerization motif, by growth on media-lacking adenine. However, the prion was rapidly lost upon relief of the selection pressure. Such observations are noteworthy but do not necessarily constitute ability to efficiently support prion propagation. Thus, [URE3] exhibited the highest dependence on Sis1 function, confirming the initial finding by Higurashi.

Interestingly, in the 2008 Higurashi paper, the authors proposed that the strong reliance on Sis1 by [URE3] they observed may explain a phenomenon first reported in 2000 by Reed Wickner's group [23]. Moriyama and colleagues reported that in addition to requiring Hsp104 for propagation, the [URE3] prion was cured by overexpression of the Hsp40 Ydj1. [URE3] was unique among the yeast prions in being able to be cured by overexpression of Ydj1. Higurashi showed that a mutated Ydj1 that could no longer interact with Hsp70 failed to cure [URE3] when overexpressed and also showed that overexpression of just the J-domain of Ydj1 or a different J-protein called Jjj1 could cure [URE3] when overexpressed [30]. Higurashi concluded that the curing first observed by Moriyama was not due to Ydj1 itself, but rather the result of having too many J-domains in the cell that perhaps interfered with prion propagation through unproductive interactions with Hsp70. This theory was strengthened by a study published by the Masison group in early 2009 [78]. Sharma and colleagues determined that Ydj1 curing of [URE3] was mediated through Hsp70 by screening for random mutations in Ydj1 that failed to cure [URE3] when overexpressed. Similar to the finding in the Higurashi study that the J-domain of Jjj1 could also cure [URE3], Sharma reported that overexpression of the J-domain of Sis1 also resulted in [URE3] destabilization. Thus, the two studies complemented each other and supported the idea that overabundant J-domains destabilize [URE3], mediated somehow through Hsp70. These studies conflicted with a study published in 2006 [79]. Working with purified components, Lian and colleagues reported that Ydj1 interfered with the ability of Ure2 to form amyloid in vitro in a concentration-dependent manner. The authors extended these results to conclude that overexpressed Ydj1 cured [URE3] prions in vivo through direct inhibition of the Ure2 amyloid growth. However, the effect of Ydj1 on Ure2 amyloid formation was mostly limited to increasing the lag time of amyloid formation along with a decrease in overall yield. When Ydj1 was added to Ure2 amyloid reactions during logarithmic growth of amyloid fibers, conditions that arguably more closely resembled the in vivo situation of overexpressing Ydj1 in a cell that contains actively growing amyloid, no effect on Ure2 amyloid formation kinetics was observed.

The Higurashi model of Ydj1-mediated curing of [URE3] was strengthened by findings in Sis1-Ydj1 chimera paper that further characterized [URE3]'s strong dependence on Sis1 [33]. When the chimeras that could not propagate [URE3] in place of normal Sis1 (those that did not have both the glycine-rich and C-terminal domains of Sis1) were overexpressed in wild-type cells, rapid loss of [URE3] was observed [33]. Removing the dimerization motif from the chimeras that contained the C-terminal domain of Sis1 resulted in amelioration of curing, suggesting that the chimeras destabilized [URE3] by dimerizing with normal Sis1 monomers that were thus unable to propagate [URE3]. The authors then reasoned that [URE3] loss was due to defects in Sis1's ability to propagate the prion and extended this idea to Ydj1-mediated curing. Perhaps, Ydj1 simply outcompeted Sis1 for interaction with the disaggregation machinery to such a level that was detrimental to [URE3]. Since [URE3] was much more sensitive to Sisi1 alteration than other prions, this may explain why overexpressed Ydj1 had no effect on them. The authors tested this hypothesis by co-overexpressing Sis1 at the same time as Ydj1. In line with their model, they observed that elevating Sis1 levels reduced Ydj1-mediated curing of [URE3] by tenfold, but had no effect on curing by expression of a dominant negative Hsp104 allele. Thus, the initial idea put forth by Higurashi regarding overexpressed Ydj1 curing of [URE3], that is, an imbalance of J-domains in the cell, was correct.

From these studies a correlation is evident that the demand on Sis1 increases with thermostability of the underlying amyloid. Based on the Kirkland, Harris and Reidy papers, one can rank the four prions by increasing dependence on Sis1 as strong [*PSI*$^+$] < weak [*PSI*$^+$] ≤ [*RNQ*$^+$] < [URE3]. A strong [*PSI*$^+$] variant is composed of a thermodynamically unstable amyloid; thus, it requires less Sis1 function than a weak variant of [*PSI*$^+$], which is composed of a more thermostable amyloid fiber. This model may be correct; however, there are parameters other than melting temperature that are more useful to understanding amyloid strength vis-à-vis a certain prion's reliance on Sis1. For example, amyloid formed from purified Ure2 had a melting temperature in the presence of SDS (T_M = 79 ± 4°C) very close to that of Sup35NM amyloid made at 37°C (T_M = 78 ± 7°C, called NM-37) [80]. In contrast Sup35NM amyloid prepared at 4°C (NM-4) had a melting temperature of 54 ± 2°C. Yet, [URE3] was more sensitive to Sis1 alteration than weak [*PSI*$^+$], which was derived from NM-37 amyloid. Since Ure2 amyloid and NM-37 have identical melting temperatures, there must be some other factor that governs dependence on Sis1. More biophysical data on these amyloids is needed to fully understand the relationship between amyloid structure and stability with dependence on Sis1. Interestingly, Ure2 does not exhibit temperature-mediated differences in thermostability the way Sup35 does, maybe because the prion-forming domain of Ure2 is less complex in terms of the types of amino acids present [80]. For example, the prion-forming domain of Ure2 contains no tyrosines, yet Sup35 has 20. Some of these tyrosines have been shown to play a role in governing formation of amyloids that give rise to strong [*PSI*$^+$] [81, 82] and aromatic residues like tyrosine have been shown to play a role in amyloid formation and stability of poly-glutamine and other amyloidogenic peptides [83, 84]. On the other hand, both [URE3] and weak [*PSI*$^+$], but not strong [*PSI*$^+$], were cured by expression of a human anti-amyloid protein called DNAJB6b [80]. This finding suggested that Ure2 and NM-37 amyloids shared a common structural characteristic that is absent in NM-4 amyloid. What is needed is a robust, reliable and reproducible in vitro assay that could be employed to probe these unknowns.

5. The present and future of Sis1 research

Sis1 is a busy molecule, as we have seen. While the reliance on different functions of Sis1 is well documented, there remains a lack of understanding as to what these functions actually are. It is likely that these functions can be thought of as fine adjustments on the primary function of assisting Hsp70 in substrate delivery to Hsp104. However, this model does not satisfactorily explain why a minimal Sis1 molecule lacking the entire substrate-binding domain is able to propagate some prions such as strong [*PSI*$^+$] [31, 32]. One explanation is that certain amyloids simply do not require direct interaction with the C-terminal domain of Sis1 and Sis1's regulation of Hsp70 (but not that of other J-proteins) is sufficient to process these amyloids. Another explanation is that the G/F region that is part of the minimal construct is sufficient to interact with some amyloids but not others. Yet, the G/F region is dispensable for propagation of strong [*PSI*$^+$] when the C-terminal domain is present, so perhaps there is some overlap in G/F and C-terminal domain functions. Obviously, what Sis1 is actually doing in the cell is still very far from clear. Of course, all of these possible explanations assume that Sis1's only role in prion maintenance is in the disaggregation reaction with Hsp70, Hsp104 and nucleotide exchange factors.

One intriguing idea that has emerged is that Sis1 may be functioning in other pathways that are important for prion stability that are not well understood. In 2008 Reed Wickner's lab reported that overexpression of Btn2 or its homolog, a previously uncharacterized open reading frame that the authors named Cur1, cured cells of [URE3] [85]. Btn2 was shown previously to be involved with endosome trafficking [86]. Kryndushkin and colleagues also observed that deletion of both *BTN2* and *CUR1* genes stabilized [URE3], increased the de novo appearance of spontaneous [URE3]s and resulted in an increase of the average number of prion seeds per cell. The authors went on to show that Ure2-GFP and Btn2-RFP co-localized during the curing [85]. In 2014 the Wickner lab reported that normal, i.e., wild type, levels of Btn2 were sufficient to cure most [URE3] prions that arose either spontaneously or via induction [87]. The authors concluded that Btn2 and Cur1 comprise an "anti-prion system" that exists to protect yeast cells from prions by binding to them and preventing their transmission to daughter cells. These conclusions conflicted with a 2012 paper from the laboratory of Simon Alberti [88]. In that study, Malinovska and colleagues argued that Btn2 cured prions indirectly, by causing redistribution of chaperones and protein-sorting factors in response to stress-induced protein aggregation. The authors did not use [URE3] for their studies, but instead a hybrid prion composed of a fusion between the prion-forming domain of Nrp1 and the C-terminal functional domain of Sup35. According to their model, Btn2 overexpression cures prions not by directly binding to prion aggregates and sequestering them in the mother cell during mitosis, as proposed by the Wickner lab, but rather by depleting the cytosol of Sis1. However, this model did not explain the findings by the Wickner lab that Btn2 co-localized with Ure2, a finding that has been reported by another group [89]. Furthermore, while the Malinovska study did demonstrate interaction between Btn2 and Sis1, their model does not explain how Btn2 and Cur1 are able to block de novo [URE3] prions at their wild-type levels, especially since there is much more Sis1 in the cell than either Btn2 or Cur1 [90]. A study by the Bukau group in 2015 added some understanding to the role of Sis1, Btn2 and Hsp42 (a small heat shock protein involved in aggregate formation and necessary for the curing of [URE3] by Btn2 overexpression [85]) in aggregate formation in various compartments that have been described [91]. These studies cursorily mentioned here merely illustrate that in addition to the disaggregation reaction, Sis1 also plays a role in protein aggregate sorting and processing that requires more work to understand. Since some of the described aggregate compartments have been shown to contain amyloidogenic proteins [92], it is not too great of a stretch to suggest that Sis1 exerts influence over prion maintenance through its role in these processes. If so, the idea that Sis1 plays a role in aggregate processing in addition to disaggregation may explain how all various prions rely on Sis1 to different degrees. Much work is still needed, such as comprehensive mutational analyses like those done for the prions, to determine the relationship between Sis1's various functions in aggregate formation and sorting. Unfortunately, the field has yet to resolve exactly what these aggregate compartments are and how they arise, since different groups all seem to have different names and markers for them (for a review of this subject, please see Ref. [93]). Perhaps, such deeper investigation into Sis1's role in these aggregates will provide the resolution or at least clarify our understanding a bit.

Acknowledgments

This research was supported by the Intramural Research Program of the National Institutes of Health and the National Institute of Diabetes and Digestive and Kidney Diseases. I thank my Laboratory of Biochemistry and Genetics colleagues for thoughtful discussions and critical reading of the manuscript.

Author details

Michael Reidy

Address all correspondence to: michael.reidy@nih.gov

Laboratory of Biochemistry and Genetics, National Institutes of Health, National Institute of Diabetes, Digestive and Kidney Diseases, Bethesda, MD, USA

References

[1] Cox BS. PSI, a cytoplasmic suppressor of super-suppressor in yeast. Heredity (Edinb). 1965;20:505–21.

[2] Cox BS. A recessive lethal super-suppressor mutation in yeast and other psi phenomena. Heredity (Edinb). 1971;26:211–32.

[3] Lacroute F. Non-Mendelian mutation allowing ureidosuccinic acid uptake in yeast. J Bacteriol. 1971;106:519–22.

[4] Aigle M, Lacroute F. Genetical aspects of [URE3], a non-mitochondrial, cytoplasmically inherited mutation in yeast. Mol Gen Genet. 1975;136:327–35.

[5] Wickner RB. [URE3] as an altered URE2 protein: evidence for a prion analog in *Saccharomyces cerevisiae*. Science. 1994;264:566–9.

[6] Wickner RB, Masison DC, Edskes HK. [PSI] and [URE3] as yeast prions. Yeast. 1995; 11:1671–85.

[7] Prusiner SB. Novel proteinaceous infectious particles cause scrapie. Science. 1982; 216:136–44.

[8] Masison DC, Wickner RB. Prion-inducing domain of yeast Ure2p and protease resistance of Ure2p in prion-containing cells. Science. 1995;270:93–5.

[9] Wickner RB, Masison DC. Evidence for two prions in yeast: [URE3] and [PSI]. Curr Top Microbiol Immunol. 1996;207:147–60.

[10] Wickner RB. Yeast and fungal prions. Cold Spring Harb Perspect Biol. 2016;8:a023531.

[11] Chernoff YO, Lindquist SL, Ono B, Inge-Vechtomov SG, Liebman SW. Role of the chaperone protein Hsp104 in propagation of the yeast prion-like factor [psi$^+$]. Science. 1995;268:880–4.

[12] Lindquist S, Patino MM, Chernoff YO, Kowal AS, Singer MA, Liebman SW, et al. The role of Hsp104 in stress tolerance and [PSI$^+$] propagation in *Saccharomyces cerevisiae*. Cold Spring Harb Symp Quant Biol. 1995;60:451–60.

[13] Derkatch IL, Bradley ME, Zhou P, Chernoff YO, Liebman SW. Genetic and environmental factors affecting the de novo appearance of the [PSI$^+$] prion in *Saccharomyces cerevisiae*. Genetics. 1997;147:507–19.

[14] Rogoza T, Goginashvili A, Rodionova S, Ivanov M, Viktorovskaya O, Rubel A, et al. Non-Mendelian determinant [ISP$^+$] in yeast is a nuclear-residing prion form of the global transcriptional regulator Sfp1. Proc Natl Acad Sci U S A. 2010;107:10573–7.

[15] Du Z, Park KW, Yu H, Fan Q, Li L. Newly identified prion linked to the chromatin-remodeling factor Swi1 in *Saccharomyces cerevisiae*. Nat Genet. 2008;40:460–5.

[16] Patel BK, Gavin-Smyth J, Liebman SW. The yeast global transcriptional co-repressor protein Cyc8 can propagate as a prion. Nat Cell Biol. 2009;11:344–9.

[17] Alberti S, Halfmann R, King O, Kapila A, Lindquist S. A systematic survey identifies prions and illuminates sequence features of prionogenic proteins. Cell. 2009;137:146–58.

[18] Suzuki G, Shimazu N, Tanaka M. A yeast prion, Mod5, promotes acquired drug resistance and cell survival under environmental stress. Science. 2012;336:355–9.

[19] Schlesinger MJ. Heat shock proteins. J Biol Chem. 1990;265:12111–4.

[20] Kampinga HH, Craig EA. The HSP70 chaperone machinery: J proteins as drivers of functional specificity. Nat Rev Mol Cell Biol. 2010;11:579–92.

[21] Chernoff YO, Ono B. Dosage-dependent modifiers of Psi-dependent omnipotent suppression in yeast. In A.J.P. Brown, M.F. Tuite, & J.E.G. McCarthy (Eds), Protein synthesis and targeting in yeast. pp. 101–7. Berlin:Springer-Verlag.

[22] Reidy M, Masison DC. Modulation and elimination of yeast prions by protein chaperones and co-chaperones. Prion. 2011;5:245–9.

[23] Moriyama H, Edskes HK, Wickner RB. [URE3] prion propagation in *Saccharomyces cerevisiae*: requirement for chaperone Hsp104 and curing by overexpressed chaperone Ydj1p. Mol Cell Biol. 2000;20:8916–22.

[24] Bardill JP, Dulle JE, Fisher JR, True HL. Requirements of Hsp104p activity and Sis1p binding for propagation of the [RNQ(+)] prion. Prion. 2009;3:151–60.

[25] Masison DC, Reidy M. Yeast prions are useful for studying protein chaperones and protein quality control. Prion. 2015;9:174–83.

[26] Luke MM, Sutton A, Arndt KT. Characterization of SIS1, a *Saccharomyces cerevisiae* homologue of bacterial dnaJ proteins. J Cell Biol. 1991;114:623–38.

[27] Reidy M, Masison DC. Yeast prions help identify and define chaperone interaction networks. Curr Pharm Biotechnol. 2014;15:1008–18.

[28] Yan W, Craig EA. The glycine-phenylalanine-rich region determines the specificity of the yeast Hsp40 Sis1. Mol Cell Biol. 1999;19:7751–8.

[29] Tsai J, Douglas MG. A conserved HPD sequence of the J-domain is necessary for YDJ1 stimulation of Hsp70 ATPase activity at a site distinct from substrate binding. J Biol Chem. 1996;271:9347–54.

[30] Higurashi T, Hines JK, Sahi C, Aron R, Craig EA. Specificity of the J-protein Sis1 in the propagation of 3 yeast prions. Proc Natl Acad Sci U S A. 2008;105:16596–601.

[31] Kirkland PA, Reidy M, Masison DC. Functions of yeast Hsp40 chaperone Sis1p dispensable for prion propagation but important for prion curing and protection from prion toxicity. Genetics. 2011;188:565–77.

[32] Harris JM, Nguyen PP, Patel MJ, Sporn ZA, Hines JK. Functional diversification of hsp40: distinct j-protein functional requirements for two prions allow for chaperone-dependent prion selection. PLoS Genet. 2014;10:e1004510.

[33] Reidy M, Sharma R, Shastry S, Roberts BL, Albino-Flores I, Wickner S, et al. Hsp40s specify functions of Hsp104 and Hsp90 protein chaperone machines. PLoS Genet. 2014;10:e1004720.

[34] Sha B, Cyr D. Purification, crystallization and preliminary X-ray crystallographic studies of *S. cerevisiae* Hsp40 Sis1. Acta Crystallogr D Biol Crystallogr. 1999;55:1234–6.

[35] Wickner RB, Dyda F, Tycko R. Amyloid of Rnq1p, the basis of the [PIN+] prion, has a parallel in-register beta-sheet structure. Proc Natl Acad Sci U S A. 2008;105:2403–8.

[36] Shewmaker F, Kryndushkin D, Chen B, Tycko R, Wickner RB. Two prion variants of Sup35p have in-register parallel beta-sheet structures, independent of hydration. Biochemistry. 2009;48:5074–82.

[37] Kryndushkin DS, Wickner RB, Tycko R. The core of Ure2p prion fibrils is formed by the N-terminal segment in a parallel cross-beta structure: evidence from solid-state NMR. J Mol Biol. 2011;409:263–77.

[38] Wickner RB, Shewmaker F, Edskes H, Kryndushkin D, Nemecek J, McGlinchey R, et al. Prion amyloid structure explains templating: how proteins can be genes. FEMS Yeast Res. 2010;10:980–91.

[39] Derkatch IL, Chernoff YO, Kushnirov VV, Inge-Vechtomov SG, Liebman SW. Genesis and variability of [PSI] prion factors in *Saccharomyces cerevisiae*. Genetics. 1996;144:1375–86.

[40] Bradley ME, Edskes HK, Hong JY, Wickner RB, Liebman SW. Interactions among prions and prion "strains" in yeast. Proc Natl Acad Sci U S A. 2002;99 Suppl 4:16392–9.

[41] Tanaka M, Chien P, Naber N, Cooke R, Weissman JS. Conformational variations in an infectious protein determine prion strain differences. Nature. 2004;428:323–8.

[42] Gorkovskiy A, Thurber KR, Tycko R, Wickner RB. Locating folds of the in-register parallel beta-sheet of the Sup35p prion domain infectious amyloid. Proc Natl Acad Sci U S A. 2014;111:E4615–22.

[43] Baxa U, Taylor KL, Wall JS, Simon MN, Cheng N, Wickner RB, et al. Architecture of Ure2p prion filaments: the N-terminal domains form a central core fiber. J Biol Chem. 2003;278:43717–27.

[44] Baxa U, Keller PW, Cheng N, Wall JS, Steven AC. In Sup35p filaments (the [PSI+] prion), the globular C-terminal domains are widely offset from the amyloid fibril backbone. Mol Microbiol. 2011;79:523–32.

[45] Stansfield I, Tuite MF. Polypeptide chain termination in *Saccharomyces cerevisiae*. Curr Genet. 1994;25:385–95.

[46] Zhouravleva G, Frolova L, Le Goff X, Le Guellec R, Inge-Vechtomov S, Kisselev L, et al. Termination of translation in eukaryotes is governed by two interacting polypeptide chain release factors, eRF1 and eRF3. EMBO J. 1995;14:4065–72.

[47] Courchesne WE, Magasanik B. Regulation of nitrogen assimilation in *Saccharomyces cerevisiae*: roles of the URE2 and GLN3 genes. J Bacteriol. 1988;170:708–13.

[48] Coschigano PW, Magasanik B. The URE2 gene product of *Saccharomyces cerevisiae* plays an important role in the cellular response to the nitrogen source and has homology to glutathione s-transferases. Mol Cell Biol. 1991;11:822–32.

[49] Blinder D, Coschigano PW, Magasanik B. Interaction of the GATA factor Gln3p with the nitrogen regulator Ure2p in *Saccharomyces cerevisiae*. J Bacteriol. 1996;178:4734–6.

[50] Brachmann A, Toombs JA, Ross ED. Reporter assay systems for [URE3] detection and analysis. Methods. 2006;39:35–42.

[51] Sondheimer N, Lindquist S. Rnq1: an epigenetic modifier of protein function in yeast. Mol Cell. 2000;5:163–72.

[52] Liebman SW, Bagriantsev SN, Derkatch IL. Biochemical and genetic methods for characterization of [PIN$^+$] prions in yeast. Methods. 2006;39:23–34.

[53] Vitrenko YA, Pavon ME, Stone SI, Liebman SW. Propagation of the [PIN$^+$] prion by fragments of Rnq1 fused to GFP. Curr Genet. 2007;51:309–19.

[54] Volkov KV, Aksenova AY, Soom MJ, Osipov KV, Svitin AV, Kurischko C, et al. Novel non-Mendelian determinant involved in the control of translation accuracy in *Saccharomyces cerevisiae*. Genetics. 2002;160:25–36.

[55] Jung G, Masison DC. Guanidine hydrochloride inhibits Hsp104 activity in vivo: a possible explanation for its effect in curing yeast prions. Curr Microbiol. 2001;43:7–10.

[56] Ferreira PC, Ness F, Edwards SR, Cox BS, Tuite MF. The elimination of the yeast [PSI$^+$] prion by guanidine hydrochloride is the result of Hsp104 inactivation. Mol Microbiol. 2001;40:1357–69.

[57] Wegrzyn RD, Bapat K, Newnam GP, Zink AD, Chernoff YO. Mechanism of prion loss after Hsp104 inactivation in yeast. Mol Cell Biol. 2001;21:4656–69.

[58] Schirmer EC, Glover JR, Singer MA, Lindquist S. HSP100/Clp proteins: a common mechanism explains diverse functions. Trends Biochem Sci. 1996;21:289–96.

[59] Lum R, Tkach JM, Vierling E, Glover JR. Evidence for an unfolding/threading mechanism for protein disaggregation by *Saccharomyces cerevisiae* Hsp104. J Biol Chem. 2004;279:29139–46.

[60] Reidy M, Miot M, Masison DC. Prokaryotic chaperones support yeast prions and thermotolerance and define disaggregation machinery interactions. Genetics. 2012;192:185–93.

[61] Kummer E, Szlachcic A, Franke KB, Ungelenk S, Bukau B, Mogk A. Bacterial and yeast AAA+ disaggregases ClpB and Hsp104 operate through conserved mechanism involving cooperation with Hsp70. J. Mol. Biol. 2016;428:4378-91.

[62] Sondheimer N, Lopez N, Craig EA, Lindquist S. The role of Sis1 in the maintenance of the [RNQ$^+$] prion. EMBO J. 2001;20:2435–42.

[63] Aron R, Higurashi T, Sahi C, Craig EA. J-protein co-chaperone Sis1 required for generation of [RNQ$^+$] seeds necessary for prion propagation. EMBO J. 2007;26:3794–803.

[64] Belli G, Gari E, Piedrafita L, Aldea M, Herrero E. An activator/repressor dual system allows tight tetracycline-regulated gene expression in budding yeast. Nucleic Acids Res. 1998;26:942–7.

[65] Tipton KA, Verges KJ, Weissman JS. In vivo monitoring of the prion replication cycle reveals a critical role for Sis1 in delivering substrates to Hsp104. Mol Cell. 2008;32:584–91.

[66] Sanchez Y, Lindquist SL. HSP104 required for induced thermotolerance. Science. 1990;248:1112–5.

[67] Schirmer EC, Ware DM, Queitsch C, Kowal AS, Lindquist SL. Subunit interactions influence the biochemical and biological properties of Hsp104. Proc Natl Acad Sci U S A. 2001;98:914–9.

[68] Flynn JM, Neher SB, Kim YI, Sauer RT, Baker TA. Proteomic discovery of cellular substrates of the ClpXP protease reveals five classes of ClpX-recognition signals. Mol Cell. 2003;11:671–83.

[69] Weibezahn J, Tessarz P, Schlieker C, Zahn R, Maglica Z, Lee S, et al. Thermotolerance requires refolding of aggregated proteins by substrate translocation through the central pore of ClpB. Cell. 2004;119:653–65.

[70] Sielaff B, Tsai FT. The M-domain controls Hsp104 protein remodeling activity in an Hsp70/Hsp40-dependent manner. J Mol Biol. 2010;402:30–7.

[71] Miot M, Reidy M, Doyle SM, Hoskins JR, Johnston DM, Genest O, et al. Species-specific collaboration of heat shock proteins (Hsp) 70 and 100 in thermotolerance and protein disaggregation. Proc Natl Acad Sci U S A. 2011;108:6915–20.

[72] DeSantis ME, Leung EH, Sweeny EA, Jackrel ME, Cushman-Nick M, Neuhaus-Follini A, et al. Operational plasticity enables hsp104 to disaggregate diverse amyloid and non-amyloid clients. Cell. 2012;151:778–93.

[73] Shorter J, Lindquist S. Hsp104 catalyzes formation and elimination of self-replicating Sup35 prion conformers. Science. 2004;304:1793–7.

[74] Inoue Y, Taguchi H, Kishimoto A, Yoshida M. Hsp104 binds to yeast Sup35 prion fiber but needs other factor(s) to sever it. J Biol Chem. 2004;279:52319–23.

[75] Shorter J. Hsp104: a weapon to combat diverse neurodegenerative disorders. Neurosignals. 2008;16:63–74.

[76] Halfmann R, Alberti S, Lindquist S. Prions, protein homeostasis and phenotypic diversity. Trends Cell Biol. 2010;20:125–33.

[77] Suh WC, Burkholder WF, Lu CZ, Zhao X, Gottesman ME, Gross CA. Interaction of the Hsp70 molecular chaperone, DnaK, with its cochaperone DnaJ. Proc Natl Acad Sci U S A. 1998;95:15223–8.

[78] Sharma D, Stanley RF, Masison DC. Curing of yeast [URE3] prion by the Hsp40 cochaperone Ydj1p is mediated by Hsp70. Genetics. 2009;181:129–37.

[79] Lian HY, Jiang Y, Zhang H, Jones GW, Perrett S. The yeast prion protein Ure2: structure, function and folding. Biochim Biophys Acta. 2006;1764:535–45.

[80] Reidy M, Sharma R, Roberts BL, Masison DC. Human J-protein DnaJB6b cures a subset of *Saccharomyces cerevisiae* prions and selectively blocks assembly of structurally related amyloids. J Biol Chem. 2016;291:4035–47.

[81] Ohhashi Y, Ito K, Toyama BH, Weissman JS, Tanaka M. Differences in prion strain conformations result from non-native interactions in a nucleus. Nat Chem Biol. 2010;6:225–30.

[82] Reymer A, Frederick KK, Rocha S, Beke-Somfai T, Kitts CC, Lindquist S, et al. Orientation of aromatic residues in amyloid cores: structural insights into prion fiber diversity. Proc Natl Acad Sci U S A. 2014;111:17158–63.

[83] Alexandrov IM, Vishnevskaya AB, Ter-Avanesyan MD, Kushnirov VV. Appearance and propagation of polyglutamine-based amyloids in yeast: tyrosine residues enable polymer fragmentation. J Biol Chem. 2008;283:15185–92.

[84] MacLea KS, Paul KR, Ben-Musa Z, Waechter A, Shattuck JE, Gruca M, et al. Distinct amino acid compositional requirements for formation and maintenance of the [PSI(+)] prion in yeast. Mol Cell Biol. 2015;35:899–911.

[85] Kryndushkin DS, Shewmaker F, Wickner RB. Curing of the [URE3] prion by Btn2p, a Batten disease-related protein. EMBO J. 2008;27:2725–35.

[86] Kama R, Robinson M, Gerst JE. Btn2, a Hook1 ortholog and potential Batten disease-related protein, mediates late endosome-Golgi protein sorting in yeast. Mol Cell Biol. 2007;27:605–21.

[87] Wickner RB, Bezsonov E, Bateman DA. Normal levels of the antiprion proteins Btn2 and Cur1 cure most newly formed [URE3] prion variants. Proc Natl Acad Sci U S A. 2014;111:E2711–20.

[88] Malinovska L, Kroschwald S, Munder MC, Richter D, Alberti S. Molecular chaperones and stress-inducible protein-sorting factors coordinate the spatiotemporal distribution of protein aggregates. Mol Biol Cell. 2012;23:3041–56.

[89] Kanneganti V, Kama R, Gerst JE. Btn3 is a negative regulator of Btn2-mediated endosomal protein trafficking and prion curing in yeast. Mol Biol Cell. 2011;22:1648–63.

[90] Ghaemmaghami S, Huh WK, Bower K, Howson RW, Belle A, Dephoure N, et al. Global analysis of protein expression in yeast. Nature. 2003;425:737–41.

[91] Miller SB, Ho CT, Winkler J, Khokhrina M, Neuner A, Mohamed MY, et al. Compartment-specific aggregases direct distinct nuclear and cytoplasmic aggregate deposition. EMBO J. 2015;34:778–97.

[92] Kaganovich D, Kopito R, Frydman J. Misfolded proteins partition between two distinct quality control compartments. Nature. 2008;454:1088–95.

[93] Miller SB, Mogk A, Bukau B. Spatially organized aggregation of misfolded proteins as cellular stress defense strategy. J Mol Biol. 2015;427:1564–74.

Chapter 5

Molecular Signature in Human and Animal Prion Disorders

Michele Fiorini, Matilde Bongianni and Gianluigi Zanusso

Additional information is available at the end of the chapter

http://dx.doi.org/10.5772/67329

Abstract

In human and animal transmissible spongiform encephalopathies (TSEs) or prion disorders, biochemical analysis of disease-associated prion protein (PrP^{TSE}) is a first-line approach for large scale routine testing and for a rapid molecular typing. This characterization is based on conformational properties of PrP^{TSE} enciphered in its secondary and tertiary structures and on glycosylation profile. Several biochemical approaches are helpful in distinguishing PrP^{TSE} forms in human prion diseases. In particular, in sporadic Creutzfedlt-Jakob disease (CJD), PrP^{TSE} is characterized by two main glycotypes conventionally named PrP^{TSE} type 1 and PrP^{TSE} type 2 based on the apparent gel migration at 19 kDa and 17.5 kDa and glycofrom ratio. Further, there are PrP^{TSE} low molecular weight fragments which correlate to distinct phenotypes of sCJD. Finally, by using two-dimensional PAGE analysis, which separates PrP^{TSE} on both isoelectric point and molecular size, we were able to detect two distinct migration pattern in PrP^{TSE} type 2, one in subjects with MM at codon 129 and another in MV, VV. We here provide an extensive PrP^{TSE} biochemical analysis in humans and animals affected with prion disorders. Further, we showed that PrP^{TSE} glycotypes observed in CJD shared similarities with PrP^{TSE} in bovine spongiform encephalopathies (BSEs). These signature similarities obtained by a biochemical analysis had been further confirmed by experimental transmission.

Keywords: prion protein, pathological prion protein, transmissible spongiform encephalopathies, prion disorders, protease-resistant PrP, biochemical phenotype, conformational assays, two-dimensional analysis, amyloid

1. Introduction

Prion diseases, or transmissible spongiform encephalopathies (TSEs), are fatal neurodegenerative disorders affecting humans and animals with a sporadic, genetic, or iatrogenic etiology [1]. The crucial event in the pathogenesis of TSEs is the conformational conversion of the normal cellular prion protein (PrP^{C}) into a pathologic isoform (PrP^{TSE}), which is self-propagating and infectious [2]. PrP^{C} is a glycosylphosphatidylinositol (GPI) anchored protein residing on the outer leaflet of the cellular membrane of most cell types in mammals. It is synthetized as 253 amino acids polypeptide before being posttranscriptionally modified by the cleavages of 22 amino acids of signal sequence at N-terminal and of 23 amino acids at the C-terminal for adding GPI anchor. The mature protein contains a disulfide bond between Cys179 and Cys214 and can be glycosylated at Asn181 and Asn197. While PrP N-terminus contains a variable number of octapeptide repeats, it is flexible and disordered, and C-terminus is more structured in a globular domain characterized by three α-helixes and two short β-sheet structures [3]. Structurally, PrP^{C} contains mainly α-helix structures, while PrP^{TSE} contains β-sheet structures [4]. These conformational changes in secondary and tertiary structures determine PrP^{TSE} specific physicochemical changes such as PK resistance, insolubility in nonionic detergents and high propensity to aggregate in oligomers of different size [5]. It has been assessed that PrP^{TSE} conformations are related to distinct prion strains, which propagate with specific transmission properties in susceptible mammals (different infectious properties, incubation times or neuropathological lesions) [6]. Aim of the present chapter is to describe different biochemical strategies to characterize molecular features and biochemical properties of prions in humans and animals.

1.1. Defining molecular features of prions by biochemical analysis, cellular and disease-associated PrP biochemical characterization

A suitable way to detect and reveal PrP^{C} and PrP^{TSE} is Western Blot analysis following electrophoretic mono-dimensional (1D) separation [7]. Electrophoretic analysis provides information about glycotype based on PrP molecular weight and glycosylation profile [8]. Two-dimensional (2D) electrophoretic analysis is a more in depth analysis to investigate the molecular features of proteins, improving the resolution since a single amino acid substitution in PrP sequence, glycosylation profile or the presence or absence of GPI anchor is sufficient for determining a shift pointing migration. The goal of 2D electrophoresis is to characterize PrP^{TSE} molecular signature typical of each prion strain, more accurate and specific than simple classical 1D electrophoretic pattern.

1.2. Conformational assays to characterize PrP^{TSE} biochemical properties in human and animal prion disorders

Several simple biochemical methods can be used to investigate conformational features of different biochemical prion strains.

1.2.1. Resistance to proteinase K treatment

Western blot analysis following PK digestion allows the detection of PK-resistant PrP, also termed PrP27-30. This method is routinely used to confirm TSEs diagnosis.

http://dx.doi.org/10.5772/67329

Biochemical strains of PrP^{TSE} can be defined also by the presence of PK resistant additional minor C-terminally truncated fragments (CTFs).

1.2.2. Detergent insolubility and separation by size of PrP^{TSE} aggregates

The high representation of β-sheet structures is a requisite of PrP^{TSE} to form insoluble aggregates in nonionic detergents. By ultracentrifugation, enriched fractions of PrP^{TSE} can be prepared and separated by different size of aggregates in sucrose gradients. This analysis allows to characterize PrP^{TSE} conformational properties in a given prion strains.

1.2.3. Conformational stability in increasing concentration of GdnHCl

Different prion strains show different conformational stability, which can be assessed by PK-resistance testing following exposure to different denaturing or nondenaturing conditions.

2. PrP conformers and disease phenotypes in human and animal TSEs

2.1. 1D analysis of molecular strains

2.1.1. Human prion disorders

2.1.1.1. Sporadic forms

In human prion disorders, several different PrP^{TSE} types have been described, based on the electrophoretic migration and the glycosylation profile of PrP27-30. This is composed of a major triplet of bands, which represent the differently glycosylated isoforms of PrP^{TSE}. Since prions are associated with distinct conformations, biochemical analyzes are useful to define prion strains.

In human sporadic CJD, PrP^{TSE} separates as two main glycotypes: PrP^{TSE} type 1 and PrP^{TSE} type 2A with an apparent gel migration of the unglycosylated isoform at 21 kDa and 19 kDa respectively (**Figure 1A**) [9]. Type-1 and 2A show similar glycosylation profile (**Figure 1B**).

In 2007, we reported on a novel PrP^{TSE} glycotype, showing a predominant unglycosylated isoform and slightly the monoglicosylated isoform, but completely lacking the diglycosylated one, named Type-U (**Figure 1A** and **B**) [10].

In 2010, an additional form of prion disease has been described, called variably protease-sensitive prionopathy (VPSPr). VPSPr is characterized not only by a distinct disease phenotype but also by a ladder-like electrophoretic profile of the PK-resistant PrP^{TSE} fragments (**Figure 1C**). The ladder-like profile consisted of five major bands migrating at approximately 26 kDa, 23 kDa, 20 kDa, 17 kDa, and 7 kDa [11].

2.1.1.2. Genetic forms

Familial prion diseases, FFI and GSS are characterized by distinct biochemical profiles, with typical migration properties, glycosylation profiles or truncated fragments expression. While fCJD and FFI show the presence of PrP27-30 differentially PK cleaved and glycosylated, in GSS PrP27-30 is absent, pathological PrP is composed of internal fragments of 8 and 11 kDa with the exception of P102L. P102L shows a peculiar pattern with the presence of both PrP27-30 and 8 kDa internal fragment. Familial prion diseases western blot is schematically reported in **Figure 1C** [12–14].

2.1.1.3. Infectious form

Following BSE transmission to humans causing variant CJD (vCJD), a new human molecular strain was defined (type 2B) with a molecular weight comparable to type 2A but with a prevalent diglycosylated isoform (**Figure 1C**) [15].

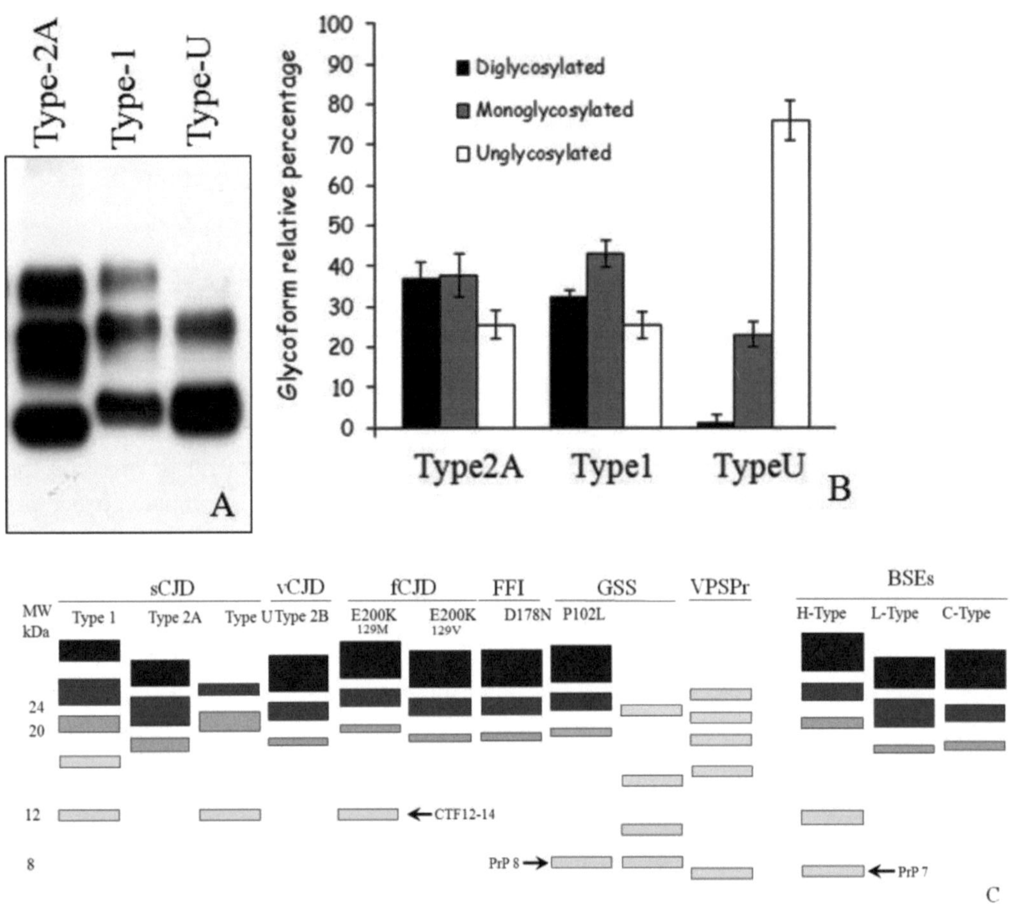

Figure 1. (A) Western blot profile of three sCJD molecular strains and their relative glycoform profile (B). (C) Schematic representation of human western blot profile of sporadic, genetic and acquired CJD molecular types.

2.1.2. Size aggregates

Since the abundance of β-sheet in the secondary structure of PrP^{TSE} confers the tendency to aggregate, ultracentrifugation procedures can be applied to discriminate different con-

http://dx.doi.org/10.5772/67329

formational states associated with different prion strains. By using ultracentrifugation in sucrose gradients and sarkosyl, insolubility and the size of PrP^{TSE} aggregates can be compared [16].

The three sporadic molecular subtypes are characterized by distinct sedimentation patterns, considering ultracentrifugation analysis before and after PK treatment (**Figure 2**). MV-1 PrP species are distributed at the beginning and at the end of the gradient, indicating the presence of small soluble forms and big insoluble aggregates; this distribution is maintained also after PK treatment. MV-2 sedimentation pattern of cellular PrP is characterized by a wide distribution all over the gradient, while after PK digestion PrP^{TSE} is detected as big insoluble aggregates at the end of the gradient. MV-U sedimentation pattern of cellular PrP is comparable to MV-1, but PrP^{TSE} species are found mainly at the bottom of the gradient as for MV-2.

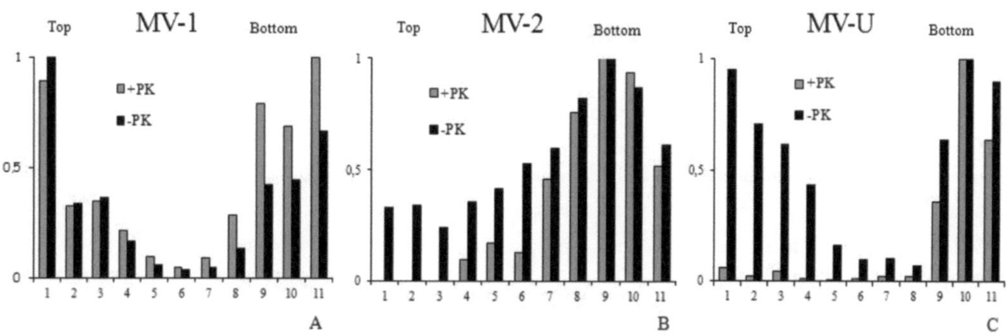

Figure 2. Fractionation of sCJD PrP aggregates. Brain homogenates from frontal cortexes of MV-1 and MV-2 and MV-U were sedimented in a 10–60% sucrose gradient. After sedimentation, half samples were digested with PK. Relative cellular (black) and PK resistant (gray) percentage of fraction distribution in MV-1 (A), MV-2 (B) and MV-U (C).

2.1.3. Conformational stability assay

Sporadic human strains can be distinguished also by testing the strength of three dimensional protein structure against denaturing conditions. This is investigated by PK treatment after exposure to increasing amounts of guanidine [17].

In **Figure 3**, it can be noted that in MV-1 and MV-2, the structure integrity is maintained until an exposition to 2 M guanidine before PK can completely digest the protein; in MV-U, a concentration of 1.5 M is enough to unfold the PrP^{TSE}. It's interesting to note that in MV-U at a 1.0 M guanidine concentration, PK digestion produces two conformers of PrP^{TSE} at different molecular weights, indicating that two molecular strains are hidden in the three dimensional conformation (unpublished data). Inoculation experiments in bank voles have shown this MV-U case contains two different strains with different incubation time and different lesion profile associated with two different molecular electrophoretic patterns after transmission (unpublished data).

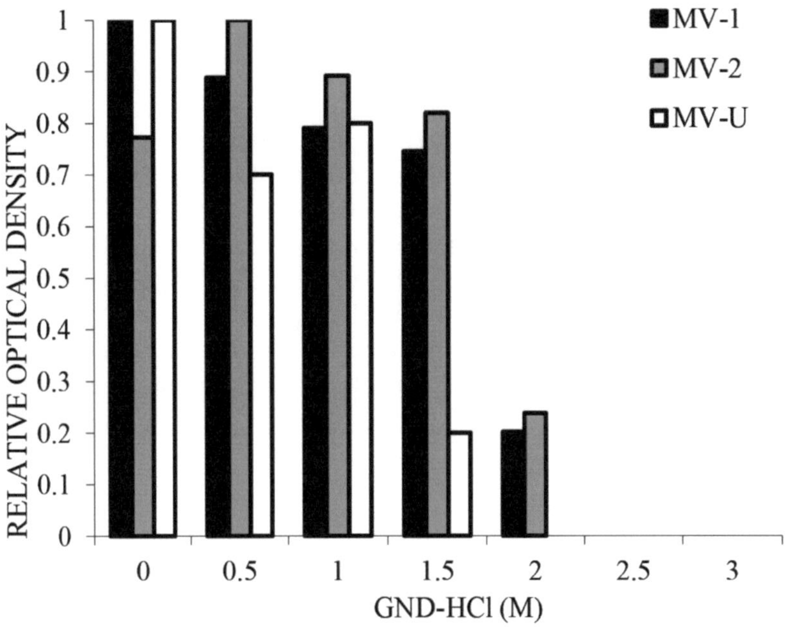

Figure 3. Relative quantification of denaturation transitions for MV-1, MV-2 and MV-U types.

2.2. 2D analysis of molecular strains

2.2.1. Molecular signature

2D analysis of PK and PNGase treated samples gives trains of spots corresponding to the nude N-ragged ended isoforms of the prion core fragment. Western blot using antibodies against the C-terminal of prions evidences also the presence of truncated fragments (CTFs) [18].

Two-dimensional immunoblot with anti-PrP antibodies gives the possibility to identify two groups of C-terminal protease-resistant PrP fragments. All sCJD cases with type 1 PrP27-30, in addition to MM subjects with type 2 PrP27-30, are characterized by the presence of CTFs of 16–17 kDa and 12–14 kDa. Conversely, brain homogenates from VV and MV patients with type 2 PrP27-30 contain CTFs migrating at 17.5–18 kDa. Therefore, we can conclude that the mechanism involved in the formation of CTFs is not influenced by codon 129 and by the type of PrP27-30.

Based on the biochemical patterns obtained by combining the PrP27-30 core fragment and lower truncated PrP species, three distinct groups or fingerprints of disease-associated PrP species in sCJD with type 1 PrP^{TSE}, MM2 subjects, and MV2/VV2 cases can be defined (**Figure 4**).

2.2.2. GPI anchor

PrP posttransductional modifications, such as the presence of GPI anchor can be easily investigated by 2D analysis [1]. 2D molecular coordinates (pI and Mw) of GPI anchor were calculated by comparing the unglycosylated PrP in wild type and anchorless transgenic mice. By 2D analysis, we can compare the 2D coordinates of known recombinant peptides with unknown samples to see if their 2D coordinates correspond to the nude peptides of are shifted by the "weight" of the GPI anchor. Since recombinant protein molecular coordinates in 2D analysis correspond exactly to the theoretical values (**Figure 5**), anchored or anchorless prions can be identified by only valuating if the measured pI and Mw correspond to the theoretical ones with or without GPI weight.

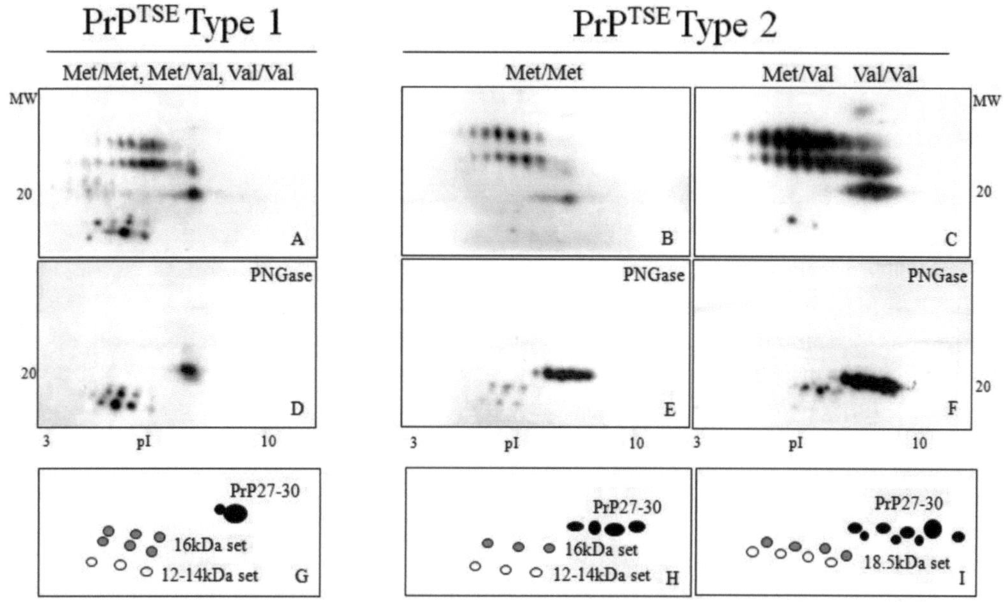

Figure 4. Two-dimensional mapping of sCJD brain homogenates after PK treatment (A–C) and deglycosylation (D–F) with anti-C–terminal antibody. Schematic diagram of PK-resistant C-terminal PrP core fragments in sCJD subtypes. (G, H, I) [17].

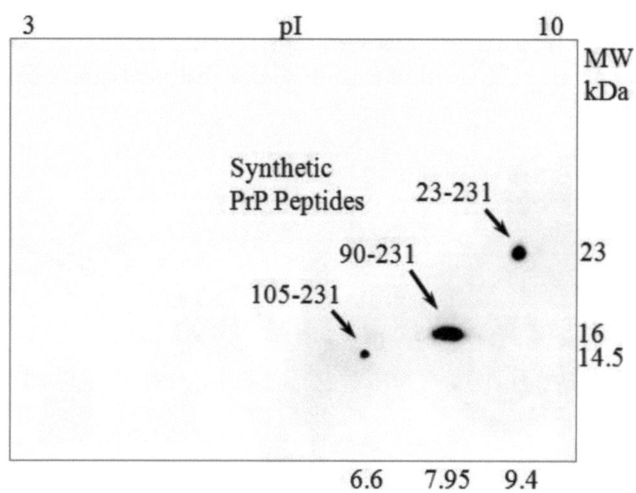

Figure 5. Two-dimensional mapping of synthetic PrP peptides [1].

Figure 6 represents a schematic picture of PrP^{TSE} core fragment after 2D analysis [1].

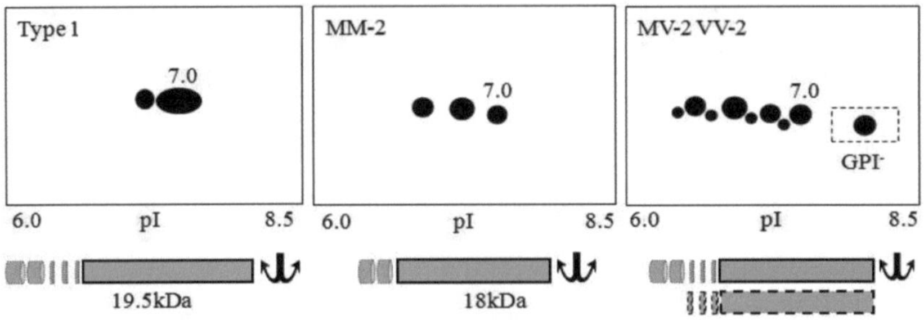

Figure 6. Schematic representation of anchored and anchorless PK-resistant PrP core fragments in sCJD subtypes.

All the sCJD molecular type 1 and 2 subtypes have all the 27–30 isoforms with a pI more acidic than pH 7 except the group MV-2/VV-2 showing an extra isoform at pI ~ 8. This last isoform has the same molecular coordinates of the synthetic peptide 90–231 and corresponds to anchorless form. All other spots identify anchored PrP^{TSE} forms, since their pI is shifted about 1 pH unit toward the acidic pole.

2.3. Cattle

2.3.1. Animal prion disorders

Since it was known, BSE was always described by the same molecular strain characterized by a diglycosylated electrophoretic pattern. In 2004, in Italy, two old cows were described by Zanusso et al. as showing a lower molecular weight of the prion core fragment and a different glycosylation pattern at western blot [19]. In 2007, other cases were found in France with classical glycosylation profile but with higher molecular weight of the prion electrophoretic profile (**Figure 7**) [20]. These new atypical molecular types where named BASE (bovine amyloidotic spongiform encephalopathy) or L-type BSE and H-type BSE considering the lower or higher western blot profile. The three molecular profiles also reflect different clinicopathological features of the diseases [21].

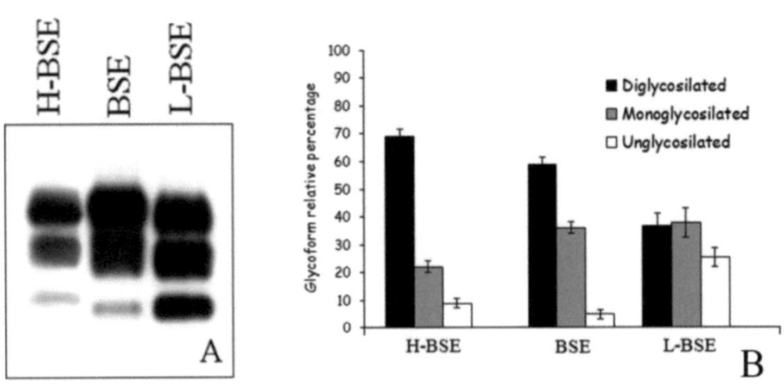

Figure 7. (A) Western blot profile of three BSE molecular strains and their relative glycoform profile (B).

2.3.1.1. *Size aggregates*

Ultracentrifugation analysis before PK treatment shows a similar sedimentation pattern in the three cattle molecular subtypes: samples present both small soluble forms and large insoluble aggregates. The treatment with PK shows PrP^{TSE} is present in the insoluble aggregates in all BSE strains (**Figure 8**); moreover, aclassical BSE shows also an additional small amount of soluble forms (**Figure 8C**).

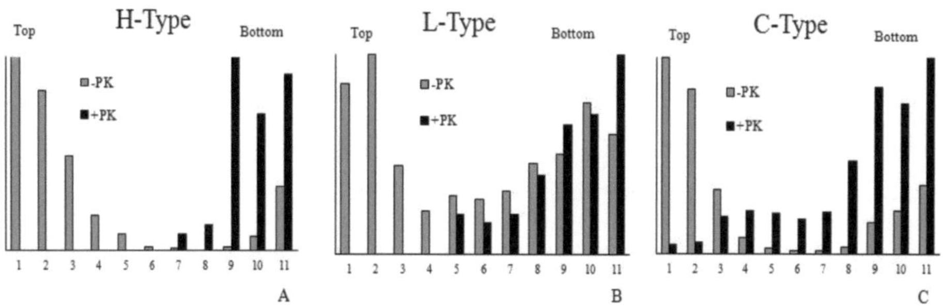

Figure 8. Fractionation of BSE PrP aggregates. Brain homogenates from frontal cortexes of H-BSE and L-BS and C-BSE were sedimented in a 10–60% sucrose gradient. After sedimentation, half samples were digested with PK. Relative cellular (gray) and PK resistant (black) percentage of fraction distribution in H-BSE (A), L-BSE (B) and C-BSE (C).

2.3.1.2. *Conformational stability assay*

Both atypical forms of BSE can be distinguished from classical BSE and also human sCJD on the basis of structure denaturation by chaotropic agents such as guanidine. While human sporadic PrP^{TSE} is digested after an exposition over 2 M guanidine, all BSE forms maintain a minimal Pk resistance until 3 M guanidine. Among BSEs, C-type is shown to be strongly resistant to Pk digestion until 2 M guanidine, while H- and L-type resistances are stable until 2.5 M (**Figure 9**).

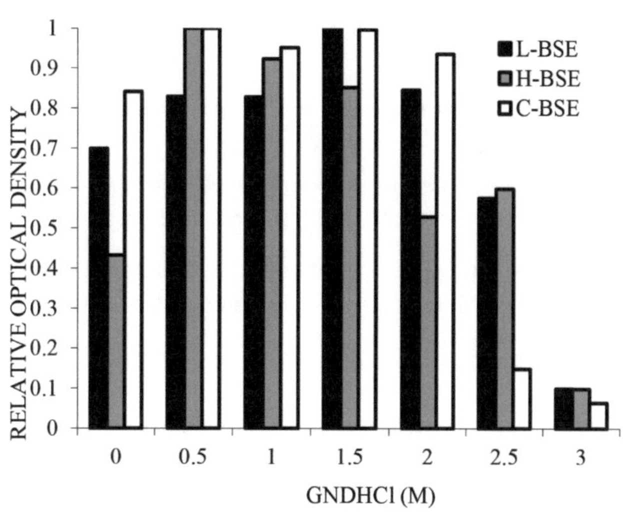

Figure 9. Relative quantification of denaturation transitions for the H-BSE, C-BSE, and L-BSE.

2.3.1.3. Molecular signature

In **Figure 10**, 2D analysis of typical and atypical BSE shows that the three forms of BSE correlate to three distinct signatures. H-type BSE shows a consistent representation of truncated fragments at 12 kDa, while C-type and L-type molecular fingerprint is mainly characterized by 27–30 PrP.

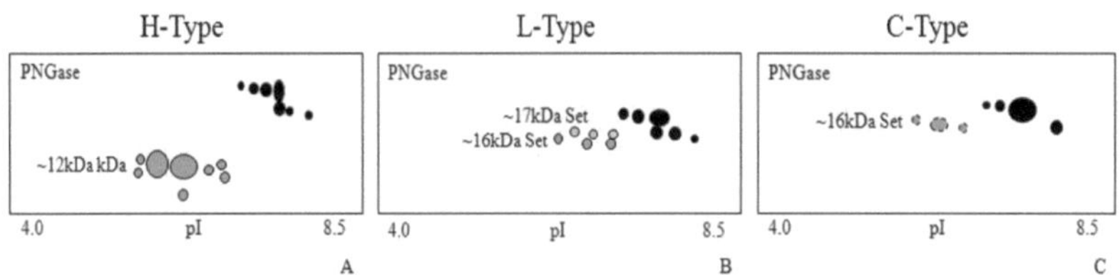

Figure 10. Two-dimensional mapping of BSE brain homogenates after PK treatment. Schematic diagram of PK-resistant C-terminal PrP core fragments in BSE strains (A–C).

2.3.1.4. GPI anchor

In the three forms of BSE, PrP27-30 core fragment is characterized by two sets of isoforms differing of ~ 1.0 unit of pI and ~2.0 kDa (**Figure 11**).

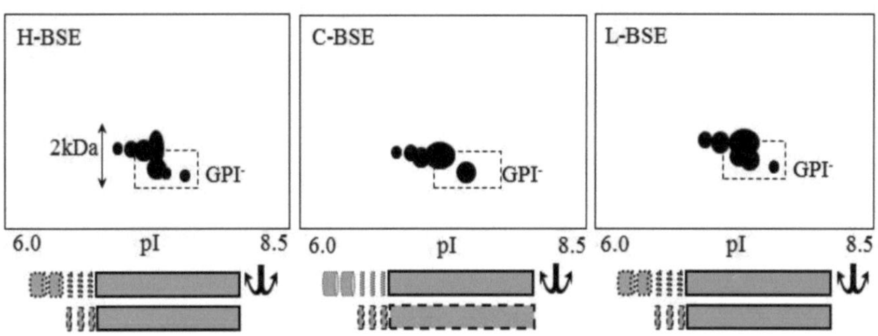

Figure 11. Schematic representation of anchored and anchorless PK-resistant PrP core fragments in BSE strains.

The comparison between theoretical and measured isoelectric points and molecular weights of core fragments indicates that the upper set represents anchored forms.

Therefore, classical BSE shows only one anchorless isoform, while in L-BSE and H-BSE, there are three anchorless isoforms with average amount comparable to the anchored ones.

2.4. Molecular similarities between human and cattle TSE forms

2.4.1. Comparison of human and cattle molecular strains by 1D analysis

In **Figure 12**, biochemical PrP^{TSE} types are matched two by two to best compare the molecular similarities. sCJD type 1 and H-type BSE share the same molecular weight; sCJD type 2A and L-type BSE show similar molecular weight and glycosylation profile; vCJD and classical BSE are characterized by a similar diglycosylated profile.

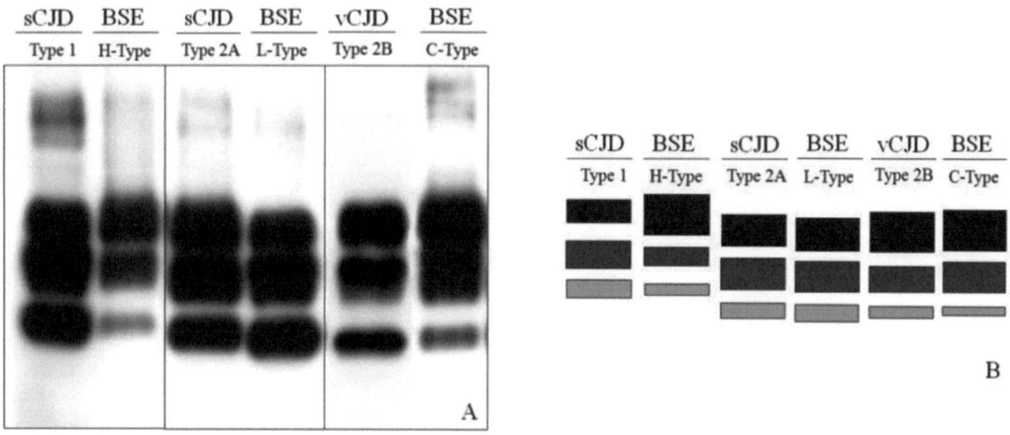

Figure 12. Western blot profile (A) and schematic representation of paired human and BSE strains (B).

2.4.2. Comparison of human and cattle molecular strains by 2D analysis

Increasing resolution power by 2D analysis, it's possible to deeply compare biochemical signatures of PrP^{TSE} between humans and cattle (**Figure 13**). PrP^{TSE} shows similar signatures in BSE-H and sCJD type 1 and is characterized by the dominance of C-terminal fragments. These patterns are distinct from those observed in other forms. Both sCJD type 2A and L-type BSE show the same set of spot at about 18 kDa, while in vCJD and L-BSE the molecular signature seems to be different.

2.4.3. Comparison of human and cattle molecular strains by 2D analysis after experimental transmission

A lot of experimental transmission studies have been performed to define prion strains from small animals such as mice or hamster to highly evolved primates such as chimpanzees or macaques. Transmission studies in transgenic mice, carrying one or more human or bovine prion gene copy, are often a useful approach to investigate the relationship among different prion strains [22].

Nevertheless primates can be considered the host nearest to humans. In fact, several interesting similarities between human and cattle strains can be enhanced by molecular analysis after transmission experiments to primates.

sCJD MM-1 and sCJD MM-1 after experimental transmission to primate share identical patterns of PrP27-30 and C-terminal fragments (CTFs) indicating that PrP^{Sc} fingerprints are conserved throughout transmission as reported in **Figure 14**. This finding confirms that primates are a good model to simulate transmission to humans of human prion strains.

In **Figure 15**, it can be noted that C-BSE shows the appearance of CTFs after first passage transmission, which maintains an identical pattern at second passage.

vCJD and vCJD passaged to primate share the same PrP^{TSE} fingerprints identical to those observed in BSE at first and second passage (**Figure 16**). This is a further confirmation of the correlation between BSE and vCJD.

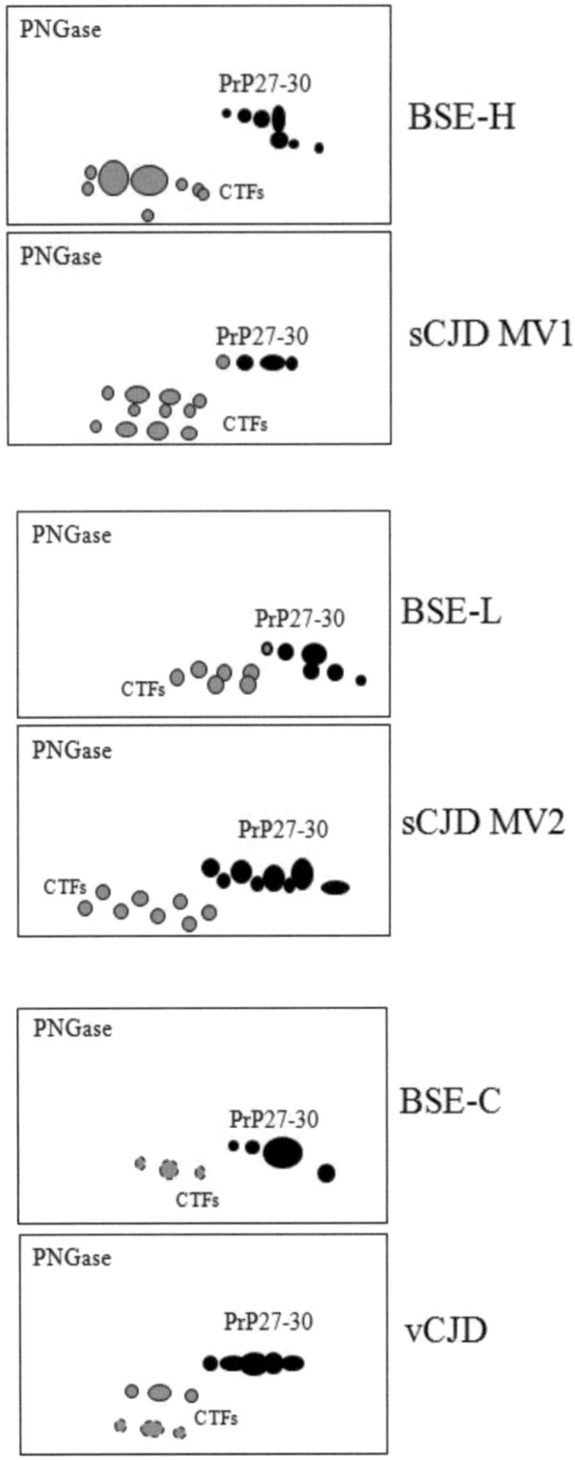

Figure 13. 2D western blot comparison between human and cattle TSE.

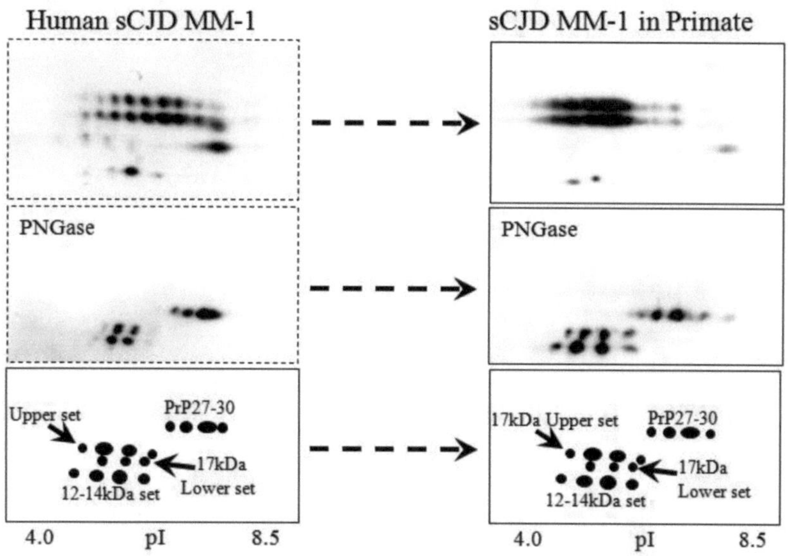

Figure 14. 2D western blot comparison between human MM-1 before and after transmission to primate.

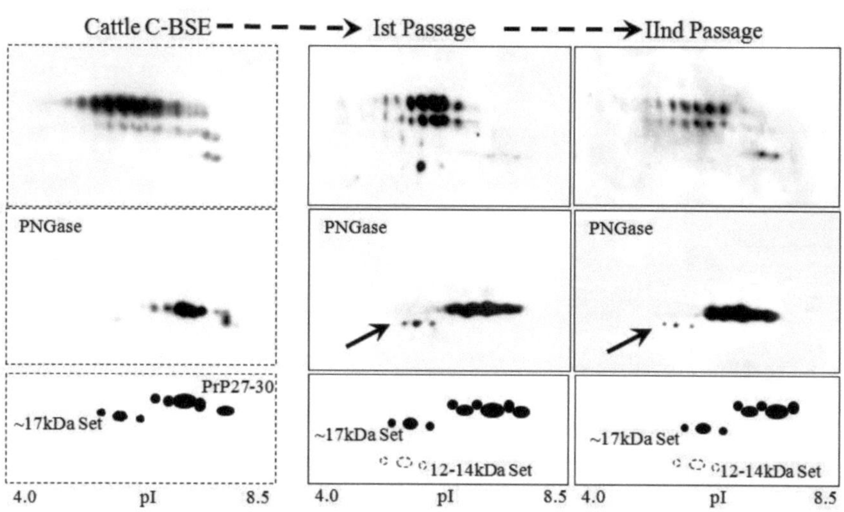

Figure 15. 2D western blot comparison between C-BSE before and after transmission at first and second passage to primate.

Figure 17 shows L-BSE PrP^{TSE} CTFs pattern in primate similar to that of L-BSE in cattle, characterized by a set of fragments migrating at 18 kDa; this set of spots are absent in BSE and vCJD passaged to primates. It's to be noted that L-BSE transmitted to primate is almost identical to human MV-2. These molecular signature similarities confirm molecular pattern previously observed for 1D immunoblot and suggests a possible molecular common origin of the two molecular strains. This correlation however needs to be deeply analyzed and confirmed.

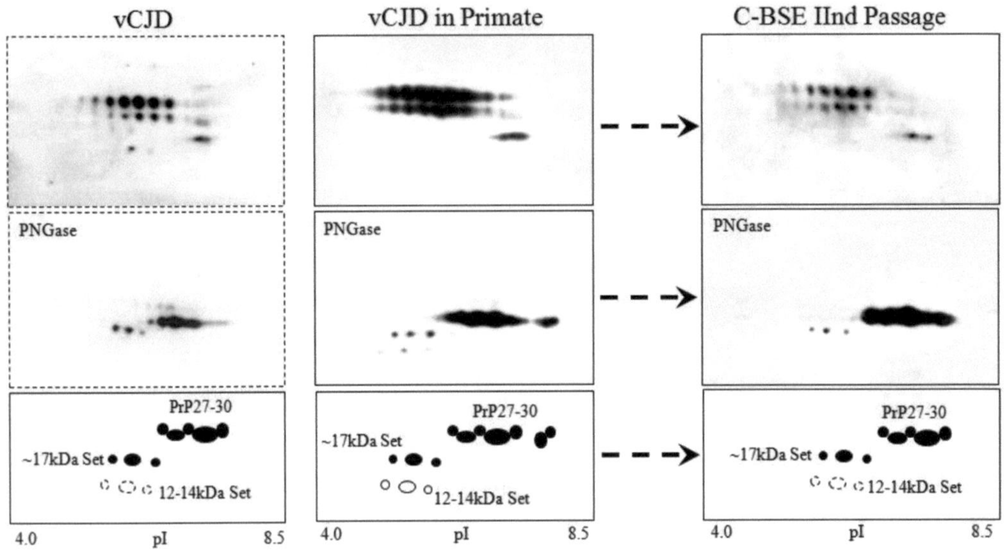

Figure 16. 2D western blot comparison between vCJD before and after transmission to primate and C-BSE after second passage to primate.

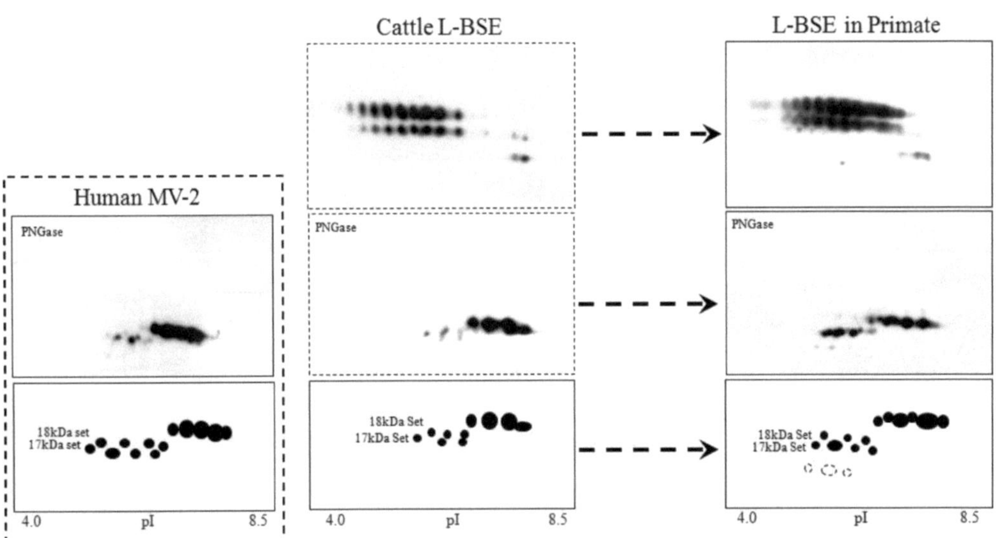

Figure 17. 2D western blot comparison between L-BSE before and after transmission to primate.

3. Conclusions

We have shown that molecular analysis of prions is a powerful approach to characterize prions.

By using several different biochemical approaches, it's possible to enhance molecular differences and similarities to define prion strains.

In particular, biochemical analysis is shown to be rapid and informative in:

- differentiation of PrP^{TSE} strains;
- correlation of molecular to clinicopoathological phenotypes;
- large scale epidemiological studies and surveillance: finding and discriminating strains (sCJD, vCJD, atypical BSEs).

Author details

Michele Fiorini*, Matilde Bongianni and Gianluigi Zanusso

*Address all correspondence to: michele.fiorini@univr.it

Department Neurosciences, Biomedicine and Movement Sciences, University of Verona, Italy

References

[1] Prusiner SB. Prions. Proc Natl Acad Sci USA. 1998;**95**(23):13363–83.

[2] Basler K, Oesch B, Scott M, Westaway D, Wälchli M, Groth DF, McKinley MP, Prusiner SB, Weissmann C. Scrapie and cellular PrP isoforms are encoded by the same chromosomal gene. Cell. 1986;**46**(3):417–28.

[3] Zanusso G, Fiorini M, Ferrari S, Meade-White K, Barbieri I, Brocchi E, Ghetti B, Monaco S. Gerstmann-Sträussler-Scheinker disease and "anchorless prion protein" mice share prion conformational properties diverging from sporadic Creutzfeldt-Jakob disease. J Biol Chem. 2014 Feb 21;289(8):4870–81. DOI: 10.1074/jbc.M113.531335

[4] McKinley MP, Prusiner SB. Biology and structure of scrapie prions. Int Rev Neurobiol. 1986;**21**:1–57.

[5] Bazan JF1, Fletterick RJ, McKinley MP, Prusiner SB. Predicted secondary structure and membrane topology of the scrapie prion protein. Protein Eng. 1987;**1**(2):125–35.

[6] Safar J, Wille H, Itri V, Groth D, Serban H, Torchia M, Cohen FE, Prusiner SB. Eight prion strains have PrPSc molecules with different conformations. Nat Med. 1998;**4**(10):1157–65.

[7] Bode L, Pocchiari M, Gelderblom H, Diringer H. Characterization of antisera against scrapie-associated fibrils (SAF) from affected hamster and cross-reactivity with SAF from scrapie-affected mice and from patients with Creutzfeldt-Jakob disease. J Gen Virol. 1985;**66**(11):2471–8.

[8] Hill AF, Joiner S, Wadsworth JD, Sidle KC, Bell JE, Budka H, Ironside JW, Collinge J. Molecular classification of sporadic Creutzfeldt-Jakob disease. Brain. 2003;**126**(6):1333–46.

[9] Parchi P, Giese A, Capellari S, Brown P, Schulz-Schaeffer W, Windl O, Zerr I, Budka H, Kopp N, Piccardo P, Poser S, Rojiani A, Streichemberger N, Julien J, Vital C, Ghetti B, Gambetti P, Kretzschmar H. Classification of sporadic Creutzfeldt-Jakob disease based on molecular and phenotypic analysis of 300 subjects. Ann Neurol. 1999;**46**(2):224–33.

[10] Zanusso G, Polo A, Farinazzo A, Nonno R, Cardone F, Di Bari M, Ferrari S, Principe S, Gelati M, Fasoli E, Fiorini M, Prelli F, Frangione B, Tridente G, Bentivoglio M, Giorgi A, Schininà ME, Maras B, Agrimi U, Rizzuto N, Pocchiari M, Monaco S. Novel prion protein conformation and glycotype in Creutzfeldt-Jakob disease. Arch Neurol. 2007;**64**(4):595–9.

[11] Zou WQ, Puoti G, Xiao X, Yuan J, Qing L, Cali I, Shimoji M, Langeveld JP, Castellani R, Notari S, Crain B, Schmidt RE, Geschwind M, Dearmond SJ, Cairns NJ, Dickson D, Honig L, Torres JM, Mastrianni J, Capellari S, Giaccone G, Belay ED, Schonberger LB, Cohen M, Perry G, Kong Q, Parchi P, Tagliavini F, Gambetti P. Variably protease-sensitive prionopathy: A new sporadic disease of the prion protein. Ann Neurol. 2010;**68**(2):162–72. DOI: 10.1002/ana.22094.

[12] Tagliavini F, Prelli F, Ghiso J, Bugiani O, Serban D, Prusiner SB, Farlow MR, Ghetti B, Frangione B.. Amyloid protein of Gerstmann-Sträussler-Scheinker disease (Indiana kindred) is an 11 kd fragment of prion protein with an N-terminal glycine at codon 58. EMBO J. 1991;**10**(3):513–9.

[13] Tagliavini F, Prelli F, Porro M, Rossi G, Giaccone G, Farlow MR, Dlouhy SR, Ghetti B, Bugiani O, Frangione B. Amyloid fibrils in Gerstmann-Sträussler-Scheinker disease (Indiana and Swedish kindreds) express only PrP peptides encoded by the mutant allele. Cell. 1994;**79**(4):695–703.

[14] Piccardo P, Dlouhy SR, Lievens PM, Young K, Bird TD, Nochlin D, Dickson DW, Vinters HV, Zimmerman TR, Mackenzie IR, Kish SJ, Ang LC, De Carli C, Pocchiari M, Brown P, Gibbs CJ Jr, Gajdusek DC, Bugiani O, Ironside J, Tagliavini F, Ghetti B. Phenotypic variability of Gerstmann-Sträussler-Scheinker disease is associated with prion protein heterogeneity. J Neuropathol Exp Neurol. 1998;**57**(10):979–88.

[15] Collinge J, Sidle KC, Meads J, Ironside J, Hill AF. Molecular analysis of prion strain variation and the aetiology of 'new variant' CJD. Nature. 1996;**383**(6602):685–90.

[16] Shaked GM, Fridlander G, Meiner Z, Taraboulos A, Gabizon R. Protease-resistant and detergent-insoluble prion protein is not necessarily associated with prion infectivity. J Biol Chem. 1999;**274**(25):17981–6.

[17] Peretz D, Scott MR, Groth D, Williamson RA, Burton DR, Cohen FE, Prusiner SB. Strain-specified relative conformational stability of the scrapie prion protein. Protein Sci. 2001;**10**(4):854–63.

[18] Zanusso G, Farinazzo A, Prelli F, Fiorini M, Gelati M, Ferrari S, Righetti PG, Rizzuto N, Frangione B, Monaco S. Identification of distinct N-terminal truncated forms of prion protein in different Creutzfeldt-Jakob disease subtypes. J Biol Chem. 2004;**279**(37):389366–42.

[19] Casalone C, Zanusso G, Acutis P, Ferrari S, Capucci L, Tagliavini F, Monaco S, Caramelli M. Identification of a second bovine amyloidotic spongiform encephalopathy: molecular similarities with sporadic Creutzfeldt-Jakob disease. Proc Natl Acad Sci USA. 2004;**101**(9):3065–70.

[20] Polak MP, Zmudzinski JF, Jacobs JG, Langeveld JP. Atypical status of bovine spongiform encephalopathy in Poland: a molecular typing study. Arch Virol. 2008;**153**(1):69–79.

[21] Lombardi G, Casalone C, D' Angelo A, Gelmetti D, Torcoli G, Barbieri I, Corona C, Fasoli E, Farinazzo A, Fiorini M, Gelati M, Iulini B, Tagliavini F, Ferrari S, Caramelli M, Monaco S, Capucci L, Zanusso G. Intraspecies transmission of BASE induces clinical dullness and amyotrophic changes. PLoS Pathog. 2008;**4**(5):e1000075. DOI: 10.1371/journal.ppat.1000075

[22] Weissmann C, Enari M, Klöhn P-C, Rossi D, Flechsig E. Transmission of prions. Proc Natl Acad Sci USA. 2002;**99**(Suppl 4):16378–83.

Section 3

Metals in Prion Disease

Chapter 6

Disruption of Metal Homeostasis and the Pathogenesis of Prion Diseases

Masahiro Kawahara, Ken-ichiro Tanaka and
Dai Mizuno

Additional information is available at the end of the chapter

http://dx.doi.org/10.5772/67327

Abstract

Prion diseases are progressive neurodegenerative diseases that are associated with the conformational conversion of normal cellular prion protein (PrP^C) into abnormal pathogenic prion protein (PrP^{Sc}). PrP^C is a metal-binding protein that is located in the synapse and possesses the ability to bind to various metals, including Cu, Zn, Mn and Fe. Moreover, increasing evidence suggests that PrP^C plays essential roles in the maintenance of metal homeostasis in the synapse. Trace elements have a crucial influence on the conformational change of PrP^C. Given that other disease-related proteins such as β-amyloid protein and its precursor protein (APP) in Alzheimer's disease also exist in the synapse and possess a metal-binding ability, an interaction between PrP and metals and between PrP and APP, may occur in the synapse; the resulting metal homeostasis may lead to the pathogenesis of prion diseases. Here, we review our studies and other new findings that inform the current understanding of the link between trace elements and physiological functions of PrP^C and the neurotoxicity of PrP^{Sc}.

Keywords: Alzheimer's disease, synapse, calcium homeostasis, zinc, copper, iron, manganese

1. Introduction

Prion diseases are fatal neurodegenerative diseases, such as scrapie in sheep, bovine spongiform encephalopathy (BSE) in cattle and Creutzfeldt-Jakob disease (CJD), Gerstmann-Sträussler-Scheinker syndrome (GSS) and Kuru in humans [1]. The common pathological hallmarks of prion diseases are the spongiform degeneration of glial cells and neurons. The accumulation of amyloidogenic prion protein (PrP) as the abnormal scrapie type isoform (PrP^{Sc}) is also observed in the brain of patients. Prion diseases are also called transmissible spongiform encephalopathies because their infection characteristics are caused by the activities of PrP^{Sc} in the pathogenetic tissues [2].

Although the molecular pathogenesis and transmission pathway of prion diseases are still controversial, it is widely accepted that the conformational conversion of normal cellular prion protein (PrP^{C}) into an abnormal PrP^{Sc} is the transmissible characteristic of prion diseases. Normal PrP^{C} is a 30–35 kDa cell surface glycoprotein anchored at the plasma membrane with a glycosylphosphatidylinositol (GPI) domain. PrP^{C} is ubiquitously expressed in the body and notably expressed in the brain. Both PrP^{C} and PrP^{Sc} have the same characteristic chemical modification of the same primary sequence. However, PrP^{C} differs from PrP^{Sc} in terms of resistance to protease digestion, a high content of β-sheet secondary structure and the propensity to form insoluble amyloid fibrils. When the misfolded PrP^{Sc} enters into the body via the ingestion of contaminated food, etc., the protease-resistant PrP^{Sc} can aggregate, resulting in fibril formation that in turn promotes other PrP^{C} molecules in the brain to misfold and aggregate. These lines of evidence suggest that the conformational change of PrP is crucial for the pathogenesis of prion diseases. Thus, prion diseases are included in the category of protein-misfolding diseases (conformational diseases), along with Alzheimer's disease (AD), triplet repeat diseases and dementia with Lewy bodies (DLB) [3]. All of these diseases share common properties, such as the deposition of disease-related proteins (amyloids) and in the exhibition of neurotoxicity. The disease-related proteins, which are termed amyloidogenic proteins, include β-amyloid protein (AβP) in AD, prion protein in prion diseases, polyglutamine in triplet repeat disease and α-synuclein in DLB. Although their primary sequences are identical, all of these proteins form insoluble fibril-like structures (amyloid fibrils) with β-pleated sheet structures. Furthermore, all of these amyloidogenic proteins possess the ability to bind trace metals [4].

In the brain, considerable amounts of trace elements such as iron (Fe), zinc (Zn), copper (Cu) and manganese (Mn) exist, as well as other ubiquitous elements such as sodium (Na), potassium (K), calcium (Ca) and magnesium (Mg). The concentration and the distribution of each metal differ across brain regions [5, 6]. These trace elements are essential for the normal brain functions. However, an excess of these metals are neurotoxic. Thus, their concentration and chemical form are strictly regulated.

Increasing evidence suggests that trace elements are involved in the neurodegenerative pathways for prion diseases [7]. There are three possible roles for trace elements in these neurodegenerative pathways [8]: (1) supporting the "loss of the normal, protective functions of PrP^{C}"; (2) supporting a "gain of toxic functions of PrP^{Sc}"; and (3) "a combination of both." Although the physiological roles of PrP^{C} are not yet fully understood despite its wide distribution, several studies suggest that PrP^{C} regulates metal homeostasis and has antioxidant and cytoprotective effects against the neurotoxicity induced by Cu^{2+} or free radicals. Therefore, the depletion of PrP^{C} and the resulting metal dyshomeostasis may trigger the neurodegenerative processes. Moreover, PrP^{Sc} and its fragment peptides cause synaptic impairment and apoptosis in neurons or astrocytes *in vitro* or *in vivo* [9, 10]. Trace

http://dx.doi.org/10.5772/67327

elements cause conformational changes in PrP and enhance its neurotoxicity. Furthermore, prion plaques in the patient brain reportedly contain low Cu and high Mn [11]. The expression level of PrP is correlated with the distribution of metals [12]. Here, we review our studies and other new findings for a current understanding of the link between trace elements and the pathogenesis of prion diseases. We also discuss the role of PrP as the regulator of metal homeostasis and the protector against neurotoxicity of β-amyloid protein (AβP) at the synapse.

2. Metal homeostasis and normal prion protein

2.1. Cu and normal prion protein

Cu is the third most abundant metal in the brain. Cu is essential for brain function and is a cofactor for numerous enzymes, including cytochrome C, superoxide dismutase, lysyl oxidase and tyrosinase. Cu is involved in Fe homeostasis as a component of ceruloplasmin. Moreover, Cu has neuroprotective activity as a component of Cu/Zn superoxide dismutase (Cu/ZnSOD), an endogenous antioxidant. Thus, Cu deficiency has adverse effects on myelination. However, Cu is a redox-active metal and exists as both oxidized Cu^{2+} and reduced Cu^{+}. Excess free Cu is toxic because it produces ROS and binds with the thiol groups of functional proteins. Cu binds to transporter proteins such as CTR1, ATP7A and ATP7B and is transported into the brain. Cu deficiency or excess due to an impairment of these transporters leads to severe neurodegenerative diseases such as Wilson's disease or Menkes disease.

Recent studies suggest that Cu has modulatory effects on neuronal information processes [13–15]. Intracellular Cu accumulates in synaptic vesicles and is then released into the synaptic clefts during neuronal excitation at the concentration about 15–100 μM. These characteristics are quite similar to Zn. The released Cu reportedly influences various receptors, including *N*-methyl-D-aspartate (NMDA)-type glutamate receptor, AMPA-type glutamate receptor and GABA receptor to modulate the neuronal activity [16].

The link between Cu and prion diseases were first reported by Brown et al. in 1997 [17]. They demonstrated that the levels of Cu in the brains of PrP-knockout mice are significantly decreased compared to those levels in normal mice. The activity of Cu-dependent enzymes was also reduced in PrP-null mice. As shown in **Figure 1**, PrP^{C} contains 208 amino acid residues and possesses a highly conserved octarepeat domain composed of multiple tandem copies of the eight-residue sequence PHGGGWGQ in its N-terminal (**Figure 1**). Jackson et al. reported that PrP^{C} binds to four Cu atoms in its octarepeat domain and binds to two Cu atoms in addition to two histidine (His) residues, His^{96} and His^{111} [18]. They also demonstrated that other metals including Zn^{2+}, Mn^{2+} and Ni^{2+} bind to these binding sites with lower affinities compared to Cu^{2+}. Extended X-ray absorption fine structure (EXAFS) spectroscopy demonstrated that Cu binds His residues in the octarepeat domain [19]. Moreover, Valensin et al. reported that His^{111} in the neurotoxic fragment PrP106-126 has the ability to bind Cu^{+} and Ag^{+} [20].

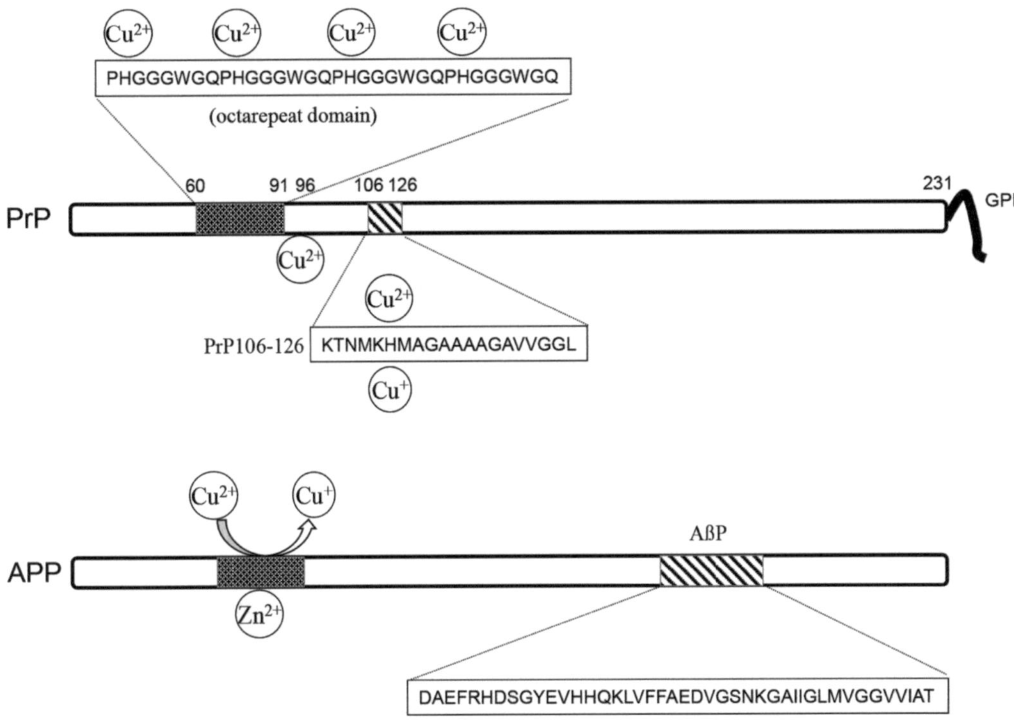

Figure 1. The structure and the metal-binding properties of prion protein and APP.

PrP^C reportedly transports Cu from the extracellular space to the intracellular space via endocytosis and thus regulates the intracellular concentrations of Cu [21]. Furthermore, PrP possesses or modulates Cu/ZnSOD activity in the brain and plays roles in the cellular resistance to oxidative stress [22]. Indeed, PrP-deficient neurons exhibit a lower glutathione activity and susceptibility to hydrogen peroxide [23]. Recent studies suggest that PrP^C regulates the excitability of NMDA-type glutamate receptor in a Cu-dependent manner [24]. Moreover, Cu^{2+} influences the gene expression and cellular trafficking of PrP [25]. PrP^{Sc}-infected cells exhibit decreased Cu^{2+} binding. The Cu-deficient condition due to a mutation of ATP7A delays the onset of prion diseases. These results indicate that the regulation of Cu homeostasis is involved in the physiological roles of PrP and its mechanism of infection and neurodegeneration.

These characteristics of PrP^C are similar to those of the AD-related protein AβP (**Figure 1**). AβP is a small peptide of 39–43 amino acid residues, which results from a cleavage of a large precursor protein (APP; amyloid precursor protein). The conformational change of AβP and its neurotoxicity play central roles in the pathogenesis of AD [26]. APP has distinct binding domains for Cu, Zn and Fe. APP binds to Cu with its N-terminal and converts Cu^{2+} into Cu^+ [27]. Cu influences the expression and the dimerization of APP and the trafficking of APP from the ER to the neurites. Moreover, Cu promotes the production of AβP.

http://dx.doi.org/10.5772/67327

2.2. Zn and normal prion protein

Other metals are also associated with prion diseases. Among them, Zn^{2+} has the next highest binding affinity to PrP^C compared to Cu^{2+}. Zn is the second most abundant element in the brain. Zn is essential for most organisms and plays important roles in various physiological functions such as mitotic cell division, immune system functioning and synthesis of proteins and DNA [28]. Moreover, Zn acts as a cofactor to more than 300 enzymes or metalloproteins. Recent studies have revealed that Zn signaling plays crucial roles as a second messenger in various human biological systems. Thus, Zn deficiency in children results in dwarfism, delayed mental and physical development, immune dysfunction and learning disabilities. Zn deficiency also produces learning disorders, taste disorders and odor disorders in adults.

The human body contains approximately 2 g of Zn. In the brain, Zn is concentrated in the regions such as cerebral cortex, amygdala, hippocampus, thalamus and olfactory cortex. Zn in the brain firmly binds to metalloproteins or enzymes. However, a substantial fraction (approximately 10% or more) of Zn either forms free Zn ions (Zn^{2+}) or is loosely bound. This Zn fraction is histochemically detectable via staining with chelating reagents [29]. In the presynaptic vesicles of excitatory glutamatergic neurons, the chelatable Zn is stored and is secreted into synaptic clefts together with glutamate during neuronal firings. The concentration of this secreted Zn is estimated to be 1–100 μM [30, 31]. Secreted Zn^{2+} modulates overall brain excitability by binding with *N*-methyl-D-aspartate (NMDA)-type glutamate receptors, GABA receptors and glycine receptors. The secreted Zn^{2+} is critical for neuronal communication, synaptic plasticity and memory formation [32]. Indeed, Zn^{2+} in the hippocampus is essential for the induction of long-term potentiation (LTP), which is a form of synaptic information storage that has become a well-known paradigm for the mechanisms underlying memory formation.

There are two factors involved in the maintenance of Zn homeostasis, metallothioneins and Zn transporters. Metallothioneins are ubiquitous metal-binding proteins with 68 amino acids that bind seven metal atoms (including Zn, Cu, Cd, etc.) via 20 cysteine residues. There are three types of metallothioneins, MT-1, MT-2 and MT-3. MT-1 and MT-2 are ubiquitously expressed throughout the entire body, whereas MT-3 is primary localized in the central nervous system.

Zn transporters also control Zn homeostasis by facilitating Zn influx and efflux [33]. There are two types of mammalian Zn transporters, ZnT transporters and Zrt-, Irt-like protein (ZIP) transporters. ZnT transporters are involved with the solute carrier (*SLC30*) gene family and decrease intracellular Zn via a facilitation of Zn efflux from cells. There are 14 types of ZnT transporters in mammals, including ZnT-1 and ZnT-3, which are colocalized with chelatable Zn in the brain. ZnT-1 is a membrane protein with six transmembrane domains and is widely distributed in mammalian cells. ZnT-1 has a pivotal role in Zn efflux and protects against excess Zn. ZnT-3 is localized to the membranes of presynaptic vesicles, transports Zn into synaptic vesicles and maintains high Zn concentrations in the vesicles.

ZIP transporters are another type of Zn transporter encoded by *SLC39* genes. ZIP transporters increase cytosolic Zn by promoting transport from extracellular to intracellular compartments.

Fourteen ZIP genes have been identified in mammals and the ZIP transporters are localized to the cell membranes or to the membranes of the Golgi apparatus or ER. These transporters control Zn influx into subcellular organs. The impairment of Zn transporters results in severe diseases such as Ehlers-Danlos syndrome.

The concentration of Zn in the brain is much higher compared to Cu; therefore, Zn^{2+} may influence PrP^C binding to Cu [34]. Bioinformatics analysis has revealed evolutionary similarities between prion genes and gene-encoding ZIP transporters [35, 36]. Among 14 transporters, the sequential similarities exist between PrP^C and ZIP5, ZIP6 and ZIP10. Taylor et al. reported that ZIP6 and ZIP10 form heteromers similar to PrP structures and influences cell migration [37]. PrP^C colocalizes with ZIP5 and forms dimers [38]. These findings strongly suggest that PrP^C plays important roles in the neuronal regulation of Zn. Watt et al. reported that PrP^C-enhanced cellular uptake of Zn via binding with the AMPA-type glutamate receptor and that PrP^C acts as Zn sensor in the synapse [39]. Indeed, PrP facilitates Zn influx into the brain, regulates Zn homeostasis and attenuates Zn-induced neurotoxicity.

2.3. Fe and prion protein

Fe is the most abundant metal in the brain as well as in the entire body. Fe is essential for numerous biological functions as an enzyme cofactor for metabolic processes such as the oxygen transport, oxidative phosphorylation and energy transfer. Fe has critical roles in specialized brain functions such as the synthesis of dopaminergic neurotransmitters and myelination. Therefore, Fe deficiency impairs learning, especially in children or infants. The Fe deficiency impairs working ability or learning ability also in adults. However, excess Fe can generate reactive oxygen species (ROS) that damage DNA, proteins and lipids and can therefore be toxic to neurons.

Fe exists in two different forms, ferrous iron (Fe^{2+}) and ferric iron (Fe^{3+}). In general, oxidized Fe^{3+} is insoluble and exists extracellularly, whereas reduced Fe^{2+} is soluble and intracellularly located. Orally administrated Fe is primarily absorbed from the gastrointestinal pathway via divalent metal transporter-1 (DMT-1) as Fe^{2+}. Once it enters the circulation, Fe^{2+} ions are oxidized into Fe^{3+} by ferroxidases such as ferritin or ceruloplasmin. Transferrin, an iron transporter protein, binds two Fe^{3+} ions. Transferrin-bound iron (Fe^{3+}) crosses the blood brain barrier (BBB) via transferrin receptors and enters into cells. Finally, Fe^{3+} is reduced into Fe^{2+} by ferrireductase and functions as a cofactor for neuronal enzymes such as tyrosine hydroxylase, which is necessary for the dopamine synthesis. Thus, Fe levels, as well as the ratio between Fe^{2+} and Fe^{3+}, are strictly regulated in normal brains.

Increasing evidence suggests that PrP^C is involved in Fe homeostasis [40]. PrP^C reportedly has ferrireductase activity and modulates the cellular uptake of Fe [41]. Tripathi et al. demonstrated that PrP induces the conversion from Fe^{3+} to Fe^{2+} and then Fe^{2+} is intracellularly transported by ZIP14/DMT-1 [42]. PrP-knockout mice exhibit altered Fe metabolism [43]. PrP is cotransported with ferritin, an iron-binding protein. Moreover, a decreased level of transferrin was observed in the cerebrospinal fluid of CJD patients [44].

2.4. Mn and prion protein

There are several studies suggesting that Mn may be a facilitator of prion diseases. Mn is an essential trace elements and crucial for various enzymes such as hydrolase, glutamine synthetase, arginase and pyruvate carboxylase [45]. However, excess Mn is neurotoxic and induces Parkinson's disease-like syndrome.

Johnson et al. investigated the levels of trace elements in prion-infected hamster brains using X-ray photoelectron emission microscopy with synchrotron radiation and found reduced Cu and increased Mn in prion protein plaques [11]. Thackray et al. reported that PrP^{C} loses its SOD-like activity when Cu is replaced with Mn [46]. Mn enhances the survival of PrP in model soils and increases its infectivity [47]. The risk of a prion disease in elk, termed chronic wasting disease, was associated with an Mg deficiency and increased Mn concentrations [48]. A recent epidemiological survey suggests a relationship between the pathogenesis of CJD and the imbalance of Mn [49]. Moreover, the impairment of Mn transporter is reportedly involved in the infection process [50].

3. Metal and PrP^{Sc} neurotoxicity

3.1. Metal-induced conformational changes of prion protein and its neurotoxicity

The conformational changes and neurotoxicity of PrP^{Sc} are central for the transmission and the pathogenesis of prion disease. To investigate the neurotoxicity of PrP^{Sc}, we and other researchers have employed synthetic fragment peptides of PrP (PrP106-126) as a model peptide of PrP^{Sc}, considering the methodological difficulties of using a whole prion protein owing to its strong infectious characteristics [51]. The structure of PrP106-126 coincides with the proposed β-sheet structures of PrP^{Sc} [52]. PrP106-126 forms aggregates with β-sheet structures as amyloid fibrils that share several characteristics of PrP^{Sc}, causes the apoptotic death of cultured neurons or glial cells and possess the ability to bind to metals including Cu^{2+} and Zn^{2+}.

We synthesized three fragment peptides: PrP77-83 (WGQPHGGGWGQPHGGG), PrP106-126 (KTNMKHMAGAAAAGAVVGGLG) and PrP144-157 (DYEDRHRENMHRY). All three peptides attenuated Cu^{2+}-induced neurotoxicity [51]. Although PrP77-83 and PrP144-157 are not neurotoxic, PrP106-126 forms β-sheet structures during the "aging" process (the incubation at 37°C for several days), as determined using the thioflavin T (ThT) fluorescence assay, far-UV circular dichroism (CD) spectroscopy and atomic force microscopy (AFM) imaging. Moreover, aged PrP106-126 exhibits enhanced neurotoxicity on primary cultured rat hippocampal neurons. Thus, we added various trace elements or metal chelators to solutions of PrP106-126 during the aging process and evaluated its conformational changes and neurotoxicity. We found that the coexistence of Zn^{2+} or Cu^{2+} during the aging process significantly attenuated the neurotoxicity of PrP106-126. Moreover, the presence of Al^{3+}, Fe^{2+} and Fe^{3+} did not result in significant changes. We also observed the oligomerization of PrP106-126 using the fluorescent changes of ThT, which binds with pleated β-sheet structures. The ThT fluorescence of solutions of aged PrP106-126 increased compared to freshly dissolved PrP106-126 solutions. The ThT fluorescence of aged PrP106-126 with Zn^{2+}, Fe^{2+}, or Fe^{3+} was significantly decreased compared to aged PrP106-126 alone. In particular, the addition of Cu^{2+} dramatically decreased ThT fluorescence to the same level as fresh PrP106-126. Furthermore, aged PrP106-126 forms amyloid fibrils with distinct straight and long morphology on mica plates, as observed using AFM, although we did not observe fiber-like structures in freshly prepared PrP106-126. Moreover, aged PrP106-126 with Cu or Zn exhibited different morphological features compared to aged PrP106-126 alone. Therefore, it is possible that Cu^{2+} and Zn^{2+} influenced the β-sheet formation of PrP106-126 and thereafter attenuated its neurotoxicity. Our results are consistent with other studies that demonstrate that Cu^{2+} inhibited the ß-sheet formation of PrP111-126 or that Cu^{2+} inhibited the conformational changes of the larger fragment [53]. Thakur et al. reported that Cu^{2+} did not induce the oligomerization of PrP at physiological temperature and that Cu^{2+} may act as an attenuator in prion diseases [54].

3.2. Molecular mechanism of the neurotoxicity induced by PrP106-126

Understanding the pathway for PrP^{Sc}-induced neurodegeneration is of particular importance for identifying substances that protect against prion diseases. PrP106-126 causes adverse effects, such as the proliferation of microglia, the induction of pro-inflammatory responses, the production of reactive oxygen species (ROS) and the activation of ER stress. Our review focuses the disruption of Ca homeostasis, because Ca^{2+} ions are required for various functions of key enzymes such as kinases, phosphatases and proteases. The disruption of neuronal Ca homeostasis and alteration of intracellular calcium Ca^{2+} levels ($[Ca^{2+}]_i$) activated, various apoptotic proteins such as calpain and caspase, leading to neuronal death. The disruption of Ca homeostasis might trigger various adverse effects that are also associated with prion diseases.

Support of this idea was first demonstrated in a study of the neurotoxicity of AβP [55–57]. In 1993, Arispe et al. demonstrated that AβP(1–40), i.e., the first 40-residues of AβP, directly incorporates into artificial lipid bilayer membranes and forms cation-selective ion channels [58]. The channels, termed "amyloid channels," are giant multilevel pores and can allow a large amount of Ca^{2+} to pass through them. Their activity can be blocked by Zn^{2+} ions. We observed the appearance of amyloid channels on membrane patches from a neuroblastoma cell line (GT1-7 cells). GT1-7 cells possess neuron-like characteristics, such as the expression of neuron-specific proteins, the expression of various channels and receptors and the extension of neuritis [59]. After the administration of AβP(1–40), the current derived from the amyloid channels appeared. The activity of amyloid channels was inhibited by the addition of Zn^{2+} and recovered by the administration of *o*-phenanthroline (a Zn chelator). Based on these findings, we proposed the hypothesis termed the "amyloid channel hypothesis." This hypothesis demonstrates that the direct binding of AβPs on membranes and the subsequent disruption of Ca^{2+} homeostasis through amyloid channels might be the primary event in AβP neurotoxicity. AβP might have a similar mechanism of toxicity as that underlies the toxicity of various antimicrobial or antifungal peptides that also exhibit channel-forming activity and cell toxicity [60]. Indeed, Soscia et al. demonstrated that AβP exerts antimicrobial activity against eight common and clinically relevant microorganisms [61]. Furthermore, the presence of pore-

http://dx.doi.org/10.5772/67327

like structures of AβPs was demonstrated in the neuronal cell membrane of the brains of AD patients and AD-model mice [62].

Increasing evidence suggests that other amyloidogenic proteins also form pores and disrupts Ca homeostasis. Lashuel et al. used electron microscopy to show that α-synuclein, a DLB-related protein with 141 amino acid residues, forms annular pore-like structures [63]. Lal et al. investigated the oligomerization and conformational changes of AβP, α-synuclein, islet amyloid peptide (amylin) and other amyloidogenic proteins using gel electrophoresis and AFM imaging [64]. Their results demonstrate that these amyloidogenic proteins form annular channel-like structures on bilayer membranes. Electrophysiological and morphological studies have revealed that PrP forms amyloid channels similar to AβP. PrP106-126 reportedly forms cation-permeable pores in artificial lipid bilayers as well as AβP [65]. Zn^{2+} also inhibited the activity of PrP channels. Kourie et al. found that PrP106-126 was directly incorporated into the lipid bilayers and formed cation-selective, Cu-sensitive ion channels and that quinacrine (a potent therapeutic drug for prion diseases) inhibited the currents induced by PrP channels [66]. Demuro et al. reported that AβP, human amylin, prion and polyglutamine increased the elevation of $[Ca^{2+}]_i$ in a conformation-dependent manner [67]. Furthermore, a recombinant PrP protein (PrP90-231) formed channels through artificial lipid bilayers [68]. PrP has microbial activity similar to AβP [69].

We observed temporal changes in $[Ca^{2+}]_i$ within GT1-7 cells using a high-resolution multisite video imaging system with fura-2 as the cytosolic free fluorescent calcium reporter probe [70]. Shortly after exposure to PrP106-126, a marked increase in $[Ca^{2+}]_i$ occurred within many neurons, as well as an increase in AβP. Moreover, scrambled PrP106-126 (a nontoxic and nonamyloidogenic analogue with the random sequence of PrP106-126) did not cause such an elevation. These findings strongly suggest that the disruption of Ca homeostasis via unregulated amyloid channels may be the molecular basis of the neurotoxicity of prion diseases and other conformational diseases.

3.3. Protective substances against PrP106-126-induced neurotoxicity

Substances that prevent the neurotoxicity of PrP^{Sc} are of particular interest for screening preventive drugs for the treatment of prion diseases. Trace elements can induce conformational changes in AβP; therefore, clioquinol (5-chloro-7-iodo-8-quinolinol), a chelator of Zn and Cu and its derivatives have been used in therapeutic trials for AD [71]. Clioquinol also affected scrapie-induced memory impairment [72] and D-(-)-penicillamine, a Cu^{2+}-specific chelator, attenuated the pathogenesis of prion diseases *in vivo* [73]. Furthermore, small peptides, such as that the β-sheet breaker peptide, inhibit the conformational changes of PrP and AβP [74]. Our survey for substances that protect against PrP106-126-induced neurotoxicity revealed that carnosine (β-alaninyl histidine) might be a candidate for treatment of prion diseases. Carnosine is a water-soluble dipeptide that is contained in mammalian muscle and brain and particularly in the olfactory bulbs [75]. Carnosine has antioxidant, anticross-linking, antiglycosylation activities and the ability to bind to metals (**Figure 2**). Carnosine inhibits the oligomerization of AβP and attenuates neurodegeneration in AD model mice [76]. We have reported that carnosine inhibits Zn^{2+}-induced neuronal death which plays a central role in the pathogenesis of vascular-type senile dementia [77]. Considering these beneficial characteristics of carnosine, carnosine may act as a neuroprotector in the brain. Based on these findings, we published a patent for carnosine as a possible target for drugs for vascular type senile dementia [78].

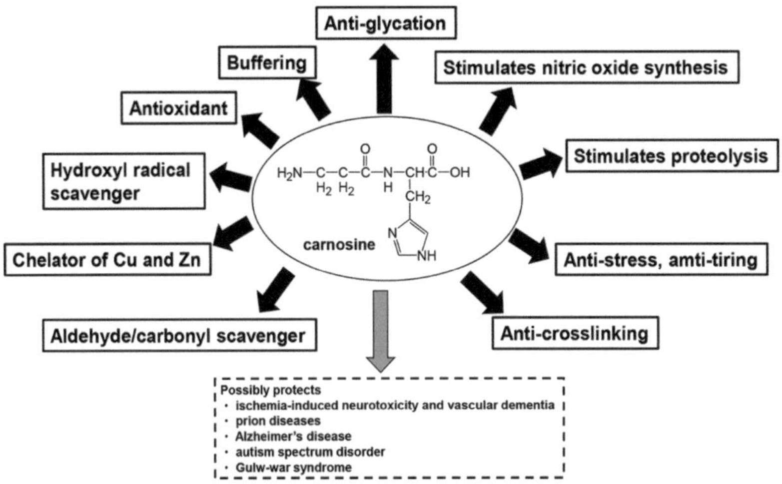

Figure 2. Structure and roles of carnosine.

4. Hypothesis: link between trace elements in the pathogenesis of prion diseases

4.1. PrP^C as a controller of metal homeostasis at the synapse

Considering the results of our study together with those of the other studies, we propose the following hypothetical mechanism regarding the role of PrP and the neurodegeneration processes underlying prion diseases (**Figure 3**). PrP^C and other various proteins including Alzheimer's APP, receptors, such as the NMDA-type glutamate receptor or AMPA-type glutamate receptor, are colocalized at the synapse. Synapses are critical nodes for the processing of neural information and the memory formation in neural networks. Thus, disorders of the synapses are the primary symptoms of neurodegenerative diseases. APP is localized to the presynaptic region of synapses and AβP is secreted into synaptic clefts in the presence of neuronal stimuli [79]. Meanwhile, PrP^C is localized to the postsynaptic membrane and is coupled to glutamate receptors [24]. Both of PrP^C and APP are metal-binding proteins and regulate metal homeostasis. The synaptic cleft is considered to be cylindrical with a radius of 120 nm and a height of 20 nm; it composes ~1% of the extracellular volume and ~20% of the total brain volume [80]. Zn and Cu are released into this small compartment at the micromolar levels. Therefore, APP and PrP^C likely interact with each other in this small compartment, which is filled with Zn and Cu.

http://dx.doi.org/10.5772/67327

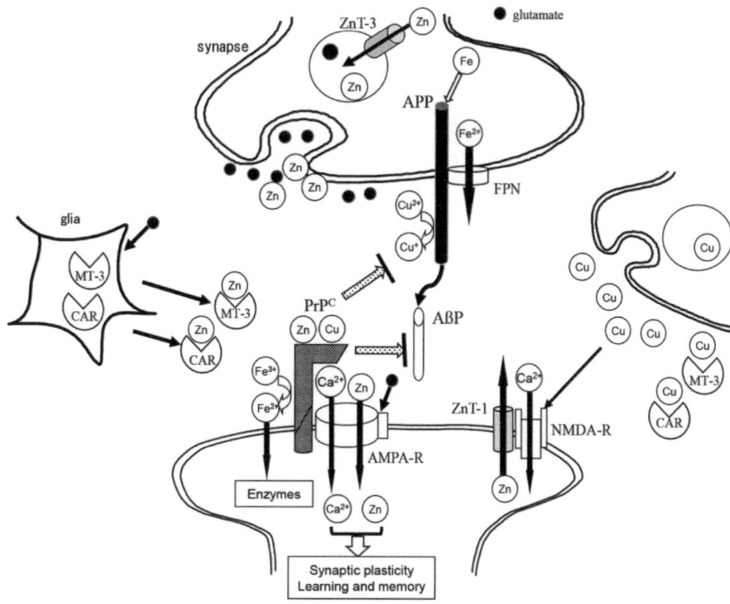

Figure 3. Hypothetical model of the physiological roles of normal prion protein at the synapse. Zn^{2+} and glutamate accumulate in synaptic vesicles and are released into synaptic clefts during neuronal excitation. Zn^{2+} regulates Ca^{2+} influx through glutamate receptors (NMDA-R, Ca-A/K), modulates neuronal information and is implicated in the maintenance of synaptic plasticity and memory formation, similar to Ca^{2+}. Zn has important roles in neural communication. Cu^{2+} is also released into synaptic vesicles and regulates various receptors, similar to Zn^{2+}. APP is present in the presynaptic domain and PrP^C is localized to the postsynaptic domain. These proteins are closely associated with the synaptic cleft and have cytoprotective roles via the regulation of metal homeostasis and protection against free radicals. PrP^C binds to the AMPA-type glutamate receptors and regulates Zn^{2+} levels similar to ZIP Zn transporters. Additionally, the ZnT-1 Zn transporter is localized to postsynaptic membranes that express NMDA-type glutamate receptors and regulates Zn homeostasis. Moreover, PrP^C has SOD activity and also regulates Cu^{2+} levels, which influence APP processing. APP converts Cu^{2+} into Cu^{+} and regulates Cu at the synapse. PrP^C has ferrireductase activity, which converts Fe^{3+} to Fe^{2+}. APP binds to ferroportin and thereby regulates Fe^{2+} efflux. MT-3 and carnosine are released from glial cells, into synaptic clefts and are also implicated in the regulation of excess Zn. Abbreviations: ZnT-1, zinc transporter 1; AMPA-R, AMPA-type glutamate receptor; NMDA-R, NMDA-type glutamate receptor; MT-3, metallothionein 3.

PrP^C regulates the cellular uptake of Cu, Zn and Fe as discussed previously. PrP^C, an analogue of ZIP transporters, is localized to the postsynaptic membrane, binding with the AMPA-type glutamate receptor, which facilitates Zn influx. The ZnT-1 transporter, which enhances Zn efflux into the extracellular compartment, is also localized to the postsynaptic membrane and regulates the activity of the NMDA-type glutamate receptor [81, 82]. Thus, synaptic Zn levels are likely controlled by both ZnT-1 and PrP^C. In comparison, MT-3 that is secreted from neurons or glia may regulate Zn homeostasis at synapses. Uchida et al. found that neuronal growth inhibitory factor (GIF) that inhibits neurite extensions and prevents neuronal death was decreased in the brains of AD patients and determined that GIF is equivalent to MT-3 [83]. Therefore, MT-3 (GIF) is implicated in AD-associated neuronal death. Considering our results and other numerous findings, carnosine may be another regulator of metal homeostasis in the synapse, similar to MT-3; carnosine is synthesized in glial cells (astrocytes and oligodendrocytes) and secreted into synaptic clefts after the glutamate response.

PrP^C also regulates the level of Fe and the ratio between Fe^{3+} and Fe^{2+} as a ferrireductase. APP binds to a Fe transporter, ferroportin and regulates Fe efflux. Furthermore, PrP^C regulates Cu, which influences the expression of APP and the production of AβP. The roles of APP and PrP^C in the maintenance of metal homeostasis are essential for normal brain function; therefore, a disruption of this homeostasis may trigger the degeneration of synapses and ultimately lead to the pathogenesis observed in AD or prion diseases. Recent studies demonstrate that PrP^C plays critical roles in the cleavage of APP and the regulation of AβP levels [84]. PrP^C reportedly attenuates the oligomerization of AβP and the neurotoxicity [85]. Considering these results together, PrP^C is crucial for neuroprotection and the regulation of various neuronal processes because it modulates SOD, protects cells from free radicals and controls AβP neurotoxicity.

However, under pathological conditions (**Figure 4**), PrP^{Sc} enters into the brain via the ingestion of contaminated food, for example and then triggers the conformational conversion of PrP^C into PrP^{Sc}. Mn may act in these pathways. The loss of neuroprotective PrP^C induces the dyshomeostasis of trace elements and ultimately leads to apoptotic death of neurons. Excess Zn or Cu influences APP, induces conformational changes of AβP and enhances its neurotoxicity. Oligomerized PrP^{Sc}, as well as AβP, form pores in synaptic membrane, causing the disruption of Ca homeostasis, ultimately leading to apoptotic neuronal death. This working hypothesis offers insight into the mechanism of prion diseases.

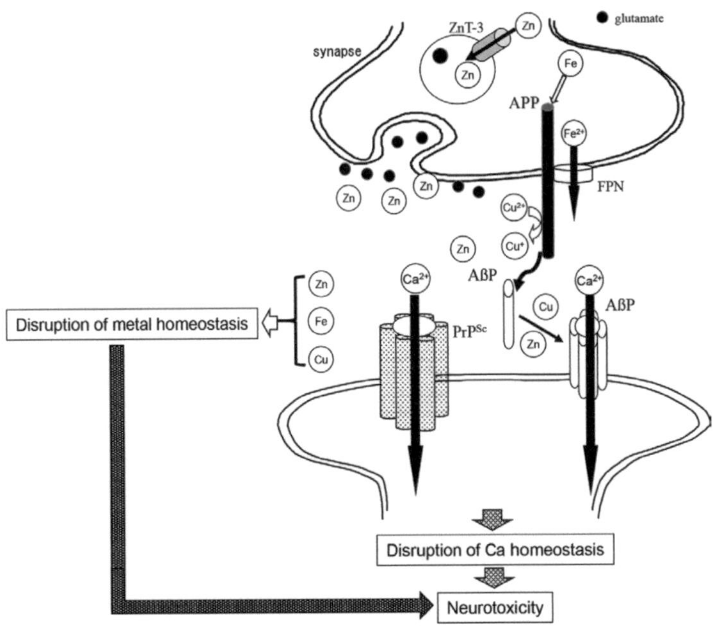

Figure 4. Hypothetical model of prion disease pathogenesis. In the pathological condition, PrP^{Sc} enters the brain and triggers the conversion of PrP^C, which depletes PrP^C and accumulates of PrP^{Sc}. The loss of the neuroprotective functions of PrP^C induces oxidative stress, enhance AβP neurotoxicity and ultimately lead to neuronal death. The accumulated PrP^{Sc} forms Ca^{2+}-permeable pores in the membrane and disrupted Ca^{2+} homeostasis. The imbalance of metals at the synapse triggers conformational changes in AβP, which enhances its neurotoxicity via the formation of Ca^{2+}-permeable pores. Subsequent Ca^{2+} dyshomeostasis leads to neuronal death.

In conclusion, our results shed light on the enigmatic roles of trace elements in the pathogenesis of prion diseases. However, further research is necessary particularly regarding the inhibitory mechanism of carnosine and the development of possible protective agents for prion diseases.

Acknowledgements

This work was partially supported by a Grant-in Aid for Scientific Research from the Ministry of Education, Culture, Sports, Science and Technology of Japan.

Author details

Masahiro Kawahara[1]*, Ken-ichiro Tanaka[1] and Dai Mizuno[2]

*Address all correspondence to: makawa@musashino-u.ac.jp

1 Department of Bio-Analytical Chemistry, Faculty of Pharmacy, Musashino University, Tokyo, Japan

2 Department of Forensic Medicine, Faculty of Medicine, Yamagata University, Yamagata-shi, Yamagata, Japan

References

[1] Prusiner SB: Prion diseases and the BSE crisis. Science. 1997; **278**: 245–251.

[2] Brundin P, Melki R, Kopito R: Prion-like transmission of protein aggregates in neurodegenerative diseases. Nat Rev Mol Cell Biol. 2010; **11**: 301–307.

[3] Carrell RW, Lomas DA: Conformational disease. Lancet. 1997; **350**: 134–138.

[4] Kawahara M: Role of calcium dyshomeostasis via amyloid channels in the pathogenesis of Alzheimer's disease. Curr Pharm Des. 2010; **16**: 2779–2789.

[5] Becker JS, Matusch A, Palm C, Salber D, Morton K & Becker S: Bioimaging of metals in brain tissue by laser ablation inductively coupled plasma mass spectrometry (LA-ICP-MS) and metallomics. Metallomics. 2010; **2**: 104–111.

[6] Dobrowolska J, Dehnhardt M, Matusch A, Zoriy M, Palomero-Gallagher N, Koscielniak P, Becker JS: Quantitative imaging of zinc, copper and lead in three distinct regions of the human brain by laser ablation inductively coupled plasma mass spectrometry. Talanta. 2008; **74**: 717–23.

[7] Mizuno D, Koyama H, Ohkawara S, Sadakane Y, Kawahara M: Involvement of trace elements in the pathogenesis of prion diseases. Curr Pharam Biotechnol. 2014;**15**:1049–57.

[8] Winklhofer KF, Tatzelt J, Haass C: The two faces of protein misfolding: gain- and loss-of-function in neurodegenerative diseases. EMBO J. 2008; **27**: 336–49.

[9] Simoneau S, Rezaei H, Salès N, Kaiser-Schulz G, Lefebvre-Roque M, Vidal C, Fournier JG, Comte J, Wopfner F, Grosclaude J, Schätzl H, Lasmézas CI: In vitro and in vivo neurotoxicity of prion protein oligomers. PLoS Pathog. 2007; **3**: e125.

[10] Fioriti L, Angeretti N, Colombo L, De Luigi A, Colombo A, Manzoni C, Morbin M, Tagliavini F, Salmona M, Chiesa R, Forloni G: Neurotoxic and gliotrophic activity of a synthetic peptide homologous to Gerstmann-Sträussler-Scheinker disease amyloid protein. J Neurosci. 2007; **27**: 1576–83.

[11] Johnson CJ, Gilbert PU, Abrecht M, Baldwin KL, Russell RE, Pedersen JA, Aiken JM, McKenzie D: Low copper and high manganese levels in prion protein plaques. Viruses. 2013; **5**: 654–62.

[12] Pushie MJ, Pickering IJ, Martin GR, Tsutsui S, Jirik FR, George GN: Prion protein expression level alters regional copper, iron and zinc content in the mouse brain. Metallomics. 2011; **3**: 206–14.

[13] D'Ambrosi N, & Rossi L: Copper at synapse: release, binding and modulation of neurotransmission. Neurochem Int. 2015; **90**: 36–45.

[14] Hopt A, Korte S, Fink H, Panne U, Niessner R, Jahn R, Herms J: Methods for studying synaptosomal copper release. J Neurosci Methods. 2003; **128**: 159–172.

[15] Kardos J, Kovács I, Hajós F, Kálmán M, Simonyi M: Nerve endings from rat brain tissue release copper upon depolarization. A possible role in regulating neuronal excitability. Neurosci Lett. 1989; **103**:139–44.

[16] Aedo F, Delgado R, Wolff D, Vergara C: Copper and zinc as modulators of neuronal excitability in a physiologically significant concentration range. Neurochem Int. 2007; **50**: 591–600.

[17] Brown DR, Qin K, Herms JW, Madlung A, Manson J, Strome R, Fraser PE, Kruck T, von Bohlen A, Schulz-Schaeffer W, Giese A, Westaway D, Kretzschmar H: The cellular prion protein binds copper in vivo. Nature. 1997; **390**: 684–7.

[18] Jackson GS, Murray I, Hosszu LL, Gibbs N, Waltho JP, Clarke AR, Collinge J: Location and properties of metal-binding sites on the human prion protein. Proc Natl Acad Sci U S A. 2001; **98**: 8531–5.

[19] McDonald A, Pushie MJ, Millhauser GL, George GN: New insights into metal interactions with the prion protein: EXAFS analysis and structure calculations of copper binding to a single octarepeat from the prion protein. J Phys Chem B. 2013; **117**:13822–41.

[20] Valensin D, Padula EM, Hecel A, Luczkowski M, Kozlowski H:Specific binding modes of Cu(I) and Ag(I) with neurotoxic domain of the human prion protein. Inorg Biochem. 2016; **155**:26–35.

[21] Vassallo N, Herms J: Cellular prion protein function in copper homeostasis and redox signaling at the synapse. J Neurochem. 2003; **86**: 538–44.

[22] Brown DR, Besinger A: Prion protein expression and superoxide dismutase activity. Biochem J. 1998; **334**: 423–9.

[23] White AR, Collins SJ, Maher F, Jobling MF, Stewart LR, Thyer JM, Beyreuther K, Masters CL, Cappai R: Prion protein-deficient neurons reveal lower glutathione reductase activity and increased susceptibility to hydrogen peroxide toxicity. Am J Pathol. 1999; **155**: 1723–30.

[24] Stys PK, You H, Zamponi GW: Copper-dependent regulation of NMDA receptors by cellular prion protein: implications for neurodegenerative disorders. J Physiol. 2012; **590**: 1357–68.

[25] Varela-Nallar L, Toledo EM, Larrondo LF, Cabral AL, Martins VR, Inestrosa NC: Induction of cellular prion protein gene expression by copper in neurons. Cell Physiol. 2006; **290**: C271–81.

[26] Kawahara M, Ohtsuka I, Yokoyama S, Kato-Negishi M, Sadakane Y: Membrane incorporation, channel formation, and disruption of calcium homeostasis by Alzheimer's ß-amyloid protein. Int. J. Alzheimer Dis. 2011; **304583**. doi: 10.4061/2011/304583.

[27] Multhaup G, Schlicksupp A, Hesse L, Beher D, Ruppert T, Masters CL, Beyreuther K: The amyloid precursor protein of Alzheimer's disease in the reduction of copper(II) to copper (I). Science. 1996; **271**:1406–9.

[28] Kawahara M, Mizuno D, Koyama H, Konoha K, Ohkawara S, Sadakane Y: Disruption of zinc homeostasis and the pathogenesis of senile dementia. Metallomics 2013; **6**: 209–212.

[29] Frederickson CJ, Bush AI: Synaptically released zinc: physiological functions and pathological effects. Biometals. 2001; **14**: 353–66.

[30] Vogt K, Mellor J, Tong G, Nicoll R: The actions of synaptically released zinc at hippocampal mossy fiber synapses. Neuron. 2000; **26**: 187–96.

[31] Kay AR: Imaging synaptic zinc: promises and perils. Trends in Neurosciences, 2006; **29**: 200–6.

[32] Tamano H, Koike Y, Nakada H, Shakushi Y, Takeda A: Significance of synaptic Zn^{2+} signaling in zincergic and non-zincergic synapses in the hippocampus in cognition. J Trace Elem Med Biol. 2016; S0946-672X(16): 30024–4.

[33] Fukada T, Kambe T: Molecular and genetic features of zinc transporters in physiology and pathogenesis. Metallomics. 2011; **3**: 662–74.

[34] Stellato F, Spevacek A, Proux O, Minicozzi V, Millhauser G, Morante S: Zinc modulates copper coordination mode in prion protein octa-repeat subdomains. Eur Biophys J. 2011; **40**: 1259–70.

[35] Schmitt-Ulms G, Ehsani S, Watts JC, Westaway D, Wille H: Evolutionary descent of prion genes from the ZIP family of metal ion transporters. PLoS One. 2009; **4**: e7208.

[36] Ehsani S, Tao R, Pocanschi CL, Ren H, Harrison PM, Schmitt-Ulms G: Evidence for retrogene origins of the prion gene family. PLoS One 2011; **6**: e26800.

[37] Taylor KM, Muraina I, Brethour D, Schmitt-Ulms G, Nimmanon T, Ziliotto S, Hogstrand C: Zinc transporter ZIP10 forms a heteromer with ZIP6 which regulates embryonic development and cell migration. Biochemical Journal. 2016; **10**: 2531–2544.

[38] Pocanschi CL, Ehsani S, Mehrabian M, Wille H, Reginold W, Trimble WS, Wang H, Yee A, Arrowsmith CH, Bozóky Z, Kay LE, Forman-Kay JD, Rini JM, Schmitt-Ulms G: The ZIP5 ectodomain co-localizes with PrP and may acquire a PrP-like fold that assembles into a dimer. PLoS One. 2013; **8**: e72446.

[39] Watt NT, Griffiths HH, Hooper NM: Neuronal zinc regulation and the prion protein. Prion. 2013; **7**: 203–8.

[40] Singh A, Mohan ML, Isaac AO, Luo X, Petrak J, Vyoral D, Singh N: Prion protein modulates cellular iron uptake: a novel function with implications for prion disease pathogenesis. PLoS One. 2009; **4**: e4468.

[41] Singh A, Haldar S, Horback K, Tom C, Zhou L, Meyerson H, Singh N: Prion protein regulates iron transport by functioning as a ferrireductase. J Alzheimers Dis. 2013; **35**: 541–52.

[42] Tripathi AK, Haldar S, Qian J, Beserra A, Suda S, Singh A, Singh N: Prion protein functions as a ferrireductase partner for ZIP14 and DMT1. Free Radic Biol Med. 2015; **84**: 322–330.

[43] Singh A, Kong Q, Luo X, Petersen RB, Meyerson H, Singh N: Prion protein (PrP) knock-out mice show altered iron metabolism: a functional role for PrP in iron uptake and transport. PLoS One. 2009; **4**: e6115.

[44] Singh A, Beveridge AJ, Singh N: Decreased CSF transferrin in sCJD: a potential pre-mortem diagnostic test for prion disorders. PLoS One. 2011; **6**: e16804.

[45] Tuschl K, Mills PB, Clayton PT: Manganese and the brain. Int Rev Neurobiol. 2013;110:277–312. doi: 10.1016/B978-0-12-410502-7.00013-2.

[46] Thackray AM, Madec JY, Wong E, Morgan-Warren R, Brown DR, Baron T, Bujdoso R: Detection of bovine spongiform encephalopathy, ovine scrapie prion-related protein (PrP^{Sc}) and normal PrP^{c} by monoclonal antibodies raised to copper-refolded prion protein. Biochem J. 2003; **370**: 81–90.

[47] Davies P, Brown DR: Manganese enhances prion protein survival in model soils and increases prion infectivity to cells. PLoS One. 2009; **4**: e7518.

[48] White SN, O'Rourke KI, Gidlewski T, VerCauteren KC, Mousel MR, Phillips GE, Spraker TR: Increased risk of chronic wasting disease in Rocky Mountain elk associated with decreased magnesium and increased manganese in brain tissue. Can J Vet. Res. 2010; **74**: 50–3.

[49] Slivarichová D, Mitrová E, Ursínyová M, Uhnáková I, Koscová S, Wsólová L: Geographic accumulation of Creutzfeldt-Jakob disease in Slovakia—environmental metal imbalance as a possible cofactor. Cent Eur J Public Health. 2011; **19**: 158–64.

[50] Pass R, Frudd K, Barnett JP, Blindauer CA, Brown DR: Prion infection in cells is abolished by a mutated manganese transporter but shows no relation to zinc. Mol Cell Neurosci. 2015; **68**:186–93.

[51] Kawahara M, Koyama H, Nagata T, Sadakane Y: Zinc, copper and carnosine attenuate neurotoxicity of prion fragment PrP106-126. Metallomics. 2011; **3**: 726–734.

[52] Bonetto V, Massignan T, Chiesa R, Morbin M, Mazzoleni G, Diomede L, Angeretti N, Colombo L, Forloni G, Tagliavini F, Salmona M: Synthetic miniprion PrP106. J Biol Chem. 2002; **277**: 31327–34.

[53] Inayathullah M, Satheeshkumar KS, Malkovskiy AV, Carre AL, Sivanesan S, Hardesty JO, Rajadas J: Solvent microenvironments and copper binding alters the conformation and toxicity of a prion fragment. PLoS One. 2013; **8**: e85160.

[54] Thakur AK, Srivastava AK, Srinivas V, Chary KV, Rao CM: Copper alters aggregation behavior of prion protein and induces novel interactions between its N- and C-terminal regions. J Biol Chem. 2011; **286**: 38533–45.

[55] Arispe N, Diaz JC, Simakova O: Abeta ion channels. Prospects for treating Alzheimer's disease with Abeta channel blockers. Biochim Biophys Acta. 2007; **1768**: 1952–65.

[56] Lashuel HA, Hartley D, Petre BM, Walz T, Lansbury PT Jr.: Neurodegenerative disease: amyloid pores from pathogenic mutations. Nature. 2002; **418**: 291.

[57] Mizuno D and Kawahara M: Oligomerization of proteins and neurodegenerative diseases, *In* Oligomerization of Chemical and Biological Compounds, (ed by Claire Lesieur, InTech d.o.o, Rijeka, Croatia) pp 279–293, ISBN 980-953-307-1130-3(2014).

[58] Arispe N, Rojas E, Pollard HB: Alzheimer disease amyloid beta protein forms calcium channels in bilayer membranes: blockade by tromethamine and aluminum. Proc Natl Acad Sci U S A. 1993; **90**: 567–71.

[59] Kawahara M, Arispe N, Kuroda Y, Rojas E: Alzheimer's disease amyloid β-protein forms Zn^{2+}-sensitive, cation-selective channels across excised membrane patches from hypothalamic neurons. Biophys J. 1997; **73**: 67–75.

[60] Kagan BL, Jang H, Capone R, Teran Arce F, Ramachandran S, Lal R, Nussinov R: Antimicrobial properties of amyloid peptides. Mol Pharm. 2012; **9**: 708–17.

[61] Soscia SJ, Kirby JE, Washicosky KJ, Tucker SM, Ingelsson M, Hyman B, Burton MA, Goldstein LE, Duong S, Tanzi RE, Moir RD: The Alzheimer's disease-associated amyloid beta-protein is an antimicrobial peptide. PLoS One. 2010; **5**: e9505.

[62] Inoue S: In situ Aß pores in AD brain are cylindrical assembly of Abeta protofilaments. Amyloid. 2008; **15**:223–33.

[63] Lashuel HA and Lansbury PT Jr.: Are amyloid diseases caused by protein aggregates that mimic bacterial pore-forming toxins? Q Rev. Biophys. 2002; **39**: 167–201.

[64] Lal R, Lin H, Quist AP: Amyloid beta ion channel: 3D structure and relevance to amyloid channel paradigm. Biochim Biophys Acta. 2007; **1768**: 1966–75.

[65] Lin MC, Mirzabekov T, Kagan BL: Channel formation by a neurotoxic prion protein fragment. J Biol Chem. 1997; **272**: 44–47.

[66] Bahadi R, Farrelly PV, Kenna BL, Curtain CC, Masters CL, Cappai R, Barnham KJ, Kourie JI: Cu^{2+}-induced modification of the kinetics of Aβ(1–42) channels. Am J Physiol Cell Physiol. 2003; **285**: C873–80.

[67] Demuro A, Mina E, Kayed R, Milton SC, Parker I, Glabe CG: Calcium dysregulation and membrane disruption as a ubiquitous neurotoxic mechanism of soluble amyloid oligomers. J Biol Chem. 2005; **280**: 17294–300.

[68] Paulis D, Maras B, Schininà ME, di Francesco L, Principe S, Galeno R, Abdel-Haq H, Cardone F, Florio T, Pocchiari M, Mazzanti M: The pathological prion protein forms ionic conductance in lipid bilayer. Neurochem Int. 2011; **59**: 168–74.

[69] Pasupuleti M, Roupe M, Rydengård V, Surewicz K, Surewicz WK, Chalupka A, Malmsten M, Sörensen OE, Schmidtchen A: Antimicrobial activity of human prion protein is mediated by its N-terminal region. PLoS One. 2009; **4**: e7358.

[70] Kawahara M, Arispe N, Rojas E, Kuroda Y: Alzheimer's β-amyloid, human islet amylin and prion protein fragment evoke intracellular free-calcium elevations by a common mechanism in a hypothalamic GnRH neuronal cell-line. J Biol Chem. 2000; **275**: 14077–83.

[71] Faux NG, Ritchie CW, Gunn A, Rembach A, Tsatsanis A, Bedo J, Harrison J, Lannfelt L, Blennow K, Zetterberg H, Ingelsson M, Masters CL, Tanzi RE, Cummings JL, Herd CM, Bush AI: PBT2 rapidly improves cognition in Alzheimer's Disease: additional phase II analyses. J Alzheimers Dis. 2010; **20**:509–16.

[72] Bareggi SR, Braida D, Pollera C, Bondiolotti G, Formentin E, Puricelli M, Poli G, Ponti W, Sala M: Effects of clioquinol on memory impairment and the neurochemical modifications induced by scrapie infection in golden hamsters. Brain Res. 2009; **1280**: 195–200.

[73] Sigurdsson EM, Brown DR, Alim MA, Scholtzova H, Carp R, Meeker HC, Prelli F, Frangione B, Wisniewski T: Copper chelation delays the onset of prion disease. J Biol Chem. 2003; **278**: 46199–202.

[74] Soto C, Kascsak RJ, Saborío GP, Aucouturier P, Wisniewski T, Prelli F, Kascsak R, Mendez E, Harris DA, Ironside J, Tagliavini F, Carp RI, Frangione B: Reversion of prion protein conformational changes by synthetic beta-sheet breaker peptides. Lancet. 2000; **355**: 192–7.

[75] Hipkiss AR: Carnosine and its possible roles in nutrition and health. Adv Food Nutr Res. 2009; **57**: 87–154.

[76] Corona C, Frazzini V, Silvestri E, Lattanzio R, La Sorda R, Piantelli M, Canzoniero LM, Ciavardelli D, Rizzarelli E, Sensi SL: Effects of dietary supplementation of carnosine on mitochondrial dysfunction, amyloid pathology and cognitive deficits in 3xTg-AD mice. PLoS One. 2011; **6**: e17971.

[77] Kawahara M, Konoha K, Nagata T, Sadakane Y: Protective substances against zinc-induced neuronal death after ischemia: carnosine a target for drug of vascular type of dementia. Recent Pat CNS Drug Discov. 2007; **2**: 145–149.

[78] Kawahara M, Konoha K, Nagata A, Sadakane Y: 2013: JP5382633.

[79] Sabo SL, Ikin AF, Buxbaum JD, Greengard P: The amyloid precursor protein and its regulatory protein, FE65, in growth cones and synapses in vitro and in vivo. J Neurosci. 2003; **23**: 5407–15.

[80] Schikorski T, Stevens CF: Quantitative ultrastructural analysis of hippocampal excitatory synapses. J Neurosci. 1997; **17**: 5858–67.

[81] Sindreu C, Bayés Á, Altafaj X, Pérez-Clausell J: Zinc transporter-1 concentrates at the postsynaptic density of hippocampal synapses. Mol Brain. 2014; **7**: 7–16.

[82] Mellone M, Pelucchi S, Alberti L, Genazzani AA, Di Luca M, Gardoni F: Zinc transporter-1: a novel NMDA receptor-binding protein at the postsynaptic density. J Neurochem. 2015; **132**:159–68.

[83] Uchida Y, Takio K, Titani K, Ihara Y, Tomonaga M: The growth inhibitory factor that is deficient in the Alzheimer's disease brain is a 68 amino acid metallothionein-like protein. Neuron 1991; **7**: 337–47.

[84] Griffiths HH, Whitehouse IJ, Hooper NM: Regulation of amyloid-β production by the prion protein. Prion. 2012; **6**: 217–22.

[85] Fluharty BR, Biasini E, Stravalaci M, Sclip A, Diomede L, Balducci C, La Vitola P, Messa M, Colombo L, Forloni G, Borsello T, Gobbi M, Harris DA: An N-terminal fragment of the prion protein binds to amyloid-β oligomers and inhibits their neurotoxicity in vivo. J Biol Chem. 2013; **288**: 7857–66.

Section 4

Genetic Resistance and Immunobiology of Prions

Chapter 7

Immunobiology of Prion Diseases

Konstantinos Xanthopoulos, Dimitra Dafou,
Eirini Kanata and Theodoros Sklaviadis

Additional information is available at the end of the chapter

http://dx.doi.org/10.5772/66447

Abstract

Prion diseases are invariably lethal neurodegenerative diseases, associated with the structural conversion of the cellular isoform of the prion protein to its pathological, disease-associated isoform. The cellular isoform of the prion protein is highly conserved and virtually ubiquitously expressed; nevertheless, its physiological role remains unclear. Mounting evidence suggests its involvement in the regulation and function of the immune system. At the same time, the immune system is heavily involved in the pathogenesis of the diseases, playing a major role in the peripheral replication of the infectious agent and spread toward the central nervous system. On the other hand, immunotherapies are among the most promising means of intervention. This chapter deals with these fascinating and sometimes contrasting aspects of prion biology, with an emphasis on the immunization protocols developed for prophylaxis and treatment of prion diseases.

Keywords: prion, immunobiology, active immunization, passive immunization, DNA vaccines, mucosal vaccination

1. Introduction

Transmissible spongiform encephalopathies (TSEs) or prion diseases are invariably lethal neurodegenerative diseases afflicting a wide variety of species, including humans [1]. The common pathogen to all TSEs is termed prion and is believed to consist solely or primarily of the disease-associated isoform (PrP^{Sc}) of the cellular prion protein (PrP^{C}). PrP^{C} is a highly conserved, GPI-anchored sialoglycoprotein encoded by the single-copy *Prnp* gene. *Prnp* is virtually ubiquitously expressed, with its expression peaking in the neuronal tissue, whereas high *Prnp* expression levels have been reported in many cells of the immune system. PrP^{Sc} is believed to propagate by inducing the conformational conversion of PrP^{C} molecules into new

PrP^{Sc} copies. The exact mechanism governing this conversion is still under dispute, but it is widely accepted that it does not involve modifications of the primary structure of the protein.

The physiological and pathological PrP isoforms display distinct conformations. The N-terminal region of PrP^C is highly unstructured, as opposed to the globular C-terminal region, which contains predominantly a-helices and only a minor region encompassing two-stranded β sheet [2]. Infrared spectroscopy and circular dichroism data indicate clear differences in the secondary structure of PrP^C and PrP^{Sc}, in which equal amounts of a-helices and β sheets can be found [3]. This conformational difference is believed to be at the basis of the biochemical differences observed between the two isoforms, namely, the partial proteinase K resistance, the reduced solubility, and the fibril-producing potential displayed by PrP^{Sc} [4]. To date, the only known difference at the chemical level is associated with the oxidation level of the methionine residues, which was found to be elevated in PrP^{Sc} compared to PrP^C [5].

The physiological role of the prion protein remains obscure. Its high level of conservation among species would indicate that PrP^C is of crucial importance to the organism; however, $PrP^{-/-}$ mice are viable, developmentally and behaviorally normal, and do not display a prominent phenotype except for the complete protection against prion diseases [6, 7]. PrP^C has since been implicated in a variety of cellular functions, including cell proliferation, differentiation and survival, protection against oxidative stress, and synaptic function (reviewed in [8, 9]). Further evidence suggests it may play a role in the immune system. In line with this, it has been recently reported that $PrP^{-/-}$ mice display lower numbers of CD4 T cells and lymphoid tissue inducer (LTi) cells as well as impaired splenic T zone structures [10]. Moreover, immune responses have been reported during prion diseases progression, suggesting the involvement of the immune system in disease pathogenesis, and immune-based approaches have yielded some of the most promising results toward protection and/or treatment of spongiform encephalopathies. In this chapter these exciting aspects of prion biology will be discussed.

2. PrP and the immune system

2.1. PrP^C expression patterns in cells of the immune system

Even though PrP^C is predominantly expressed in the central and peripheral nervous system [11, 12], elevated protein expression levels have also been reported in many cells of the immune system. In long-term hematopoietic stem cells (HSCs), PrP^C expression levels are raised and PrP^C has been suggested as a marker for these cells [13]. PrP^C expression is retained throughout maturation either toward the myeloid [14] or the lymphoid lineage [15, 16]. Interestingly, along the granulocyte maturation lineage, PrP^C expression is downregulated [17].

Among cells of the lymphoid lineage, T cells, monocytes, and natural killer (NK) cells express higher PrP^C levels compared to B lymphocytes [18]. PrP^C expression levels are regulated and can vary greatly across different T-cell subtypes: $CD8^+$ cells display higher expression levels than $CD4^+$ cells, and between $CD4^+$ cells, $CD25^+$ expresses 4.5-fold higher *Prnp* levels than $CD25^-$ cells [19], while $CD45RO^+$ memory T lymphocytes express higher PrP^C levels compared to naïve CD45RA$^+$ T lymphocytes [16]. It would thus appear that PrP^C expression levels in cells of the immune system are dynamic, indicating that PrP^C may play a role in the immune system.

2.2. PrP^C function in the immune system

Despite evidence that PrP^C may be associated with the function of the immune system, its role remains unclear. PrP$^{-/-}$ mice do not display gross overt effects, at least under normal conditions. However, evidence indicates that when PrP$^{-/-}$ mice are subject to immunological stress their phenotype may deviate from normal. To test whether PrP^C may act as a regulator of cellular immunity, the effect PrP^C deficiency may have on the course of experimental autoimmune encephalomyelitis (EAE) was assessed [20]. EAE is an inflammatory demyelinating disease of the central nervous system (CNS), triggered by the injection of brain extracts, proteins of the CNS such as the myelin basic protein and the myelin oligodendrocyte glycoprotein (MOG) or peptides from these proteins to experimental animals, usually mice and rats. EAE is widely used as an animal model for multiple sclerosis and acute disseminated encephalomyelitis but is also considered the prototype for T-cell–mediated autoimmune disease in general [21]. It was found that PrP$^{-/-}$ mice displayed a more aggressive disease onset and no clinical improvement during the chronic phase of the disease. These clinical findings were in agreement with the increased cytokine gene expression in MOG-primed PrP$^{-/-}$ cells and indicate that PrP^C could be involved in the attenuation of T-cell-dependent neuroinflammation.

Similar results were obtained when *Prnp* expression was silenced via treatment with small interfering ribonucleic acid (siRNA) targeting *Prnp*. In this case, siRNA administration led to effective *Prnp* silencing in the lymphoid tissue, but not the central nervous system. In agreement to the results obtained with PrP$^{-/-}$ mice, siRNA-mediated *Prnp* silencing led to marked worsening of EAE [22]. In a series of elegant experiments, it was shown that the central nervous system autoimmune disease was modulated at all stages of the disease and that PrP^C regulates activation of T lymphocytes mediated by the T-cell receptor (TCR), differentiation, and survival, thus identifying PrP^C as a regulator of cellular immunological homeostasis. The proposed immunomodulatory properties when considered in conjunction with (i) the protein's expression patterns, which overlap with immune-privileged organs and (ii) the observation that only minor phenotypes can be associated with PrP$^{-/-}$ mice under physiological conditions, but rather striking ones under stress and particularly under inflammation in immune-privileged organs, has led to the hypothesis that PrP^C may be involved in immune quiescence, protecting immune-privileged organs, such as the brain [23].

3. Prion disease pathogenesis and the immune system

The central event in the pathogenesis of all forms of transmissible spongiform encephalopathies is the conversion of PrP^C to the more thermodynamically stable PrP^{Sc} by PrP^{Sc} via a mechanism which remains at large obscure [24]. Regrettably, the actual conversion mechanism is not the only missing piece of the prion disease pathogenesis puzzle, and not much is known on how the infectious agent enters the host or how it is transported from the periphery to the central nervous system. A series of experiments using animal models of TSEs have provided interesting data on pathogenesis.

Parenteral—usually intracranial or intraperitoneal—administration of the pathogen to hamsters or mice is among the most widely used animal TSE models. Such models are particularly useful, since most of the naturally acquired TSE cases both in humans and animals are contracted via peripheral—through the alimentary tract—exposure to the pathogen [25]. While these models provide a wealth of information regarding pathogenesis, it later became evident that different mechanisms are involved in the pathogenesis of prion infection following the intraperitoneal or the oral route of infection [26], and other factors such as the pathogen strain and the host species and/or strain can also have a major impact on the mechanisms involved [27]. For example, in a recent study in sheep with different *Prnp* polymorphisms, which confer different levels of resistance to prion infection, it was observed that following intracranial administration of the pathogen, sheep with a "resistant" genetic polymorphism did not accumulate the pathogen in lymphoid tissues [28]. Even more strikingly, it has recently been reported that the role of the immune system might be limited in case of genetic prion disease. In a murine model of late onset genetic Creutzfeldt-Jakob disease, PrP^{Sc} has not been detected in the lymph nodes or the spleens of the transgenic mice at all ages and stages of disease, indicating that in this case conversion of PrP^{C} to PrP^{Sc} occurs predominantly or even exclusively within the CNS [29].

Prion pathogenesis can be divided into phases, some of which may take place in parallel: (i) peripheral prion exposure and uptake, (ii) peripheral pathogen replication, (iii) migration through the peripheral nervous system to the CNS, and (iv) centrifugal spread from the CNS back to the periphery [25, 27]. Despite PrP^{Sc} can be detected in various sites following peripheral exposure, especially in the lymphatic system, signs of pathology, including neurodegeneration, spongiosis, and gliosis are only found within the CNS. It is important to stress that as the means available evolve, our understanding of the phenomena taking place also improves. For instance, detection of PrP^{Sc} in the brains of some peripherally challenged hamsters as early as 4 and 9 days following challenge was recently reported [30].

M cells, which are epithelial cells specialized for transepithelial transport found in the follicle-associated epithelia of the small and large intestines, tonsils and adenoids [31], were shown capable of transcytosing the TSE infectious agent *in vivo* [32]. In addition to M cells, other epithelial cells may be involved in the uptake of the pathogen in a ferritin-mediated mechanism [33]. The pathogen is first detected in gut-associated lymphoid tissue (GALT), including Peyer's patches and mesenteric lymph nodes [26]. Evidence from in vitro studies indicates that the GALT in the small rather than the large intestine plays a major role in PrP^{Sc} accumulation and eventually neuroinvasion [34].

It is not yet clear how the pathogen is transported from the entry site to the lymphoid tissue. It has been hypothesized that following pathogen uptake by M cells, the infectious agent can be transported to the M cells' intraepithelial pocket, where it can be processed by macrophages, B- and T- lymphocytes residing within this pocket or the dendritic cells, macrophages, and lymphocytes situated immediately beneath the intraepithelial pocket [35]. Of these cells, macrophages and dendritic cells appear the most plausible candidates for effective transport of the pathogen. In line with this assumption, PrP accumulations were detected in various types of macrophages following TSE infection [36–38]. However, the role macrophages undertake remains obscure, as *in vivo* experiments have shown that macrophages may also be involved in clearing the pathogen [39, 40]. It seems that the role of the macrophages following prion infection depends on the infectious dose and the agent strain [41]. Macrophages may also be important for the delivery of the infectious agent to the neural cells, and in this case, cell death may play an important role. In recent *in vitro* studies, it was determined that coculture of killed, PrP^{Sc}-infected macrophages with N2a-3 neuroblastoma cells accelerated PrP^{Sc} transmission to the neuronal cells [42]. Dendritic cells on the other hand can be ideally located to transport the pathogen following uptake by the M cells, and some of them have already been shown to be able to transport PrP^{Sc} without degrading it [43, 44].

B lymphocytes were initially identified as the cells involved in replication of the TSE infectious agent [45], but this hypothesis was later revised, and the role of B lymphocytes in prion pathogenesis was associated with the regulated maturation of follicular dendritic cells (FDCs) [46]. Initial experiments with splenectomized or thymectomized mice indicated the dispensable role of T lymphocytes in the replication of the agent [47], whereas fractionation [48] and irradiation [49] experiments indicated that replication of the pathogen depends on radioresistant cells, localized within the stromal compartment of the spleen. FDCs fulfill all these criteria, and their crucial role for replication of the pathogen was confirmed in a series of experiments, in which depletion of mature FDCs led to prolongation of the incubation period of the disease [46, 50–53]. FDCs are of stromal origin, reside in the primary B lymphocytes follicles and germinal centers of lymphoid tissues, and are non-phagocytic and non-migratory. As a result of their large surface area and longevity, FDCs are capable of trapping and retaining antigen in its native state for months to years. FDCs retain antigens in the form of immune complexes, consisting of antigen-complement components and/or antibody and trap these complexes either through complement receptors CR1 and CR2 or through FcRIIb and FcεRII antibody receptors [35]. In agreement with the role FDCs undertake in prion pathogenesis and the involvement of complement components and receptors in antigen trapping by FDCs, it was found that the absence of complement components (C1q, C2, C3, and factor B) and cellular complement receptor can have an adverse effect on the accumulation of PrP^{Sc} in the spleen [54, 55]. However, the inability to completely inhibit disease progression via depletion of mature FDCs [46, 51], in addition to observations confirming that propagation of prion diseases is possible even in the absence of mature FDCs [41, 56–58], indicates that possibly a different cell type—most probably MOMA-1-positive macrophages [41]—is responsible for replication of the pathogen. These differences in the cell types required for pathogenesis were attributed to the dose and agent strain [41].

Peripheral replication of the pathogen precedes neuroinvasion, during which the pathogen is transported within the CNS. Both the enteric and autonomic nervous systems are believed to participate in the transport of the infectious agent [36, 59, 60]. The exact mechanism governing transport of the pathogen to the CNS remains unidentified, and has been reported to be both PrP^{C}-dependent [61, 62] and independent [63]. Interestingly, it was reported that the transfer speed of intraperitoneally administered prions relies to the distance between FDCs and splenic nerve endings [64, 65].

The immune system is greatly implicated in the peripheral pathogenesis of prion diseases but fails to provide protection. Until recently, no response against the prion pathogen has been described, and this was linked to tolerance effects due to widespread expression of the physiological isoform of the prion protein throughout the body, which prevents the host from mounting a humoral or cellular immune response against PrP^{Sc} following infection [66]. On the contrary, $PrP^{-/-}$ mice mount a robust immune response against PrP, indicating the immunogenicity of the protein. Lately it was shown that TSE infection can have adverse effects on the maturation cycle of FDCs, causing an abnormality in immune function [67]. Given the crucial role the immune system plays in the peripheral pathogenesis of prion diseases, it could be argued that it promotes rather than protects against prion pathogenesis. In agreement with this, increased susceptibility to intraperitoneal challenge with TSE agents following repetitive immunization was recently reported [68].

4. Harnessing the immune system against prion diseases

Since the immune system plays an ambivalent role in prion disease pathogenesis, the question emerged whether suppressing the immune system would be the most appropriate approach [69]. Targeting the FDCs was already proven a viable approach, providing partial protection in an animal model of prion diseases and minimizing the infectivity of the peripheral tissue of the afflicted animals [46, 50–52]. Disruption of the FDCs also appears to be the protective mechanism against TSEs following repetitive CpG administration [70]. CpG had previously been administered as a stimulator of innate immunity and was shown effective at providing partial protection in an animal model of TSEs [71]. In this case CpG was administered to stimulate the macrophages and enhance phagocytosis of the pathogen. Indeed, repetitive administration provided partial protection against TSEs [71], but as it was later shown, this protection was due to disruption of the lymphoid follicles rather than stimulation of the macrophages [70]. Interestingly, disruption of the FDCs has also been observed following immunization of wild-type mice with recombinant murine PrP aggregates and is at least in part responsible for the observed partial protection when the immunized mice were challenged with a murine strain of TSEs [72].

The first indications that the immune system might prove effective against prion diseases stemmed from *in vitro* experiments, where it was shown that treatment of TSE-infected cell cultures with monoclonal anti-PrP antibodies could effectively inhibit PrP^{Sc} replication and on some occasions clear infectivity [73–75]. Proof of principle that immunization against prion diseases can be effective against prion diseases was provided later using transgenic mice, capable of producing anti-PrP antibodies. These mice, in contrast to wild-type controls, failed to succumb to disease following challenge with a mouse-adapted scrapie strain [76]. Similarly, passive immunization of wild-type mice, by administration of anti-PrP antibodies was found to provide protection against prion diseases [77].

From this initial series of experiments, valuable conclusions emerged, most importantly, that immunization is an efficient means of therapy rather than protection, against prion diseases. Moreover, the safety of these procedures was confirmed, since immunization against a self-antigen could always give rise to autoimmunity. Given the identical primary structure PrP^C and PrP^{Sc} share, adverse reactions stemming from the reaction of the anti-PrP antibodies with PrP^C could be expected. Autoimmunity was not induced by these immunization approaches, and furthermore the "dispensable" role of the prion protein for the appearance of a physiological phenotype was already known from studies on $PrP^{-/-}$ animals [6], as well as from transgenic animals with conditional depletion of the prion protein [78] and provided an extra layer of security. However, other findings raised some concerns over the safety of administration of anti-PrP antibodies, since it was found that intracerebral administration of anti-PrP monoclonal antibodies can give rise to cross-linking of PrP molecules on adjacent neurons and eventually cell death, triggered possibly by the initiation of death signaling [79]. These effects are clearly not associated with autoimmunity, but rather with impaired cell signaling.

4.1. Passive immunization approaches

The first indications that passive immunization could prove useful at protecting against prion diseases emerged from studies in which mice genetically modified to produce an anti-PrP monoclonal antibody (6H4μ) were fully protected against prion diseases [76]. In a more classical approach, monoclonal anti-PrP antibodies (ICSM18 and ICSM35) were administered intraperitoneally to wild-type mice briefly after intraperitoneal inoculation with the pathogen or when the first clinical signs appeared. When the antibodies were administered after the inoculation, animals receiving the antibodies survived approximately 300 days more than control mice, and the accumulation of infectivity in the peripheral tissue was markedly reduced [77]. Intraperitoneal administration of a different antibody (6D11) immediately after intraperitoneal administration of the pathogen also proved its protective efficacy, since mice receiving the antibody survived longer by approximately 36.9% compared to control mice. In a recent study, a pharmacokinetic and pharmacodynamic analysis following intraperitoneal administration of various anti-PrP antibodies was carried out. The ability of an antibody to form long-lasting complexes with PrP^C was found to positively correlate with its efficacy in delaying peripheral accumulation of PrP^{Sc} and, in agreement with this, intraperitoneal administration of the monoclonal antibody BAR216 led to a statistically significant prolongation of survival of the mice [80].

The therapeutic efficacy of intracerebral administration of anti-PrP monoclonal antibodies was evaluated in two recent studies. In the first one, monoclonal antibody 4H11 ($F(ab')_2$ and IgG) was intraventricularly administered to transgenic mice overexpressing PrP using osmotic pumps from d85 to d100 following intraperitoneal challenge with a mouse-adapted bovine spongiform encephalopathy (BSE) strain. The mice were not protected by this regimen, and they succumbed to disease concomitantly with the control mice. Furthermore, mice treated with the antibodies developed neuronal cell death, associated with administration of the antibodies. In addition to previously reported results [79], linking cell death to PrP cross-linking events, in this study, emerged that PrP cross-linking is not the only mechanism mediating cell death; "coating" the whole cell surface PrP with antibodies or antibodies fragments could induce other toxic signals [81]. In the second study, intraventricular administration of antibodies 106, 110, 31C6, and 44B1 to wild-type mice was not linked with neuronal cell death; however, only a minor prolongation of survival and in one of the two tested animal models was achieved following administration of the monoclonal antibodies [82]. Differences in the epitopes recognized by the antibodies used in these two studies as well as the use of PrP overexpressing versus wild-type mice could account for the different results obtained regarding neuronal cell death. Of note, neuronal cell death has been challenged in another, more recent study, and it would be safe to assume that toxic effects are associated with the epitope and the dosage of the antibodies used [83].

A completely different passive immunization approach was used in two other studies; based on the discovery of the non-integrin 37/67 kDa lamin receptor (LRP/LR) as an interaction partner for both isoforms of PrP [84–86], polyclonal anti-LRP/LR [87] or single-chain Fv anti-LRP/LR antibodies [88] were intraperitoneally administered to wild-type mice as protective means in a mouse model of prion diseases. On both occasions, peripheral PrP^{Sc} accumulation was reduced; however, partial protection was only achieved with the polyclonal antibodies. This difference in the efficacy was attributed to differences in the pharmacokinetics and dosage regimen; polyclonal antibodies have a half-life of approximately 14 days in the blood, whereas the single-chain antibodies have a half-life of only 12 h. Moreover, the polyclonal antibodies were administered for 12 weeks, starting 1 week before administration of the pathogen, whereas the single-chain antibodies for 8 weeks. Passive immunization approaches are summarized in **Table 1**.

4.2. Active immunization approaches

Although passive immunization does protect against prion diseases, it provides a narrow window for intervention, i.e., antibodies must be administered shortly after exposure to the pathogen. In this regard, active immunization against the prion protein, which provides protection against the diseases similarly to a conventional vaccine, could prove a much more useful approach. Nevertheless, the prion protein-associated tolerance effects which prevent the immune system from mounting an immune response against the prion protein hinder development of such approaches [66].

Despite the tolerance effects, initiation of a humoral immune response against the prion protein was achieved, albeit with mediocre results in terms of protection against the disease. In the first reports, wild-type mice were immunized with recombinant murine prion protein mixed with complete Freund's adjuvant (CFA) and challenged with a mouse-adapted scrapie strain either concomitantly with the immunization (rescue treatment) or following its completion (prophylactic treatment). Although the mice developed antibodies against the prion protein, only mice of the prophylactic treatment group were partially protected against the pathogen; mice of this group succumbed to disease with a delay of approximately 16d compared to control mice [89].

4.2.1. Peptide-based active immunization

Numerous strategies were implemented to overcome the tolerance effects and promote generation of anti-prion antibodies. The most obvious approach was to use prion peptides properly modified to enhance the antigenicity of the protein (summarized in **Table 2**). Following this rationale, wild-type animals were immunized with prion protein peptides [90–93], PrP

http://dx.doi.org/10.5772/66447

Antibody name	Antibody type and target	Epitope	Administration protocol	*In vitro* assay	*In vivo* assay	Reference
ICSM18, ICSM35	Monoclonal, PrP	ICSM18: 143–153aa ICSM35: 93–105aa	Intraperitoneal administration twice weekly starting 7 or 30 days after administration of the pathogen or at onset of the clinical symptoms	NP	Prolonged survival interval in a mouse model of prion disease when the antibodies were administered prior to the appearance of clinical symptoms	[77]
6D11	Monoclonal, PrP	97–110aa	One intravenous administration immediately after administration of the pathogen followed by consecutive intraperitoneal administrations (twice per week for 4 or 8 weeks)	Prevention of infection and clearance of infection in already prion-infected cell lines	Prolongation of incubation period in a mouse model of prion disease	[115]
BAR236	Monoclonal, PrP	Linear epitope unidentified	Intraperitoneal (3 weekly administrations, starting 1 week after administration of the pathogen)	NP	Prolongation of survival interval in a mouse model of prion disease	[80]
4H11	Monoclonal or F(ab')$_2$ fragments, PrP	Epitope within octarepeat region (59–89aa)	Intraventricular (osmotic pump delivering antibody for 16 days starting 85 days after administration of the pathogen)	Inhibition of PrP^{Sc} propagation in an already prion-infected cell line. Recognition of PrP on the cell surface by FACS	Intraventricular administration of the antibody did not prolong survival interval in a mouse model of prion disease	[81]
106, 110, 31C6, 44B1	Monoclonal, anti-PrP	106: 88–90aa 110: 83–89aa 31C6: 143–149aa 44B1: discontinuous epitope within aa 155–231 aa	Intraventricular (osmotic pump delivering antibody for 14 days starting 60, 90, or 120 days after administration of the pathogen)	NP	Small (8%) prolongation of survival interval in a mouse model of prion diseases, even when administration of antibodies commences after appearance of first symptoms (120 days after administration of the pathogen)	[82]
pAb W3	Polyclonal anti-LRP/LR	Undefined	Intraperitoneal (12 weekly administrations starting 1 week before administration of the pathogen)	NP	Prolongation of survival interval, but not of incubation period in a mouse model of prion disease	[87]
S18	scFV, LRP	272–280aa	Intraperitoneal (8 weekly administrations starting 1 day before administration of the pathogen)	S18 prevents interaction of the recombinant human PrP with recombinant human LRP	Reduction of splenic PrP^{Sc}, but no prolongation of survival interval in a mouse model of prion disease	[88]

Antibody name	Antibody type and target	Epitope	Administration protocol	*In vitro* assay	*In vivo* assay	Reference
W226	Monoclonal, scFV	Undefined	Intraperitoneal administration twice weekly starting 2 or 28 days after administration of the pathogen or at onset of the clinical symptoms	Clearance of PrP^{Sc} in ScN2a cells	Minor delay of incubation time in immunized versus control mice	[116]
EB8, DC2, DE10, EF2	Monoclonal	EB8: 26–34aa; DC2: 35–46aa; DE10: 44–52aa and EF2: 47–52aa	NP	Clearance of PrP^{Sc} in ScGT2 cells	NP	[117]

Table 1. Summary of studies based on passive immunization against prion diseases.

dimers [94–96], or PrP aggregates [72]. In addition to homologous prion protein immunization [89], which provided proof of principle that active immunization can have a protective role against prion diseases, immunization with heterologous prion peptides also provided rather encouraging results [97]. In an attempt to enhance the immunogenicity of the prion peptides, various adjuvants, including Freund's adjuvant, Montanide IMS-1313, TiterMax, CpG, anti-OX40 antibodies—antibodies against the signaling molecule CD134, which recently has been shown to break T cell tolerance—and keyhole limpet hemocyanin, were used [95, 98], as well as different vaccine formulations, including encapsulation of the CpG-antigen complex in polylactide-coglycolide microspheres [96]. Interestingly, an early report indicates that immunization with complete Freund's adjuvant alone can provide partial protection in a mouse model of prion diseases through an unidentified mechanism [99]. Based on the extremely strong adjuvant effect exerted by heat-shock proteins, PrP molecules chemically cross-linked [100] or fused [72] to recombinant bacterial heat-shock proteins were also used to immunize wild-type mice and lead to the production of antibodies that recognized recombinant PrP.

Despite the widely accepted notion that PrP^{Sc} is not immunogenic and that the immune system does not provide protection against PrP^{Sc} in wild-type animals, when highly purified proteinase K-resistant PrP^{Sc}, originating from murine brains afflicted with an animal model of prion diseases was coadministered with CpG [101] or administered immobilized on Dynabeads coated with antibodies against PrP [102] a humoral immune response, which providing partial protection in animal model of prion diseases was elicited.

Although the protective role of the aforementioned, peptide-based approaches was not investigated on all occasions, it became evident that using various approaches the self-tolerance effects can be overcome and immune reactions against the prion protein can be obtained. However, it appears that protection against TSEs is restricted to antibodies capable of recognizing the native cell-surface PrP^C [95]. This requirement was met by antibodies known to provide protection against TSEs, e.g., ICSM18 [77] and 6H4 [76], whereas other antibodies

http://dx.doi.org/10.5772/66447

capable of recognizing recombinant PrP but unable to provide protection against TSEs also failed to recognize native PrP^C [72, 95].

4.2.2. *DNA vaccines*

In addition to peptide-based vaccines, DNA vaccines were also used to promote immune responses against the prion protein. In this case, nucleic acid encoding for the prion protein is administered to animals, wherein the nucleic acid is translated to the corresponding protein and an immune response is initiated. The first attempt at raising anti-PrP antibodies using DNA vaccines was only successful in $PrP^{-/-}$ mice, whereas the same approach failed to give rise to anti-PrP antibodies in wild-type mice [103]. Induction of anti-PrP antibodies using DNA vaccines in wild-type mice was triggered when the mice were immunized with a DNA construct coding for the murine prion protein fused to the lysosomal targeting signal from lysosomal integral membrane protein type II (LIMPII). Immunization with this construct leads to a remarkable delay on the onset of disease symptoms, which was not followed by a similar prolongation of survival interval. This discrepancy in the obtained results was attributed to immunopathology mediated by PrP-specific antibodies induced by the DNA vaccine used and constitutes the first report of adverse effects following active prion immunization [104].

In a different approach, DNA vaccines were used to prime wild-type mice, followed by peptide immunizations to further boost immune responses. Although this approach was successful when $PrP^{-/-}$ mice were immunized, very low antibody titers and only marginal protection were achieved when tested on wild-type mice [105]. In a recent report, wild-type mice were immunized with cDNA coding for human PrP^C fused to a T-cell stimulatory peptide. These mice developed a strong humoral immune response against the native protein, and although a bioassay was not carried out, the produced antibodies were capable of recognizing the native conformation of murine PrP^C, which—as already mentioned—constitutes a strong indicator of protective efficiency against prion diseases [106]. Studies based on DNA vaccines are summarized in **Table 3**.

4.2.3. *Immunization with PrP-displaying viral constructs*

A different approach to overcome the tolerance effects and stimulate the production of anti-PrP antibodies in wild-type mice is the expression of the prion protein on the surface of viral particles (summarized in **Table 4**). Virus-like particles (VLPs) are much better B lymphocytes immunogens than monovalent proteins and would be expected to trigger a stronger humoral immune response by passing tolerance.

In a first attempt, retroviral particles displaying the C-terminal portion of murine PrP were used to immunize wild-type mice. These mice developed anti-PrP antibodies, capable of recognizing the native form of PrP^C, thus displaying strong therapeutic potential [107]. A similar approach was used to insert the 9-amino-acid-, prion-pathogenesis associated-peptide pertaining to the murine/rat prion protein into the L1 major capsid protein of bovine papillomavirus type 1. These VLPs were used to immunize both wild-type rats and rabbits. The anti-sera

Antigen	Animals immunized	Humoral response	T-cell responses	*In vitro* assays	*In vivo* assays	Reference
Various murine PrP peptides	Wild-type mice	+	NP	NP	Reduction of proteinase K-resistant prion protein in a scrapie-infected tumor transplant	[93]
Recombinant murine PrP chemically cross-linked to bacterial heat-shock proteins	Wild-type mice	+	NP	NP	NP	[100]
Recombinant murine PrP	Wild-type mice	+	NP	NP	Prolongation of survival interval in a mouse model of prion disease	[89]
Recombinant murine PrP dimer	Wild-type mice, rabbits	+	NP	Polyclonal sera produced reduced PrP^{Sc} synthesis in prion-infected cell lines	NP	[94]
Recombinant murine prion peptide 105–125 linked to keyhole limpet hemocyanin and recombinant murine prion 90–230	Wild-type mice	+	NP	NP	Prolongation of survival interval in a mouse model of prion disease	[92]
Mouse prion peptides 31–50 and 211–230	Wild-type mice	NP	NP	NP	Prolongation of survival interval in a mouse model of prion disease, even when only the adjuvant Complete Freund's Adjuvant (CFA) is administered	[99]
Various murine prion peptides and adjuvants	Wild-type mice	+	ND	FACS to detect binding of the produced antibodies on native PrP	Statistically insignificant prolongation of survival time in a mouse model of prion disease	[95]
Murine prion peptides 39–67, 98–127, 143–172, and 158–187 with CFA or CpG	Wild-type mice	+	+	NP	NP	[98]

Antigen	Animals immunized	Humoral response	T-cell responses	*In vitro* assays	*In vivo* assays	Reference
Hamster prion peptides 105–128, 119–146, and 142–179	Wild-type hamsters	+	NP	NP	Prolongation of survival interval in a hamster model of prion diseases	[91]
Recombinant murine, ovine, and bovine prion protein	Wild-type mice	Detected following immunization with ovine and bovine recombinant PrP	NP	NP	Prolongation of survival interval in a mouse model of prion diseases following immunization with the bovine-recombinant protein	[97]
Recombinant murine PrP dimer and CpG encapsulated in polylactide-coglycolide microspheres	Wild-type mice	+	+	NP	NP	[96]
Murine scrapie-associated fibrils and CpG	Transgenic and wild-type mice	+	NP	NP	Prolongation of the survival interval of the wild-type mice in a mouse model of prion disease when CpG was used	[101]
Murine scrapie-associated fibrils immobilized on Dynabeads	Wild-type mice	+	NP	NP	Prolongation of survival interval in a mouse model of prion diseases with the bovine-recombinant protein	[102]
Cervid prion peptide sequences 168–182 and 145–164	Deer	+	NP	NP	Delay of incubation time in immunized versus control mice	[118]
Prion disease-derived brain material	Camelid	+	NP	Permanent abrogation of prion replication in a prion-permissive cell line	NP	[119]
rPrP aggregates, solubilized rPrP, DnaK-fused PrP	Mouse	+	NP	FACS to detect binding of the produced antibodies on native PrP	Statistically significant prolongation of survival time in a mouse model of prion disease	[72]

Table 2. Summary of studies on peptide-based active immunization against prion diseases.

Vaccine	Immunized animals	Humoral response	T-cell responses	*In vitro* assays	*In vivo* assays	Reference
DNA vaccine encoding either murine PrP or murine PrP fused to ubiquitin or to a lysosomal targeting signal	Wild-type mice	+	+	NP	Prolongation of asymptomatic period and accumulation of disease associated PrP, but not of survival interval. Death of the immunized mice was attributed to neurodegeneration associated with production of anti-PrP antbodies	[104]
DNA vaccine encoding murine PrP linked to helper T-cell epitopes Combination of DNA and peptide immunization	$PrP^{-/-}$ and wild-type mice	Achieved in $PrP^{-/-}$ mice, very low titer in wild-type mice	Detected in $PrP^{-/-}$ mice but not wild-type mice	FACS to detect binding of the produced antibodies on native PrP positive with $PrP^{-/-}$ mice sera, negative with wild-type mice sera. $PrP^{-/-}$ mice sera reduced PrP^{Sc} levels in prion-infected cell lines	Not effective	[105]
DNA vaccine encoding human PrP fused or not to a tetanus toxin stimulatory T-cell epitope and PrP protein boost	Wild-type mice	+	NP	FACS to detect binding of the produced antibodies on native PrP	NP	[106]
DNA vaccine encoding human PrP fused to ubiquitin, lysosomal integral membrane protein type II lysosome-targeting signal or an ER-targeting signal in conjunction with PrP vaccination	Wild-type mice	+	+	NP	NP	[120]

Table 3. Summary of studies on DNA vaccination against prion diseases.

Vaccine	Immunized animals	Humoral response	T-cell responses	*In vitro* assay	*In vivo* assay	Reference
Murine PrP or C-terminal murine PrP expressed on recombinant retroviral virus-like particles	$PrP^{-/-}$ and wild-type mice	+	NP	FACS to detect binding of the produced antibodies on native PrP	NP	[107]
Murine/rat prion 9/mer inserted into the L1 major capsid protein of bovine papillomavirus type 1	Wild-type rabbits and rats	+	NP	FACS to detect binding of the produced antibodies on native PrP, immunoprecipitation Rabbit immune sera inhibited de novo synthesis of PrP^{Sc} in prion-infected cells	NP	[108]
Priming with adenovirus 5 expressing the human PrP gene followed by boosting with the human PrP plasmid	$PrP^{-/-}$ and wild-type mice	+	+	FACS to detect binding of the produced antibodies on native PrP	Marginal prolongation of survival interval of the immunized mice	[109]

Table 4. Studies on active immunization approaches, using PrP-displaying virus constructs.

collected from both immunized species recognized native PrP^{Sc}, and importantly immune serum from the immunized rabbit prevented synthesis of PrP^{Sc} in scrapie-infected cell lines [108]. In a more recent approach, dendritic cells transduced with adenoviruses encoding the human prion protein were used to immunize wild-type mice. These mice developed antibodies against the murine prion protein as well, which provided partial protection against TSEs, as shown by the reduction in splenic PrP^{Sc} accumulation and prolongation of survival interval in a murine model of TSEs [109].

4.2.4. Mucosal immunization

To date, the only active immunization strategy providing complete protection against prion diseases is mucosal immunization. To trigger mucosal immunization, either transgenic, live-attenuated *Salmonella typhimurium* or cholera toxin is used. Both the attenuated *S. typhimurium* and the cholera toxin induce the production of IgA, which is the main immunoglobulin found in mucous secretions and is particularly abundant in the secretions of the gastrointestinal tract.

To induce mucosal immunization, a live-attenuated *S. typhimurium* vaccine strain engineered to express one [110] or two copies [110–112] of mouse [110, 112] or deer [111] PrP was administered orally to mice and deer, respectively. In a different approach, a murine PrP fragment was coadministered with cholera toxin either orally or intranasally [113]. The immunized animals were then orally challenged with a murine model of TSEs or chronic wasting disease (CWD)—infected brain homogenate to evaluate the protective potential of the immunization. Although both approaches promoted the generation of anti-PrP IgA, protection afforded by the

Vaccine	Immunized animals	Humoral response	T-cell responses	*In vitro* assay	*In vivo* assay	Reference
Orally administered *S. typhimurium* LVR01 expressing one or two copies of mouse PrP	Wild-type mice	+	NP	NP	Significant prolongation of survival interval in a mouse model of prion disease	[110, 112]
Intranasally, intragastrically, or intraperitoneally administered murine PrP90–231 and cholera toxin	Wild-type mice	+	NP	NP	Marginal prolongation of survival interval in a mouse model of prion disease following intranasal administration	[113]
Orally administered *S. typhimurium* LVR01 expressing two copies of elk PrP	White-tailed deers	+	NP	NP	Significant prolongation of survival interval in an elk model of prion disease. One immunized animal remained asymptomatic	[111]

Table 5. Mucosal vaccination approaches.

immunized animals varied greatly. Animals immunized with the attenuated PrP-expressing *Salmonella* survived significantly longer than control animals, and most importantly some of them were completely protected, remaining disease-free [110–112]. On the other hand, the cholera toxin was used to induce production of IgA, mice were only partially protected against oral exposure to the infectious agent, and modest prolongation of the survival interval was observed, without any mice remaining symptoms-free [113]. Studies dealing with mucosal immunization are summarized in **Table 5**.

Although mucosal immunization is only effective following oral exposure, it is important to remember that the gut is the major route of entry for prion diseases such as CWD in white-tailed deer, BSE in cattle, and variant Creutzfeldt-Jakob disease and kuru in humans. Furthermore, mucosal vaccination can be properly designed to induce a primarily humoral immune response and is unlikely to produce a significant immune response within the brain, thus minimizing the risk of appearance of adverse reactions [112].

5. Future perspectives

Despite fervent research and some very encouraging results, many facets of the involvement of the immune system in prion pathogenesis remain obscure, and a powerful immunoprotective tool has yet to emerge. Passive immunization with anti-prion antibodies and mucosal immunization were the only two approaches to provide satisfactory results but have a series of limitations associated with the narrow window of intervention and the route of infection. However, immune-based therapeutics both in their more classical immunization-based form or more modern, immunomodulatory form [114] hold great promise for prion diseases and other protein-misfolding diseases.

Author details

Konstantinos Xanthopoulos[1], Dimitra Dafou[2], Eirini Kanata[1] and Theodoros Sklaviadis[1]*

*Address all correspondence to: sklaviad@pharm.auth.gr

1 Department of Pharmaceutical Sciences, School of Health Sciences, Aristotle University of Thessaloniki, Thessaloniki, Greece

2 Department of Genetics, Development and Molecular Biology, School of Biology, Aristotle University of Thessaloniki, Thessaloniki, Greece

References

[1] Prusiner, S.B., *Novel proteinaceous infectious particles cause scrapie*. Science, 1982. **216**(4542): pp. 136–144.

[2] Riek, R., et al., *NMR characterization of the full-length recombinant murine prion protein, mPrP(23-231)*. FEBS Lett, 1997. **413**(2): pp. 282–288.

[3] Caughey, B.W., et al., *Secondary structure analysis of the scrapie-associated protein PrP 27-30 in water by infrared spectroscopy*. Biochemistry, 1991. **30**(31): pp. 7672–7680.

[4] Prusiner, S.B., *Prions*. Proc Natl Acad Sci U S A, 1998. **95**(23): pp. 13363–13383.

[5] Canello, T., et al., *Methionine sulfoxides on PrPSc: a prion-specific covalent signature*. Biochemistry, 2008. **47**(34): pp. 8866–8873.

[6] Bueler, H., et al., *Normal development and behaviour of mice lacking the neuronal cell-surface PrP protein*. Nature, 1992. **356**(6370): pp. 577–582.

[7] Manson, J.C., et al., *129/Ola mice carrying a null mutation in PrP that abolishes mRNA production are developmentally normal*. Mol Neurobiol, 1994. **8**(2–3): pp. 121–127.

[8] Aguzzi, A., Baumann, F., and Bremer, J., *The prion's elusive reason for being*. Annu Rev Neurosci, 2008. **31**: pp. 439–477.

[9] Linden, R., et al., *Physiology of the prion protein*. Physiol Rev, 2008. **88**(2): pp. 673–728.

[10] Kim, S., et al., *Prion protein-deficient mice exhibit decreased CD4 T and LTi cell numbers and impaired spleen structure*. Immunobiology, 2016. **221**(1): pp. 94–102.

[11] Chesebro, B., et al., *Identification of scrapie prion protein-specific mRNA in scrapie-infected and uninfected brain*. Nature, 1985. **315**(6017): pp. 331–333.

[12] Oesch, B., et al., *A cellular gene encodes scrapie PrP 27-30 protein*. Cell, 1985. **40**(4): pp. 735–746.

[13] Zhang, C.C., et al., *Prion protein is expressed on long-term repopulating hematopoietic stem cells and is important for their self-renewal*. Proc Natl Acad Sci U S A, 2006. **103**(7): pp. 2184–2189.

[14] Burthem, J., et al., *The normal cellular prion protein is strongly expressed by myeloid dendritic cells*. Blood, 2001. **98**(13): pp. 3733–3738.

[15] Cashman, N.R., et al., *Cellular isoform of the scrapie agent protein participates in lymphocyte activation*. Cell, 1990. **61**(1): pp. 185–192.

[16] Li, R., et al., *The expression and potential function of cellular prion protein in human lymphocytes*. Cell Immunol, 2001. **207**(1): pp. 49–58.

[17] Dodelet, V.C. and Cashman, N.R., *Prion protein expression in human leukocyte differentiation*. Blood, 1998. **91**(5): pp. 1556–1561.

[18] Durig, J., et al., *Differential constitutive and activation-dependent expression of prion protein in human peripheral blood leucocytes*. Br J Haematol, 2000. **108**(3): pp. 488–495.

[19] Isaacs, J.D., Jackson, G.S., and Altmann, D.M., *The role of the cellular prion protein in the immune system*. Clin Exp Immunol, 2006. **146**(1): pp. 1–8.

[20] Tsutsui, S., et al., *Absence of the cellular prion protein exacerbates and prolongs neuroinflammation in experimental autoimmune encephalomyelitis*. Am J Pathol, 2008. **173**(4): pp. 1029–1041.

[21] Miller, S.D. and Karpus, W.J., *Experimental autoimmune encephalomyelitis in the mouse*. Curr Protoc Immunol, 2007. **Chapter 15**: p. Unit 15 1.

[22] Hu, W., et al., *Pharmacological prion protein silencing accelerates central nervous system autoimmune disease via T cell receptor signalling*. Brain, 2010. **133**(Pt 2): pp. 375–388.

[23] Bakkebo, M.K., et al., *The cellular prion protein: a player in immunological quiescence*. Front Immunol, 2015. **6**: p. 450.

[24] Riesner, D., *Biochemistry and structure of PrP(C) and PrP(Sc)*. Br Med Bull, 2003. **66**: pp. 21–33.

[25] Beekes, M. and McBride, P.A., *The spread of prions through the body in naturally acquired transmissible spongiform encephalopathies*. FEBS J, 2007. **274**(3): pp. 588–605.

[26] Prinz, M., et al., *Oral prion infection requires normal numbers of Peyer's patches but not of enteric lymphocytes*. Am J Pathol, 2003. **162**(4): pp. 1103–1111.

[27] Aguzzi, A. and M. Heikenwalder, *Pathogenesis of prion diseases: current status and future outlook*. Nat Rev Microbiol, 2006. **4**(10): pp. 765–775.

[28] Greenlee, J.J., et al., *Lack of prion accumulation in lymphoid tissues of PRNP ARQ/ARR sheep intracranially inoculated with the agent of scrapie*. PLoS One, 2014. **9**(9): p. e108029.

[29] Friedman-Levi, Y., et al., *Genetic prion disease: no role for the immune system in disease pathogenesis?*. Hum Mol Genet, 2014. **23**(15): pp. 4134–4141.

[30] Chen, B., Soto, C., and Morales, R., *Peripherally administrated prions reach the brain at subinfectious quantities in experimental hamsters*. FEBS Lett, 2014. **588**(5): pp. 795–800.

[31] Kraehenbuhl, J.P. and Neutra, M.R., *Epithelial M cells: differentiation and function*. Annu Rev Cell Dev Biol, 2000. **16**: pp. 301–332.

[32] Heppner, F.L., et al., *Transepithelial prion transport by M cells*. Nat Med, 2001. **7**(9): pp. 976–977.

[33] Mishra, R.S., et al., *Protease-resistant human prion protein and ferritin are cotransported across Caco-2 epithelial cells: implications for species barrier in prion uptake from the intestine*. J Neurosci, 2004. **24**(50): pp. 11280–11290.

[34] Donaldson, D.S., Else, K.J., and Mabbott, N.A., *The gut-associated lymphoid tissues in the small intestine, not the large intestine, play a major role in oral prion disease pathogenesis*. J Virol, 2015. **89**(18): pp. 9532–9547.

[35] Mabbott, N.A. and MacPherson, G.G., *Prions and their lethal journey to the brain*. Nat Rev Microbiol, 2006. **4**(3): pp. 201–211.

[36] Beekes, M. and McBride, P.A., *Early accumulation of pathological PrP in the enteric nervous system and gut-associated lymphoid tissue of hamsters orally infected with scrapie*. Neurosci Lett, 2000. **278**(3): pp. 181–184.

[37] Herrmann, L.M., et al., *CD21-positive follicular dendritic cells: a possible source of PrPSc in lymph node macrophages of scrapie-infected sheep*. Am J Pathol, 2003. **162**(4): pp. 1075–1081.

[38] Jeffrey, M., et al., *Sites of prion protein accumulation in scrapie-infected mouse spleen revealed by immuno-electron microscopy*. J Pathol, 2000. **191**(3): pp. 323–332.

[39] Carp, R.I. and Callahan, S.M., *In vitro interaction of scrapie agent and mouse peritoneal macrophages*. Intervirology, 1981. **16**(1): pp. 8–13.

[40] Sassa, Y., Inoshima, Y., and Ishiguro, N., Bovine macrophage degradation of scrapie and BSE PrP(Sc). Vet Immunol Immunopathol, 2009. **133**(1): pp. 33–39.

[41] Prinz, M., et al., *Lymph nodal prion replication and neuroinvasion in mice devoid of follicular dendritic cells*. Proc Natl Acad Sci U S A, 2002. **99**(2): pp. 919–924.

[42] Takahashi, K., Inoshima, Y., and Ishiguro, N., *Role of cell death in the propagation of PrP(Sc) in immune cells*. Arch Virol, 2015. **160**(3): pp. 693–699.

[43] Huang, F.P., et al., *Migrating intestinal dendritic cells transport PrP(Sc) from the gut*. J Gen Virol, 2002. **83**(Pt 1): pp. 267–271.

[44] Mohan, J., Hopkins, J., and Mabbott, N.A., *Skin-derived dendritic cells acquire and degrade the scrapie agent following in vitro exposure*. Immunology, 2005. **116**(1): pp. 122–133.

[45] Klein, M.A., et al., *A crucial role for B cells in neuroinvasive scrapie*. Nature, 1997. **390**(6661): pp. 687–690.

[46] Montrasio, F., et al., *Impaired prion replication in spleens of mice lacking functional follicular dendritic cells*. Science, 2000. **288**(5469): pp. 1257–1259.

[47] Fraser, H. and Dickinson, A.G., *Studies of the lymphoreticular system in the pathogenesis of scrapie: the role of spleen and thymus*. J Comp Pathol, 1978. **88**(4): pp. 563–573.

[48] Clarke, M.C. and Kimberlin, R.H., *Pathogenesis of mouse scrapie: distribution of agent in the pulp and stroma of infected spleens*. Vet Microbiol, 1984. **9**(3): pp. 215–225.

[49] Fraser, H. and Farquhar, C.F., *Ionising radiation has no influence on scrapie incubation period in mice*. Vet Microbiol, 1987. **13**(3): pp. 211–223.

[50] Mabbott, N.A., et al., *Temporary inactivation of follicular dendritic cells delays neuroinvasion of scrapie*. Nat Med, 2000. **6**(7): pp. 719–720.

[51] Mabbott, N.A., et al., *Follicular dendritic cell dedifferentiation by treatment with an inhibitor of the lymphotoxin pathway dramatically reduces scrapie susceptibility*. J Virol, 2003. **77**(12): pp. 6845–6854.

[52] Mohan, J., Bruce, M.E., and Mabbott, N.A., *Follicular dendritic cell dedifferentiation reduces scrapie susceptibility following inoculation via the skin*. Immunology, 2005. **114**(2): pp. 225–234.

[53] Mabbott, N.A., et al., *Temporary blockade of the tumor necrosis factor receptor signaling pathway impedes the spread of scrapie to the brain*. J Virol, 2002. **76**(10): pp. 5131–5139.

[54] Klein, M.A., et al., *Complement facilitates early prion pathogenesis*. Nat Med, 2001. **7**(4): pp. 488–492.

[55] Mabbott, N.A., et al., *Temporary depletion of complement component C3 or genetic deficiency of C1q significantly delays onset of scrapie*. Nat Med, 2001. **7**(4): pp. 485–487.

[56] Oldstone, M.B., et al., *Lymphotoxin-alpha- and lymphotoxin-beta-deficient mice differ in susceptibility to scrapie: evidence against dendritic cell involvement in neuroinvasion*. J Virol, 2002. **76**(9): pp. 4357–4363.

[57] Shlomchik, M.J., et al., *Neuroinvasion by a Creutzfeldt-Jakob disease agent in the absence of B cells and follicular dendritic cells*. Proc Natl Acad Sci U S A, 2001. **98**(16): pp. 9289–9294.

[58] Manuelidis, L., et al., *Follicular dendritic cells and dissemination of Creutzfeldt-Jakob disease*. J Virol, 2000. **74**(18): pp. 8614–8622.

[59] Baldauf, E., Beekes, M., and Diringer, H., *Evidence for an alternative direct route of access for the scrapie agent to the brain bypassing the spinal cord*. J Gen Virol, 1997. **78** (Pt 5): pp. 1187–1197.

[60] McBride, P.A., et al., *Early spread of scrapie from the gastrointestinal tract to the central nervous system involves autonomic fibers of the splanchnic and vagus nerves*. J Virol, 2001. **75**(19): pp. 9320–9327.

[61] Race, R., Oldstone, M., and Chesebro, B., *Entry versus blockade of brain infection following oral or intraperitoneal scrapie administration: role of prion protein expression in peripheral nerves and spleen*. J Virol, 2000. **74**(2): pp. 828–833.

[62] Glatzel, M. and Aguzzi, A., *PrP(C) expression in the peripheral nervous system is a determinant of prion neuroinvasion*. J Gen Virol, 2000. **81**(Pt 11): pp. 2813–2821.

[63] Kunzi, V., et al., *Unhampered prion neuroinvasion despite impaired fast axonal transport in transgenic mice overexpressing four-repeat tau*. J Neurosci, 2002. **22**(17): pp. 7471–7477.

[64] Prinz, M., et al., *Positioning of follicular dendritic cells within the spleen controls prion neuroinvasion*. Nature, 2003. **425**(6961): pp. 957–962.

[65] von Poser-Klein, C., et al., *Alteration of B-cell subsets enhances neuroinvasion in mouse scrapie infection*. J Virol, 2008. **82**(7): pp. 3791–3795.

[66] Mabbott, N.A., *Prospects for safe and effective vaccines against prion diseases*. Expert Rev Vaccines, 2015. **14**(1): pp. 1–4.

[67] McGovern, G., Mabbott, N., and Jeffrey, M., *Scrapie affects the maturation cycle and immune complex trapping by follicular dendritic cells in mice*. PLoS One, 2009. **4**(12): p. e8186.

[68] Bremer, J., et al., *Repetitive immunization enhances the susceptibility of mice to peripherally administered prions*. PLoS One, 2009. **4**(9): p. e7160.

[69] Aguzzi, A. and Sigurdson, C.J., *Antiprion immunotherapy: to suppress or to stimulate?*. Nat Rev Immunol, 2004. **4**(9): pp. 725–736.

[70] Heikenwalder, M., et al., *Lymphoid follicle destruction and immunosuppression after repeated CpG oligodeoxynucleotide administration*. Nat Med, 2004. **10**(2): pp. 187–192.

[71] Sethi, S., et al., *Postexposure prophylaxis against prion disease with a stimulator of innate immunity*. Lancet, 2002. **360**(9328): pp. 229–230.

[72] Xanthopoulos, K., et al., *Immunization with recombinant prion protein leads to partial protection in a murine model of TSEs through a novel mechanism*. PLoS One, 2013. **8**(3): p. e59143.

[73] Enari, M., Flechsig, E., and Weissmann, C., *Scrapie prion protein accumulation by scrapie-infected neuroblastoma cells abrogated by exposure to a prion protein antibody*. Proc Natl Acad Sci U S A, 2001. **98**(16): pp. 9295–9299.

[74] Peretz, D., et al., *Antibodies inhibit prion propagation and clear cell cultures of prion infectivity*. Nature, 2001. **412**(6848): pp. 739–743.

[75] Perrier, V., et al., *Anti-PrP antibodies block PrPSc replication in prion-infected cell cultures by accelerating PrPC degradation*. J Neurochem, 2004. **89**(2): pp. 454–463.

[76] Heppner, F.L., et al., *Prevention of scrapie pathogenesis by transgenic expression of anti-prion protein antibodies*. Science, 2001. **294**(5540): pp. 178–182.

[77] White, A.R., et al., *Monoclonal antibodies inhibit prion replication and delay the development of prion disease*. Nature, 2003. **422**(6927): pp. 80–83.

[78] Mallucci, G., et al., *Depleting neuronal PrP in prion infection prevents disease and reverses spongiosis*. Science, 2003. **302**(5646): pp. 871–874.

[79] Solforosi, L., et al., *Cross-linking cellular prion protein triggers neuronal apoptosis in vivo.* Science, 2004. **303**(5663): pp. 1514–1516.

[80] Feraudet-Tarisse, C., et al., *Immunotherapeutic effect of anti-PrP monoclonal antibodies in TSE mouse models: pharmacokinetic and pharmacodynamic analysis.* J Gen Virol, 2010. **91**(Pt 6): pp. 1635–1645

[81] Lefebvre-Roque, M., et al., *Toxic effects of intracerebral PrP antibody administration during the course of BSE infection in mice.* Prion, 2007. **1**(3): pp. 198–206.

[82] Song, C.H., et al., *Effect of intraventricular infusion of anti-prion protein monoclonal antibodies on disease progression in prion-infected mice.* J Gen Virol, 2008. **89**(Pt 6): pp. 1533–1544.

[83] Klohn, P.C., et al., *PrP antibodies do not trigger mouse hippocampal neuron apoptosis.* Science, 2012. **335**(6064): p. 52.

[84] Gauczynski, S., et al., *The 37-kDa/67-kDa laminin receptor acts as the cell-surface receptor for the cellular prion protein.* EMBO J, 2001. **20**(21): pp. 5863–5875.

[85] Morel, E., et al., *Bovine prion is endocytosed by human enterocytes via the 37 kDa/67 kDa laminin receptor.* Am J Pathol, 2005. **167**(4): pp. 1033–1042.

[86] Gauczynski, S., et al., *The 37-kDa/67-kDa laminin receptor acts as a receptor for infectious prions and is inhibited by polysulfated glycanes.* J Infect Dis, 2006. **194**(5): pp. 702–709.

[87] Zuber, C., et al., *Anti-LRP/LR antibody W3 hampers peripheral PrPSc propagation in scrapie infected mice.* Prion, 2007. **1**(3): pp. 207–212.

[88] Zuber, C., et al., *Single chain Fv antibodies directed against the 37 kDa/67 kDa laminin receptor as therapeutic tools in prion diseases.* Mol Immunol, 2008. **45**(1): pp. 144–151.

[89] Sigurdsson, E.M., et al., *Immunization delays the onset of prion disease in mice.* Am J Pathol, 2002. **161**(1): pp. 13–17.

[90] Arbel, M., Lavie, V., and Solomon, B., *Generation of antibodies against prion protein in wild-type mice via helix 1 peptide immunization.* J Neuroimmunol, 2003. **144**(1–2): pp. 38–45.

[91] Magri, G., et al., *Decrease in pathology and progression of scrapie after immunisation with synthetic prion protein peptides in hamsters.* Vaccine, 2005. **23**(22): pp. 2862–2868.

[92] Schwarz, A., et al., *Immunisation with a synthetic prion protein-derived peptide prolongs survival times of mice orally exposed to the scrapie agent.* Neurosci Lett, 2003. **350**(3): pp. 187–189.

[93] Souan, L., et al., *Modulation of proteinase-K resistant prion protein by prion peptide immunization.* Eur J Immunol, 2001. **31**(8): pp. 2338–2346.

[94] Gilch, S., et al., *Polyclonal anti-PrP auto-antibodies induced with dimeric PrP interfere efficiently with PrPSc propagation in prion-infected cells.* J Biol Chem, 2003. **278**(20): pp. 18524–18531.

[95] Polymenidou, M., et al., *Humoral immune response to native eukaryotic prion protein correlates with anti-prion protection.* Proc Natl Acad Sci U S A, 2004. **101** Suppl 2: pp. 14670–14676.

[96] Kaiser-Schulz, G., et al., *Polylactide-coglycolide microspheres co-encapsulating recombinant tandem prion protein with CpG-oligonucleotide break self-tolerance to prion protein in wild-type mice and induce CD4 and CD8 T cell responses*. J Immunol, 2007. **179**(5): pp. 2797–2807.

[97] Ishibashi, D., et al., *Immunization with recombinant bovine but not mouse prion protein delays the onset of disease in mice inoculated with a mouse-adapted prion*. Vaccine, 2007. **25**(6): pp. 985–992.

[98] Rosset, M.B., et al., *Breaking immune tolerance to the prion protein using prion protein peptides plus oligodeoxynucleotide-CpG in mice*. J Immunol, 2004. **172**(9): pp. 5168–5174.

[99] Tal, Y., et al., *Complete Freund's adjuvant immunization prolongs survival in experimental prion disease in mice*. J Neurosci Res, 2003. **71**(2): pp. 286–290.

[100] Koller, M.F., Grau, T., and Christen, P., *Induction of antibodies against murine full-length prion protein in wild-type mice*. J Neuroimmunol, 2002. **132**(1–2): pp. 113–116.

[101] Spinner, D.S., et al., *CpG oligodeoxynucleotide-enhanced humoral immune response and production of antibodies to prion protein PrPSc in mice immunized with 139A scrapie-associated fibrils*. J Leukoc Biol, 2007. **81**(6): pp. 1374–1385.

[102] Tayebi, M., Collinge, J., and Hawke, S., *Unswitched immunoglobulin M response prolongs mouse survival in prion disease*. J Gen Virol, 2009. **90**(Pt 3): pp. 777–782.

[103] Krasemann, S., et al., *Induction of antibodies against human prion proteins (PrP) by DNA-mediated immunization of PrP0/0 mice*. J Immunol Methods, 1996. **199**(2): pp. 109–118.

[104] Fernandez-Borges, N., et al., *DNA vaccination can break immunological tolerance to PrP in wild-type mice and attenuates prion disease after intracerebral challenge*. J Virol, 2006. **80**(20): pp. 9970–9976.

[105] Nitschke, C., et al., *Immunisation strategies against prion diseases: prime-boost immunisation with a PrP DNA vaccine containing foreign helper T-cell epitopes does not prevent mouse scrapie*. Vet Microbiol, 2007. **123**(4): pp. 367–376.

[106] Alexandrenne, C., et al., *Electrotransfer of cDNA coding for a heterologous prion protein generates autoantibodies against native murine prion protein in wild-type mice*. DNA Cell Biol, 2010. **29**(3): pp. 121–131.

[107] Nikles, D., et al., *Circumventing tolerance to the prion protein (PrP): vaccination with PrP-displaying retrovirus particles induces humoral immune responses against the native form of cellular PrP*. J Virol, 2005. **79**(7): pp. 4033–4042.

[108] Handisurya, A., et al., *Vaccination with prion peptide-displaying papillomavirus-like particles induces autoantibodies to normal prion protein that interfere with pathologic prion protein production in infected cells*. FEBS J, 2007. **274**(7): pp. 1747–1758.

[109] Rosset, M.B., et al., *Dendritic cell-mediated-immunization with xenogenic PrP and adenoviral vectors breaks tolerance and prolongs mice survival against experimental scrapie*. PLoS One, 2009. **4**(3): p. e4917.

[110] Goni, F., et al., *Mucosal vaccination delays or prevents prion infection via an oral route.* Neuroscience, 2005. **133**(2): pp. 413–421.

[111] Goni, F., et al., *Mucosal immunization with an attenuated Salmonella vaccine partially protects white-tailed deer from chronic wasting disease.* Vaccine, 2015. **33**(5): pp. 726–733.

[112] Goni, F., et al., *High titers of mucosal and systemic anti-PrP antibodies abrogate oral prion infection in mucosal-vaccinated mice.* Neuroscience, 2008. **153**(3): pp. 679–686.

[113] Bade, S., et al., *Intranasal immunization of Balb/c mice against prion protein attenuates orally acquired transmissible spongiform encephalopathy.* Vaccine, 2006. **24**(9): pp. 1242–1253.

[114] Sacquin, A., et al., *Prolongation of prion disease-associated symptomatic phase relates to CD3+ T cell recruitment into the CNS in murine scrapie-infected mice.* Brain Behav Immun, 2012. **26**(6): pp. 919–930.

[115] Sadowski, M.J., et al., *Anti-PrP Mab 6D11 suppresses PrP(Sc) replication in prion infected myeloid precursor line FDC-P1/22L and in the lymphoreticular system in vivo.* Neurobiol Dis, 2009. **34**(2): pp. 267–278.

[116] Petsch, B., et al., *Biological effects and use of PrPSc- and PrP-specific antibodies generated by immunization with purified full-length native mouse prions.* J Virol, 2011. **85**(9): pp. 4538–4546.

[117] Didonna, A., et al., *Characterization of four new monoclonal antibodies against the distal N-terminal region of PrP(c).* PeerJ, 2015. **3**: p. e811.

[118] Pilon, J.L., et al., *Immunization with a synthetic peptide vaccine fails to protect mule deer (Odocoileus hemionus) from chronic wasting disease.* J Wildl Dis, 2013. **49**(3): pp. 694–698.

[119] David, M.A., Jones, D.R., and Tayebi, M., *Potential candidate camelid antibodies for the treatment of protein-misfolding diseases.* J Neuroimmunol, 2014. **272**(1–2): pp. 76–85.

[120] Han, Y., et al., *Immune responses in wild-type mice against prion proteins induced using a DNA prime-protein boost strategy.* Biomed Environ Sci, 2011. **24**(5): pp. 523–529.

Chapter 8

Genetic Resistance to Prion Diseases

Yalçın Yaman and Cemal Ün

Additional information is available at the end of the chapter

http://dx.doi.org/10.5772/66916

Abstract

Prions are abnormal isoforms of the host-encoded cellular prion proteins which are misfolding in its three-dimensional structure acquire pathogenicity. Prions cause transmissible spongiform encephalopathy (TSEs) in humans and some animal species including sheep, goats, cattle, cat, deer and elk. TSEs, also called "prion diseases," cause irreversible neurodegeneration in the central nervous system and are always fatal. Cellular prion proteins are encoded by prion protein gene (*PRNP*) in mammals; moreover, it is known that the variations in the *PRNP* gene have influence on the resistance and/or incubation period of the TSEs. It is well-documented that after exposure to the pathogenic prions, development of some TSEs depend on the host *PRNP* genotype, for example, scrapie in sheep, bovine spongiform encephalopathy (BSE) in cattle, Creutzfeldt-Jakob disease (CJD) and kuru in humans, as well. In this chapter, genetic resistance to prion diseases will be reviewed.

Keywords: TSE, prion disease, PRNP, genetic resistance

1. Introduction

It is known that conformational changes in prion protein cause Creutzfeldt-Jakob disease (CJD) in humans, scrapie disease in sheep and goats [1, 2], bovine spongiform encephalopathy (BSE) in cattle, feline spongiform encephalopathy in cat, and wasting disease in deer and elk.

Polymorphisms inside the prion protein-coding gene (*PRNP*) in humans and also in some mammalian species have been appeared to impact disease susceptibility and pathologies [3]. In human population, kuru and CJD are profoundly related with polymorphism in codon 129. All CDJ affected individuals are known to be homozygous for methionine amino acid in codon 129 while at the same codon heterozygote individuals seem most resistant to kuru [4, 5]. Also, it is known that there is a high correlation between the polymorphisms in codons

136, 154, and 171 of the PRNP gene and the level of susceptibility to scrapie in sheep [3, 6, 7]. In cattle, numerous studies were carried out for discovering a relationship amongst BSE and polymorphisms in cattle genome [8–12]. The studies about BSE-affected animals in Germany and USA represented the influence of *PRNP* promoter polymorphisms on BSE susceptibility in cattle [13, 14]. The impacts of insertion-deletion (indel) polymorphisms within a location 1.6 kbp upstream of exon 1 and inside intron 1 (23-bp and 12-bp, respectively) on BSE susceptibility are determined by further analyses in cattle [15–17]. Despite the fact that cattle with the -/-23 bp promoter genotype and the –/12 bp intron 1 genotype have both been significantly connected with BSE, it could not be reached any consensus on which genotype is most identified with BSE [13, 15, 16, 18]. In addition, indel polymorphisms that affect the sensitivity of classical BSE appear not to be pertinent to other transmissible spongiform encephalopathies in cattle [19]. Until now, the incidence of *PRNP* gene promoter polymorphisms has been identified in some cattle in Asia [20, 21], Europe [13, 16, 18, 22] and America [14, 23].

2. Resistance in humans

There exist various types of human prion disease such as Creutzfeldt-Jakob disease (CJD), fatal familial insomnia (FFI), and Gerstmann Sträussler-Scheinker syndrome (GSS). Related to the cause of the illness they exist in three main forms: Genetic, sporadic and acquired. Genetic form of the disease is caused by a mutation in prion protein-coding gene (*PRNP*), whereas acquired form occurs by the transmission of disease from an animal or another human disease. The cause of sporadic form is not clear up to now [24–26].

The human prion-coding gene consists of two exons and the second one contains the whole open reading frame. It is known that a valine amino acid at position 129 of the human prion protein provide resistancy to the Creutzfeldt-Jakob disease. Both Valin129Valin and Methionine129Methionine genotypes are resistant to the disease, whereas Methionine129Methionine genotypes are susceptible [27, 28]. Another polymorphism at codon 219 was reported to be related with development of Creutzfeldt-Jakob disease in Japanese population [29].

3. Resistance in small ruminants

Scrapie is a neurodegenerative disease of sheep and goats. As with other transmissible spongiform encephalopathies (TSE) which affect humans and animal species, scrapie is always fatal and characterized by long incubation periods ranging from months to years, vacuolation, neuronal loss and astrocytosis in the central nervous system (CNS) and has no inflammatory or immune responses [30]. The earliest reports of the scrapie based on middle of 1700s in Britain. Various terms such as "scrapie," "scratchie," "rubbers," "rickets" and "goggles" were used to indicate the disease [31].

It is thought that scrapie first occurred in the United Kingdom in the eighteenth century and following decades, particularly after World War II, the disease spread by importation of the infected animals. Scrapie has reported nearly all over the world, for example, Iceland (1878), Canada (1938), USA (1947), Australia (1952), Norway (1958), India (1961), Republic of South Africa (1966), Kenya (1970), Germany (1973), Brazil (1978), Yemen (1979), Sweden (1988), Cyprus (1989) and Japan (1990), reviewed in reference [30].

Scrapie has been known for over 250 years; therefore, it is regarded to be prototype of the TSEs [30]. Earlier, researchers thought that it was a hereditary disease, but later, according to the results of the experimental transmission studies, they were considered that "Scrapie was a natural infection and gained from ground". After seven years of working with several thousand breeding ewes within several hundred ewes were affected classical scrapie, H. B. Parry postulated some hypothesis that scrapie had a hereditary feature in a simple Mendelian autosomal recessive manner, development of the disease determined by genotype of the individuals, and it was not a natural infection. They observed that in high-incidence flocks, many scrapie diseased individuals had affected parent or progeny [32, 33]. Later studies revealed the evidences that scrapie is a transmissible infection [34] which is caused by a kind of proteins called "prion" [35], and development and/or incubation period of the disease under genetic control [36–40].

3.1. Resistance in sheep

Sheep and goat prion protein-coding gene (*PRNP*) which encodes the cellular prion protein located on chromosome 13 [41]. The gene structure of the sheep *PRNP* was determined by [40], they demonstrated that sheep *PRNP* encoded 256 amino acids and highly homologous with the *PRNP* gene of the other species. Furthermore, the authors suggest that arginine/glutamine substitution in the 171th position of the sheep *PRNP* might have affected the scrapie incubation period. According to the results of many subsequent study polymorphisms of 136th, 154th and 171th codons of ovine *PRNP* had a strong influence on susceptibility or resistance to the scrapie [8, 42–45].

Commonly encoded amino acids at three codons are as follows: alanine (A) or valine (V) at codon 136, arginine (R) or histidine (H) at codon 154 and glutamine (G), histidine (H) or arginine (R) at codon 171 and out of possible other combinations, common *PRNP* alleles are A136R154R171, A136R154Q171, A136R154H171, A136H154Q171 and V136R154Q171, (respectively, ARR, ARQ, ARH, AHQ and VRQ for short) [45, 46]. While ARR alleles related to resistance, VRQ is regarded as the most susceptible alleles. Until now, only three scrapie cases were reported in ARR homozygous sheep which are one case from Japan [47] and two cases from France and Germany [48]. Some studies on PrP genotype and their relevance to scrapie in scrapie diseased sheep are presented in **Table 1**.

There is no report about direct transmission from sheep to human in natural condition, nevertheless, scrapie can be transmitted interspecies by experimentally [59–61], furthermore, the cattle prion disease, Bovine spongiform encephalopathy (BSE) which is transmitted to human and causes a variant of Creutzfeldt-Jakob disease (vCJD) [62], originated from the usage of scrapie contaminated material in cattle nutrition [63]. Even, in a more recent study, natural scrapie isolate was successfully transmitted to a primate (cynomolgus macaque) suggesting that scrapie has zoonotic potential to primates including human [64]. Epidemiological connection with scra-

Risk groups	PrP Genotypes	Norway $n = 32$ [49]	England $n = 21$ [50]	England $n = 59$ [51]	France $n = 437$ [52]	France $n = 245$ [53]	Ireland $n = 154$ [54]	Italy $n = 34$ [55]	The Netherlands $n = 34$ [45]	Iceland $n = 101$ [56]	Greece $n = 216$ [57]	Japan $n = 15$ [47]	Canada $n = 249$ [58]
1	ARR/ARR	0.000	0.000	0.000	0.000	0.000	0.000	0.000	0.000	0.000	0.000	0.066	0.000
2	ARR/AHQ	0.000	0.000	0.000	0.000	0.000	0.000	0.000	0.000	0.000	0.005	0.000	0.000
	ARR/ARH	0.000	0.000	0.000	0.000	0.000	0.000	0.000	0.000	0.000	0.014	0.000	0.000
	ARR/ARQ	0.063	0.000	0.000	0.005	0.008	0.000	0.000	0.000	0.000	0.120	0.066	0.000
3	ARQ/ARH	0.000	0.000	0.000	0.000	0.041	0.162	0.000	0.000	0.000	0.000	0.000	0.000
	ARQ/AHQ	0.000	0.000	0.017	0.016	0.004	0.000	0.059	0.000	0.000	0.176	0.000	0.004
	AHQ/AHQ	0.063	0.000	0.017	0.002	0.004	0.000	0.000	0.000	0.000	0.000	0.000	0.000
	ARH/ARH	0.000	0.000	0.000	0.000	0.004	0.006	0.000	0.000	0.000	0.005	0.000	0.000
	AHQ/ARH	0.000	0.000	0.000	0.000	0.000	0.000	0.000	0.000	0.000	0.000	0.000	0.000
	ARQ/ARQ	0.031	0.143	0.136	0.210	0.371	0.422	0.941	0.088	0.465	0.509	0.867	0.916
4	ARR/VRQ	0.000	0.095	0.254	0.020	0.070	0.006	0.000	0.029	0.000	0.000	0.000	0.012
5	AHQ/VRQ	0.000	0.000	0.000	0.007	0.008	0.000	0.000	0.000	0.000	0.000	0.000	0.004
	ARH/VRQ	0.000	0.286	0.051	0.000	0.037	0.026	0.000	0.441	0.000	0.000	0.000	0.000
	ARQ/VRQ	0.156	0.476	0.407	0.470	0.371	0.363	0.000	0.353	0.406	0.000	0.000	0.052
	VRQ/VRQ	0.688	0.000	0.119	0.280	0.086	0.013	0.000	0.088	0.129	0.079	0.000	0.012

Table 1. PrP genotype frequencies of the scrapie-infected sheep in various countries.

pie, BSE and vCJD emerged public health concerns and lead to establishing scrapie eradication programs, including increasing the genetic resistance to scrapie in scrapie epidemic countries.

In 2001, Great Britain has established the "National Scrapie Plan" (NSP) intending to increase the frequencies of resistance alleles by selective breeding and eventually eradicate scrapie from British sheep herds. According to disease-associated alleles, five risk groups were designated from R1 to R5 where is R1 referring at the lowest risk and R5 at highest risk [65]. NSP scrapie risk groups can be seen in **Table 2**.

Reported case per year and estimated of the case number per million sheep according to risk groups in the United Kingdom (UK) are given in **Table 3**.

European Union (EU) Commission has issued a regulation in 2003 that required the establish of a selective breeding program for resistance to TSE in each sheep breed of member states [66]; therefore, European member states have been implementing breeding programs based on elimination of the most susceptible alleles while increasing resistant allele frequencies. For example, as a result of intensive genetic selection programs, particularly in high genetic merit flocks, ARR allele frequencies increased from 50 to 69% in the UK, 49 to 85% in France, 38 to 70% in the Netherlands and 47 to 70% in Italy [67].

Risk groups	Genotype of individuals	Degree of resistance/susceptibility
R1	ARR/ARR	Sheep that are most resistant to scrapie
R2	ARR/AHQ	Sheep that are resistant to scrapie, but will need careful selection when used further breeding
	ARR/ARH	
	ARR/ARQ	
R3	ARQ/ARH	Sheep that have little resistance and will need careful selection when used for further breeding
	ARQ/AHQ	
	AHQ/AHQ	
	ARH/ARH	
	AHQ/ARH	
	ARQ/ARQ	
R4	ARR/VRQ	Sheep that are susceptible to scrapie and should not be used for breeding because of carrying VRQ allele
R5	AHQ/VRQ	Sheep that are highly susceptible to scrapie and should not be used for breeding
	ARH/VRQ	
	ARQ/VRQ	
	VRQ/VRQ	

Table 2. PrP genotypes and allocation of them into scrapie risk groups (adapted from reference [65]).

Risk groups	Case per year (n)	Percentage of sheep	Case per year per million (n)
R1	0	21.3	0
R2	2.3	35.7	0.7
R3	104.9	23.9	57.8
R4	12	9.6	6.3
R5	381.8	9.6	1175.6

Table 3. Estimates of the number of reported cases of scrapie per million sheep of each risk groups in the UK (adapted from reference [46]).

Given the importance of the disease, a lot of genotyping studies on sheep *PRNP* have carried out in the almost all over the world such as; in New Zealand and Australia [68], Brazil [69], Israel, Palestine, and Jordan [70], Turkey [71], Egypt and Saudi Arabia [72] and East Asia [73], whether scrapie have reported or never been reported.

3.2. Resistance in goats

First natural scrapie case in goats was defined in 1942 [74]. Although goat scrapie has rare incidence compared with sheep, a surveillance program between 2002 and 2009 was performed according to the EU commission direction and over 3000 scrapie cases were reported in goats [75]. Scrapie cases occurring in natural condition in goats have been reported, particularly throughout Europe [76–78]. Transmission of the scrapie from naturally affected sheep to goats which rearing together has often been observed [77, 79–81], in addition, transmission from goat to goat has been known [76].

In contrast to sheep, limited data are available related to scrapie resistance and *PRNP* alleles. Genotyping studies on goats *PRNP* have given various results in terms of disease susceptibility or resistance. Assessment of *PRNP* alleles in scrapie infected and non-infected goats presented in **Table 4**.

As provided in **Table 4**, some relationships between caprine *PRNP* polymorphisms and scrapie resistance were defined. Encoding of serine instead of glycine at codon 127 has decreased the probability of clinical manifestation of the disease [86]. Isoleucine-methionine dimorphism at codon 142 has found to be associated both experimental [88] and natural infection [86, 89]; furthermore, it is reported that [89] the presence of methionine-isoleucine as heterozygous at codon 142 has been provided resistance only in proline-proline homozygous animal at codon 240. Encoding of arginine at codon 143 has provided limited protection to natural scrapie [80]. While the presence of asparagine instead of Serine or Aspartic acid at codon 146 has been found to be related to susceptibility to natural infection [78], it also has reported that the presence of Serine as heterozygous at the same codon has associated with the extended incubation period in oral challenging [90]. According to the results of various studies, arginine-histidine dimorphism at codon 154 has provided limited resistance [78, 80, 83, 89]. The presence of glutamine/arginine as heterozygous at codon 211 has been found to

http://dx.doi.org/10.5772/66916

Codons	AA substitution	Association to disease	References
18	W-R		[82]
21	V-A		[80]
23	L-P		[80]
37	G-V		[83, 84]
49	G-S		[80]
101	Q-R		[82]
110	T-P		[83, 84]
127	G-S	Incubation period/resistance	[85, 86]
133	L-Q		[93]
137	M-I		[93]
139	R-S		[87]
142	I-M	Incubation period	[84, 86, 88, 89]
142	I-T		[84]
143	H-R	Limited resistance	[80, 88]
145	G-D		[87]
146	N-S or D	Resistance	[78, 90]
151	R-H		[78]
154	R-H	Limited resistance	[78, 80, 83, 89]
168	P-Q		[80]
194	T-P		[84]
201	F-L		[86]
208	R-Q		[91]
211	R-G		[85]
211	R-Q	Lower susceptibility	[84, 89]
219	T-I		[92]
220	Q-H		[80]
222	Q-K	Resistance	[83, 89, 90, 93]
232	G-W		[82]
240	S-P	Resistance (connected with codon 142)	[88, 89]

Abbreviations of the amino acids: A, alanine; D, aspartic acid; F, phenylalanine; G, glycine; H, histidine; I, isoleucine; K, lysine; L, leucine; M, methionine; N, asparagine; P, proline; Q, glutamine; R, arginine; S, serine; T, threonine; V, valine; W, tryptophan.

Table 4. The *PRNP* polymorphisms of scrapie-infected/noninfected goats and association of polymorphisms with scrapie resistance.

be related to lower susceptibility [89], and the presence of lysine at codon 222 has been associated with resistance to both natural [83, 89, 93] and oral [90] or intracerebral challenging [94].

Apart from these polymorphisms, an allele of caprine *PRNP*, which encodes shorter cellular prion protein, has been reported. An experimental transmission to a goat carrying this allele as heterozygote has died after an unusually long incubation period [95]. In addition, a novel 28 bp insertion in the promoter region of caprine *PRNP* was found by [96] in healthy Chinese native goat breeds. Although there is no information with respect to disease resistance, some associations between this insertion/deletion polymorphism and production trait were reported.

Influences of the remaining codons over scrapie resistance or susceptibility in goats are not known yet. Currently available data on genetic resistance to scrapie are considered insufficient to establish selective breeding programs in goats.

3.3. Atypical scrapie in sheep and goats

Norwegian researchers have recognized a novel type of scrapie case in 1998 which has unusual histopathological features comparing with classical scrapie. The geographical distribution of the disease indicated that it might be spontaneous scrapie, not a contagious disease. This atypical form of scrapie designated as Nor98 by the authors [97]. Later studies conducted on archived tissue specimens revealed that atypical scrapie is not a new disease and has been existed at least from late 1980s in the UK herds [98, 99]. In the following years, many atypical scrapie cases were reported in sheep and/or goats from [100–103], North America [104] and New Zealand [105], as well.

Atypical cases have appeared to relate with the *PRNP* genotypes considered relatively resistant to classical scrapie. Sheep which are carrier of AHQ allele have found to be more susceptible to atypical scrapie; moreover, unlike classical scrapie, it was demonstrated that the presence of phenylalanine at codon 141 strongly associated with atypical cases [51, 53, 100, 106–109]. Interestingly, according to results of case control studies, while VRQ allele which is the most classical scrapie have found to be related to low incidence in atypical scrapie [51, 53, 108], the most resistant ARR allele associated with higher incidence [53, 107, 109]. Distribution of *PRNP* genotypes and roles of codon 141 on atypical scrapie resistance demonstrated in **Table 5**.

Although there is very limited data about relationship atypical scrapie and *PRNP* genotypes in goats, it has been reported that the presence of histidine at codon 154 may associated with atypical cases in goats, as well [103, 109].

European selective breeding programs against to classical scrapie in sheep already eliminating the AHQ and AFRQ alleles which have demonstrated to relate with atypical scrapie susceptibility; however, the major problem about ARR (resistant to classical scrapie but susceptible to atypical scrapie) and VRQ (susceptible to classical scrapie but resistant to atypical scrapie) alleles remains to be solved.

Risk groups for classical scrapie	Genotype of individuals	*n* = 38 [106]	*n* = 69 [51]	*n* = 51 [109]	*n* = 248 [53]
R1	ARR/ARR		0.129	0.118	0.181
R2	ARR/AHQ	0.132	0.217	0.039	0.097
	ARR/ARH		0.014		0.012
	ARR/ARQ		0.029	0.039	0.040
	ARR/**AFRQ**	0.105	0.101	0.314	0.218
R3	ARQ/ARH				
	AFRQ/ARH				0.004
	ARQ/AHQ	0.053	0.174	0.020	0.052
	AFRQ/AHQ	0.211	0.072		0.044
	AHQ/AHQ	0.211	0.145	0.039	0.024
	ARH/ARH			0.020	0.004
	AHQ/ARH	0.026		0.020	0.008
	ARQ/ARQ	0.053			0.008
	ARQ/**AFRQ**	0.079	0.014	0.176	0.173
	AFRQ/AFRQ	0.132	0.087	0.137	0.113
R4	ARR/VRQ				
R5	AHQ/VRQ			0.020	0.004
	ARH/VRQ				0.004
	ARQ/VRQ				
	AFRQ/VRQ		0.014	0.059	0.012
	VRQ/VRQ				

Table 5. *PRNP* genotypes according to codons 136, 154 and 171 (and codon 141 if the presence of phenylalanine residue) and association with atypical scrapie.

4. Resistance in cattle

Bovine spongiform encephalopathy (BSE), the cattle prion disease, belongs to animal TSE's which has been characterized histopathological changes in the CNS as with scrapie. It is newly diagnosed prion disease, which has been never known until 1986 [110]. BSE became epidemic during the 1980s in the UK as a result of the changing rendering process and allowing to enter the prion contaminated product to cattle nutrition, and it is estimated that the exposure began in the early 1980s [110]. Having transmitted to human and causing a new variant of Creutzfeldt-Jakob disease (CJD) [62] which is a human prion disease acquired from consumption of the meat products of the BSE diseased cattle [111], BSE has been regarded by the World Health Organization [112] as zoonotic. Unlike CJD, vCJD has diagnosed in younger people in the UK [113], latter in France [114]. Up to 2003, 135 vCJD cases have reported from the UK and 6 cases from France (reviewed in reference [115]).

BSE could transmit to sheep and goats by experimental routes [116] and development of the disease seemed to be affected by the *PRNP* genotype of the individual [88, 117]; furthermore, it was reported that BSE in goats can be occur in natural conditions [118, 119].

Because of the zoonotic potential and the ability to spread between species of the BSE, it has raised the public health concerns and enforced to governments to take control and preventive measures; moreover, researchers have intensified to reveal the genetic background of the disease.

Early studies on association between *PRNP* genotype of cattle and development of the BSE have focused on two known polymorphisms; the HindII restriction site and an octapeptide repeated sequence in the coding region of the cattle *PRNP*, but no relationship between these genotypes and BSE infection has found [120, 121]; however, although lack of detailed genetic information, some clues were obtained suggesting that BSE might be in linkage with host *PRNP* genotype [9].

In the following years, hundreds of nucleotide changes and insertions/deletions (indel) were identified in bovine *PRNP* [13, 122, 123, 124], including a 12 base pair (bp) indel within the intron 1 and a 23 bp indel within the promoter region [13, 122]. Case control studies showed that distribution of these two indel polymorphisms were different between healthy and BSE affected cattle and insertion alleles presumably connected with disease resistance [13]; moreover, it has demonstrated that insertion alleles related to the lower prion protein level compared with deletion alleles and may differentiate of the BSE incubation period [15]. Further studies have supported the relationship between BSE resistance and 23 bp/12 bp indel genotypes that are given in **Table 6**.

Although the clear association has been shown between *PRNP* indel genotypes and BSE incidence, there are some paradoxical situations at breed level, for example, it was reported that although Brown breeds have higher allelic frequency of insertion alleles, at the same time, these breeds have higher prevalence of BSE [17]. However, beside of the primary measures for prevention from circulation of BSE agents and exposure to both animal and human, selective breeding can offer a secondary strategy to eliminate the BSE.

Apart from classical BSE, two more types of the disease have been diagnosed by histopathological examinations; H-type and L-type, both of two types classified as atypical BSE and have been observing sporadically. While H-type BSE characterized with higher molecular mass [126], L-type BSE which is also named as bovine amyloidotic spongiform encephalopathy (BASE), characterized with lower molecular mass and has diverse glycopattern of pathogenic prion proteins [127].

It is reported that *PRNP* 23 and 12 bp indel polymorphism do not provide the genetic resistance, neither to naturally occurring atypical BSE nor to experimentally inoculated other TSEs [16]. Although very limited data, several atypical cases with extremely rare [128] glutamate to lysine mutation in codon 211 (E211K), which is homologous with human E200K mutation in

http://dx.doi.org/10.5772/66916

	23 bp indel genotypes								
	Healthy cattle				BSE-affected cattle				
Breed	*n*	**in/in**	**in/del**	**del/del**	*n*	**in/in**	**in/del**	**del/del**	**References**
Pooled German breeds	48	0.210	0.440	0.350	43	0.050	0.440	0.510	[13]
UK Holstein	276	0.047	0.489	0.464	363	0.013	0.410	0.554	[16]
German Holstein	313	0.147	0.473	0.380	127	0.079	0.465	0.457	[16]
German Brown	87	0.448	0.414	0.138	43	0.140	0.651	0.209	[16]
German Fleckvieh	136	0.103	0.434	0.463	106	0.066	0.396	0.538	[16]
Pooled German and Switzerland breeds	574	0.160	0.470	0.370	670	0.090	0.470	0.450	[17]
Pooled Japanese breeds	464	0.071	0.440	0.489	6	0.000	0.333	0.467	[20]
Pooled Czech breeds	81	0.235	0.543	0.222	26	0.077	0.538	0.385	[125]
	12 bp indel genotypes								
	Healthy cattle				**BSE-affected cattle**				
Breed	*n*	**in/in**	**in/del**	**del/del**	*n*	**in/in**	**in/del**	**del/del**	**References**
Pooled German breeds	48	0.210	0.560	0.230	43	0.090	0.470	0.440	[13]
UK Holstein	270	0.111	0.519	0.370	350	0.051	0.454	0.494	[16]
German Holstein	309	0.220	0.498	0.282	125	0.144	0.456	0.400	[16]
German Brown	90	0.744	0.222	0.033	43	0.419	0.512	0.070	[16]
German Fleckvieh	137	0.153	0.453	0.394	106	0.085	0.462	0.453	[16]
Pooled German and Switzerland breeds	574	0.230	0.460	0.310	670	0.170	0.490	0.340	[17]
Pooled Japanese breeds	476	0.095	0.468	0.437	6	0.000	0.333	0.467	[20]
Pooled Czech breeds	81	0.358	0.444	0.198	26	0.231	0.462	0.308	[125]

Table 6. The distribution of the *PRNP* 23 bp indel and 12 bp indel genotypes according to breeds, in both healthy and BSE-affected cattle.

the *PRNP* gene, has determined, suggesting that association to atypical BSE resistance may be exist [129, 130], but could not confirm by following studies [131, 132]. Transmissibility of the H-type atypical BSE to cattle which is carrying the E211K mutation was demonstrated [133], on the other hand, some evidences have obtained that the E211K is a germ line mutation, thus, may cause inherited BSE that can be transmitted genetically [130].

5. Resistance in water buffaloes

During the BSE epidemic in 1980s, it can be assumed that BSE and/or scrapie contaminated by-products most likely have entered in to water buffalo (Bubalus bubalis) nutrition systems, as well. EU member states have approximately 409 thousand of buffaloes, where 90% of those have been reared in Italy [134]. Between 2001 and 2005, 128 BSE cases in cattle have been reported from Italy [135]. Along with cattle, bison, sheep, goats and some exotic ruminants, water buffaloes have been considered as TSE-related risk factors [136]; nevertheless, no BSE or any other TSE has ever been reported in water buffaloes [137] neither in Italy nor the rest of the world.

Only few studies on indel polymorphisms of the water buffalo *PRNP* gene have conducted to compare with cattle *PRNP*. According to the results, 12 and 23 bp indel polymorphisms have been existed in water buffalo, as well. Furthermore, insertion alleles which are relate to BSE resistance have observed more frequent than those in cattle [138–141] that is given in **Table 7**.

As seen in **Table 7**, almost all buffalo breeds, except Thai river buffalo, are carrying mostly insertion alleles either at 23 or 12 bp indel loci. This may be an explanation for why buffaloes putatively resistant to BSE.

			23 bp indel alleles		12 bp indel alleles		References
Country	**Breed**	*n*	**In %**	**Del %**	**In %**	**Del %**	
Turkey	Anatolian Buffalo	106	92	8	86	14	[138]
Pakistan	Nili Buffalo	66	94	6	86	14	[139]
	Ravi Buffalo	39	97	3	83	17	
	Azikheli Buffalo	20	100	0	95	5	
	Kundhi Buffalo	34	97	3	88	12	
	Nili Ravi Buffalo	122	94	6	87	13	
Indonesia	River Buffalo	14	100	0	100	0	[142]
Thai	River Buffalo	45	53	47	84	16	
Germany	River Buffalo	11	100	0	100	0	[140]
Poland	River Buffalo	29	100	0	100	0	
Turkey	Anatolian Buffalo	89	100	0	100	0	[141]
	Murrah Buffalo	20	100	0	100	0	

Table 7. 23 and 12 bp allele frequencies of healthy water buffaloes reared in Asian and European states.

The SPRN gene, which belongs to the prion protein gene family, encodes the shadow protein. Shadow protein shares characteristic features with cellular prion protein, suggesting the existence of a functional relation with prion proteins [143]. A comparative study revealed that the SPRN gene has species-specific indel polymorphisms in cattle and buffaloes and causes different promoter activity and expression levels [144]. Furthermore, according to the results of more recent study, molecular structure of buffalo cellular prion protein is different from cattle, but similar to those of rabbits, dog and horse which are considered low susceptible to TSEs [145]. These molecular and structural differences may be another explanation with regard to TSEs resistance in buffaloes.

Author details

Yalçın Yaman[1] and Cemal Ün[2]*

*Address all correspondence to: cemaluen@gmail.com

1 Department of Biometry and Genetics, Sheep Research Institute, Bandirma, Balıkesir, Turkey

2 Department of Biology, Faculty of Science, Ege University, İzmir, Turkey

References

[1] Prusiner SB, Prions. Proceedings of the National Academy of Sciences USA. 1998; **95**:13363–13383.

[2] Hopp P, Ulvund MJ, Jarp J. A case-control study on scrapie in Norwegian sheep flocks. Preventive Veterinary Medicine. 2001;**51**:183–198.

[3] Bucalossi C, Cosseddu G, D'Agostino C, Di Bari MA, Chiappini B, Conte M, Rosone F, De Grossi L, Scavia G, Agrimi U, Nonno R, Vaccari G. Assessment of the genetic susceptibility of sheep to scrapie by protein misfolding cyclic amplification and comparison with experimental scrapie transmission studies. Journal of Virology. 2011;85(16):8386–92. doi:10.1128/JVI.00241-11

[4] Mead S, Stumpf MP, Whitfield J, Beck JA, Poulter M, Campbell T, Uphill JB, Goldstein D, Alpers M, Fisher EM, Collinge J. Balancing selection at the prion protein gene consistent with prehistoric kuru like epidemics. Science. 2003;**300**:640–643. doi:10.1126/science.1083320

[5] Peden AH, Head MW, Ritchie DL, Bell JE, Ironside JW. Preclinical vCJD after blood transfusion in a PRNP codon 129 heterozygous patient. Lancet. 2004;**364**:527–529. doi:10.1016/S0140-6736(04)16811-6

[6] Tranulis MA. Influence of the prion protein gene, PrnP, on scrapie susceptibility in sheep. Acta Pathologica, Microbiologica et Immunologica Scandinavica. 2002;**101**:33–42.

[7] Tongue SC, Wilesmith JW, Cook CJ. Frequencies of prion protein (PrP) genotypes and distribution of ages in 15 scrapie-affected flocks in Great Britain. Veterinary Record. 2004;**154**: 9–16.

[8] Goldmann W, Hunter N, Benson G, Foster JD, Hope J. Different scrapie-associated fibril proteins (PrP) are encoded by lines of sheep selected for different alleles of the sip gene. Journal of General Virology. 1991a;**72**:2411–2417. doi:10.1099/0022-1317-72-10-2411

[9] Neibergs HL, Ryan AM, Womack JE, Spooner RL, Williams JL. Polymorphism analysis of the prion gene in BSE-affected and unaffected cattle. Animal Genetics. 1994;**25**(5):313–17.

[10] Hunter N, Foster JD, Goldmann W, Stear MJ, Hope J, Bostock C. Natural scrapie in a closed flock of Cheviot sheep occurs only in specific PrP genotypes. Archives of Virology 1996;**141**:809–824. doi:10.1007/BF01718157

[11] Walawski K, Czarnik U. Prion protein octapeptide-repeat polymorphism in Polish Black and White cattle. Journal of Applied Genetics. 2003;**44:**191–195.

[12] Heaton MP, Leymaster KA, Freking BA, Hawk DA, Smith TP, Keele JW, Snelling WM, Fox JM, Chitko-McKown CG, Laegreid WW. Prion gene sequence variation within diverse groups of U.S. sheep, beef cattle, and deer. Mammalian Genome. 2003;**14**:765–777. doi:10.1007/s00335-003-2283-y

[13] Sander P, Hamann H, Pfeiffer I, Wemheuer W, Brenig B, Groschup MH, Ziegler U, Distl O, Leeb T. Analysis of sequence variability of the bovine prion protein gene (*PRNP*) in German cattle breeds. Neurogenetics. 2004;**5**(1):19–25. doi:10.1007/s10048-003-0171-y

[14] Seabury CM, Womack JE, Pedrahita J, Derr JN. Comparative PRNP genotyping of U.S. cattle sires for potential association with BSE. Mammalian Genome. 2004;**15**(10):828–833. doi:10.1007/s00335-004-2400-6

[15] Sander P, Hamann H, Drögemüller C, Kashkevich K, Schiebel K, Leeb T. Bovine prion protein gene (*PRNP*) promoter polymorphisms modulate *PRNP* expression and may be responsible for differences in bovine spongiform encephalopathy susceptibility. Journal of Biological Chemistry 2005;**280**(45):37408–14. doi:10.1074/jbc. M506361200

[16] Juling K, Schwarzenbacher H, Williams JL, Fries R. A major genetic component of BSE susceptibility. BMC Biology. 2006;**4**:33. doi:10.1186/1741-7007-4-33

[17] Haase B, Doherr MG, Seuberlich T, Drögemüller C, Dolf G, Nicken P, Schiebel K, Ziegler U, Groschup MH, Zurbriggen A, Leeb T. *PRNP* promoter polymorphisms are associated with BSE susceptibility in Swiss and German cattle. BMC Genetics. 2007;**8**:15. doi:10.1186/1471-2156-8-15

[18] Kashkevich K, Humeny A, Ziegler U, Groschup MH, Nicken P, Leeb T, Fischer C, Becker CM, Schiebel K. Functional relevance of DNA polymorphisms within the promoter region of the prion protein gene and their association to BSE infection. FASEB Journal. 2007;**21**:1547–1555.

[19] Brunelle BW, Hamir AN, Baron T, Biacabe AG, Richt JA, Kunkle RA, Cutlip RC, Miller JM, Nicholson EM. Polymorphisms of the prion gene promoter region that influence classical bovine spongiform encephalopathy susceptibility are not applicable to other transmissible spongiform encephalopathies in cattle. Journal of Animal Science. 2007;**85**(12):3142–47. doi:10.2527/jas.2007-0208

[20] Nakamitsu S, Miyazawa T, Horiuchi M, Onoe S, Ohoba Y, Kitagawa H, Ishiguro N. Sequence variation of bovine prion protein gene in Japanese cattle (Holstein and Japanese Black). The Journal of Veterinary Medical Science. 2006;**68**(1):27–33. doi:JST.JSTAGE/jvms/68.27

[21] Jeong BH, Lee YJ, Kim NH, Carp RI, Kim YS. Genotype distribution of the prion protein gene (PRNP) promoter polymorhisms in Korean cattle. Genome. 2006;**49**:1539–1544. doi:10.1139/g06-110

[22] Czarnik U, Zabolewicz T, Strychalski J, Grzybowski G, Bogusz M, Walawski K. Deletion/insertion polymorphism of the prion protein gene (PRNP) in Polish Holstein-Friesian cattle. Journal of Applied Genetics. 2007;**48**(1):69–71. doi:10.1007/BF03194659

[23] Kerber AR, Hepp D, Passos DT, Weimer TA. Polymorphisms of two indels at the PRNP gene in three beef cattle herds. Biochemical Genetics. 2007;**46**:1–7. doi:10.1007/s10528-007-9113-y

[24] Creutzfeldt HG. Über eine eigenartige herdförmige Erkrankung des Zentralnervensystems. Z Gesamte Neurol Psychiatr. 1920;**57**:1–19.

[25] Gajdusek DC, Zigas V. Degenerative disease of the central nervous system in New Guinea. The endemic occurrence of "kuru" in the native population. The New England Journal of Medicine. 1957;**257**:974–978.

[26] Richardson EP, Masters CL. The nosology of Creutzfeldt-Jakob disease and conditions related to the accumulation of PrPCJD in the nervous system. Brain Pathology. 1995;**5**:33–4.

[27] Palmer MS, Dryden AJ, Hughes JT, Collinge J. Homozygous prion protein genotype predisposes to sporadic Creutzfeldt-Jakob disease. Nature. 1991;**352**:340–342. doi:10.1038/352340a0

[28] Windl O, Dempster M, Estibeiro JP, Lathe R, de Silva R, Esmonde T, Will R, Springbett A, Campbell TA, Sidle KC, Palmer MS, Collinge J. Genetic basis of Creutzfeldt-Jakob disease in the United Kingom: a systematic analysis of predisposing mutations and allelic variation in the *PRNP* gene. Human Genetics. 1996;**98**:259–264.

[29] Shibuya S, Higuchi J, Shin RW, Tateishi J, Kitamoto T. Protective prion protein polymorphisms against sporadic Creutzfeldt-Jakob disease. Lancet. 1998;**351**:419.

[30] Detwiler LA. Scrapie. Revue Scientifique Et Technique-Office International Des Epizooties. 1992;**11**(2):491–537.

[31] M'Gowan JP. Investigation into the disease of sheep called "Scrapie" (Traberkrankheit [or] La Tremblante): with reference to its association with sarcosporidiosis. William Blackwood & Sons; 1914. 116P.

[32] Parry HB. Scrapie: a transmissible hereditary disease of sheep. Nature. 1960;**185**:441–43.

[33] Parry HB. Scrapie: a transmissible and hereditary disease of sheep. Heredity. 1962; **17**:75–105.

[34] Dickinson AG, Stamp JT, Renwick CC. Maternal and lateral transmission of scrapie in sheep. Journal of Comparative Pathology. 1974;**84**(1):19–25. doi:10.1016/0021-9975(74)90023-1

[35] Prusiner SB. Novel proteinaceous infectious particles cause scrapie. Science. 1982;**216**(4542):136–44. doi:10.1126/science.6801762

[36] Dickinson AG, Meikle VM, Fraser H. Identification of a gene which controls the incubation period of some strains of scrapie agent in mice. Journal of Comparative Pathology. 1968;**78**(3):293–99. doi:10.1016/0021-9975(68)90005-4

[37] Foster J, Dickinson A. The unusual properties of CH1641, a sheep-passaged isolate of scrapie. Veterinary Record 1988;**123**:5–8. doi:10.1136/vr.123.1.5

[38] Hope J, Hunter N. Scrapie-associated fibrils, PrP protein and the sinc gene. Ciba Foundation Symposium. 1988;**135**:146–63.

[39] Hunter N, Foster JD, Dickinson AG, Hope J. Linkage of the gene for the scrapie-associated fibril protein (PrP) to the sip gene in Cheviot Sheep. Veterinary Record. 1989;**124**(14):364–66.

[40] Goldmann W, Hunter N, Foster JD, Salbaum JM, Beyreuther K, Hope J. Two alleles of a neural protein gene linked to scrapie in sheep. Proceedings of the National Academy of Sciences of the United States of America. 1990;**87**(7):2476–80.

[41] Iannuzzi L, Palomba R, Di Meo GP, Perucatti A, Ferrara L. Comparative FISH-Mapping of the prion protein gene (*PRNP*) on cattle, river buffalo, sheep and goat chromosomes. Cytogenetics and Cell Genetics. 1998;**81**:202–4. doi:10.1159/0000 15030

[42] Clouscard C, Beaudry P, Elsen JM, Milan D, Dussaucy M, Bounneau C, Schelcher F, Chatelain J, Launay JM, Laplanche JL. Different allelic effects of the codons 136 and 171 of the prion protein gene in sheep with natural scrapie. Journal of General Virology. 1995;**76**:2097–2101.

[43] Laplanche JL, Chatelain J, Westaway D, Thomas S, Dussaucy M, Brugere-Picoux J, Launay M. PrP polymorphisms associated with natural scrapie discovered by denaturing gradient gel electrophoresis. Genomics. 1993;**15**(1):30–37. doi:10.1006/geno. 1993.1006

[44] Hunter N, Goldmann W, Benson G, Foster JD, Hope J. Swaledale sheep affected by natural scrapie differ significantly in PrP genotype frequencies from healthy sheep and those selected for reduced incidence of scrapie. Journal of General Virology 1993;**74**:1025–31. doi:10.1099/0022-1317-74-6-1025

[45] Belt PB, Muileman IH, Schreuder BE, Bos-de Ruijter J, Gielkens AL, Smits MA. Identification of five allelic variants of the sheep PrP gene and their association with natural scrapie. Journal of General Virology 1995; **76**: 509–17. doi:10.1099/0022-1317-76-3-509

[46] Baylis M, Chihota C, Stevenson E, Goldmann W, Smith A, Sivam K, Tongue S, Gravenor MB. Risk of scrapie in British sheep of different prion protein genotype. Journal of General Virology. 2004;**85**:2735–40. doi:10.1099/vir.0.79876-0

[47] Ikeda T, Horiuchi M, Ishiguro N, Muramatsu Y, Kai-Uwe GD, Shinagawa M. Amino acid polymorphisms of PrP with reference to onset of scrapie in Suffolk and Corriedale sheep in Japan. Journal of General Virology. 1995;**76**:2577–81. doi:10.1099/0022-1317-76-10-2577

[48] Groschup MH, Lacroux C, Buschmann A, Lühken G, Mathey J, Eiden M, Lugan S, Hoffmann C, Espinosa JC, Baron T, Torres JM, Erhardt G, Andreoletti O. Classic scrapie in sheep with the ARR/ARR prion genotype in Germany and France. Emerging Infectious Diseases. 2007;**13**(8);1201–7. doi:10.3201/eid1308.070077

[49] Tranulis MA, Osland A, Bratberg B, Ulvund MJ. Prion protein gene polymorphisms in sheep with natural scrapie and healthy controls in Norway. Journal of General Virology. 1999;80:1073–77. doi:10.1099/0022-1317-80-4-1073

[50] Baylis M, Goldmann W, Houston F, Cairns D, Chong A, Ross A, Smith A, Hunter N, McLean AR. Scrapie epidemic in a fully PrP-genotyped sheep flock. The Journal of General Virology. 2002;**83**:2907–14. doi:10.1099/0022-1317-83-11-2907

[51] Saunders GC, Cawthraw S, Mountjoy SJ, Hope J, Windl O. PrP genotypes of atypical scrapie cases in Great Britain. Journal of General Virology. 2006;**87**:3141–49. doi:10.1099/vir.0.81779-0

[52] François D, Elsen JM, Barillet F, Lajous D, Eychenne F, Palhière I. Breeding sheep for scrapie resistance CIHEAM. 2003;**55**:29–35.

[53] Fediaevsky A, Calavas D, Gasqui P, Moazami-Goudarzi K, Laurent P, Arsac J-N, Ducrot C, Moreno C. Quantitative estimation of genetic risk for atypical scrapie in french sheep and potential consequences of the current breeding programme for resistance to scrapie on the risk of atypical scrapie. Genetics Selection Evolution 2010;**42**(1):1–7. doi:10.1186/1297-9686-42-14

[54] O'Doherty E, Healy A, Aherne M, Hanrahan JP, Weavers E, Doherty M, Roche JF, Gunn M, Sweeney T. Prion Protein (PrP) gene polymorphisms associated with natural scrapie cases and their flock-mates in Ireland. Research in Veterinary Science. 2002;**73**(3):243–50. doi:10.1016/S0034-5288(02)00073-5

[55] Acutis PL, Sbaiz L, Verburg F, Riina MV, Ru G, Moda G, Caramelli M, Bossers A. Low frequency of the scrapie resistance-associated allele and presence of lysine-171 allele of the prion protein gene in Italian Biellese ovine breed. The Journal of General Virology. 2004;**85**:3165–72. doi:10.1099/vir.0.80053-0

[56] Thorgeirsdottir S, Sigurdarson S, Thorisson HM, Georgsson G, Palsdottir A. PrP gene polymorphism and natural scrapie in Icelandic Sheep. Journal of General Virology. 1999;**80**:2527–34.

[57] Billinis C, Psychas V, Leontides L, Spyrou V, Argyroudis S, Vlemmas I, Leontides S, Sklaviadis T, Papadopoulos O. Prion protein gene polymorphisms in healthy and scrapie-affected sheep in Greece. The Journal of General Virology. 2004;**85**:547–54. doi:10.1099/vir.0.19520-0

[58] Harrington NP, O'Rourke KI, Feng Y, Rendulich J, Difruscio C, Balachandran A. Prion genotypes of scrapie-infected Canadian Sheep 1998-2008. Canadian Journal of Veterinary Research. 2010;**74**(3):228–232.

[59] Gibbs CJ, Gajdusek DC. Transmission of scrapie to the cynomolgus monkey (*Macaca fascicularis*). Nature. 1972;**236**(5341):73–74. doi:10.1038/236073a0

[60] Bruce M, Chree A, McConnell I, Foster J, Pearson G, Fraser H. Transmission of bovine spongiform encephalopathy and scrapie to mice: strain variation and the species barrier. Philosophical Transactions of the Royal Society of London. Series B, Biological Sciences. 1994;**343**(1306):405–11. doi:10.1098/rstb.1994.0036

[61] Kimberlin RH, Walker CA. Evidence that the transmission of one source of scrapie agent to hamsters involves separation of agent strains from a mixture. Journal of General Virology. 1978;**39**(3):487–96. doi:10.1099/0022-1317-39-3-487

[62] Bruce ME, Will RG, Ironside JW, McConnell I, Drummond D, Suttie A, McCardle L, Chree A, Hope J, Birkett C, Cousens S, Fraser H, Bostock CJ. Transmissions to mice indicate that 'new variant' CJD is caused by the BSE agent. Nature. 1997;**389**(6650):498–501. doi:10.1038/39057

[63] Nathanson N, Wilesmith J, Griot C, Bovine spongiform encephalopathy (BSE): Causes and consequences of a common source epidemic. American Journal of Epidemiology. 1997;**145**(11):959–69. doi:10.1093/aje/kwi188

[64] Comoy EE, Mikol J, Luccantoni-Freire S, Correia E, Lescoutra-Etchegaray N, Durand V, Dehen C, Andreoletti O, Casalone C, Richt JA, Greenlee JJ, Baron T,.Benestad SL, Brown P, Deslys J-P. 2015. Transmission of scrapie prions to primate after an extended silent incubation period. Nature. 2015;**5**;11573 Scientific Reports doi:10.1038/srep11573

[65] DEFRA. National Scrapie Plan for Great Britaint. 2001;1 (July):1–28.

[66] Commission Decision, "Laying down minimum requirements for the establishment of breeding programmes for resistance to transmissible spongiform encephalopathies in sheep." Official Journal 2003/100/E:L41–45.

[67] EFSA. Scientific opinion on the scrapie situation in the EU after 10 years of monitoring and control in sheep and goats. EFSA Journal, 2014;**12**(7). doi:10.2903/j.efsa. 2014.3781

[68] Hunter N, Cairns D. Scrapie-free merino and poll dorset sheep from Australia and New Zealand have normal frequencies of scrapie-susceptible PrP genotypes. Journal of General Virology. 1998;**79**:2079–82. doi:10.1099/0022-1317-79-8-2079

[69] Ianella P, McManus CM, Caetano AR, Paiva SR. *PRNP* Haplotype and genotype frequencies in Brazilian sheep: Issues for conservation and breeding programs. Research in Veterinary Science. 2012;**93**(1):219–25. doi:10.1016/j.rvsc.2011.06.025

[70] Gootwine E, Abdulkhaliq A, Jawasreh KIZ, Valle Zárate A. Screening for polymorphism at the prion protein (PrP) locus (*PRNP*) in Awassi and Assaf populations in Israel, the Palestinian Authority and Jordan. Small Ruminant Research. 2008:**77**(1):80–83. doi:10.1016/j.smallrumres.2008.02.008

[71] Yaman Y, Soysal M, Ün C. Evaluation of the genetic resistance status to classical and atypical scrapie in Karacabey merino rams. Turkish Journal of Veterinary and Animal Sciences. 2015;**39**:736–40. doi:10.3906/vet-1507-36

[72] Lühken G, Lipsky S, Peter C, Erhardt E. Prion protein polymorphisms in autochthonous European sheep breeds in respect to scrapie eradication in affected flocks. Small Ruminant Research. 2008:**75**(1):43–47. doi:10.1016/j.smallrumres.2007.07.010

[73] Tsunoda K, Namikawa T, Sato K, Hasnath MA, Nyunt MM, Rajbandary HB, Loc CB, Zanchiv Ts, Chang H, Sun W, Dorji T. Prion protein polymorphisms and estimation of risk of scrapie in East Asian sheep. Biochemical Genetics. 2010;**48**(1–2): 13–25. doi:10.1007/s10528-009-9287-6

[74] Chelle PL. A case of trembling in the goat. Academie Veterinaire de France Bulletin. 1942;**15**:294–295.

[75] EFSA. Scientific opinion on genetic TSE resistance in goats in all European Union. EFSA Journal. 2009;**7**(11):1–42. doi:10.2903/j.efsa.2009.1371

[76] Wood JN, Done SH, Pritchard GC, Wooldridge MJ. Natural scrapie in goats: Case histories and clinical signs. Veterinary Record. 1992;**131**(4):66–68. doi:10.1136/vr.131.4.66

[77] Sofianidis G, Psychas V, Billinis C, Spyrou V, Argyroudis S, Papaioannou N, Vlemmas I. Histopathological and immunohistochemical features of natural goat scrapie. Journal of Comparative Pathology. 2006;**135**(2–3):116–29. doi:10.1016/j.jcpa. 2006.06.004

[78] Papasavva-Stylianou P, Kleanthous M, Toumazos P, Mavrikiou P, Loucaides P. Novel polymorphisms at codons 146 and 151 in the prion protein gene of Cyprus goats, and their association with natural scrapie. Veterinary Journal. 2007;**173**(2):459–62. doi:10.1016/j.tvjl.2005.09.013

[79] Brotherston JG, Renwick CC, Stamp JT, Zlotnik I, Pattison IH. Spread of scrapie by contact to goats and sheep. Journal of Comparative Pathology. 1968;**78**:9–17. doi:10.1016/0021-9975(68)90107-2

[80] Billinis C, Panagiotidis CH, Psychas V, Argyroudis S, Nicolaou A, Leontides S, Papadopoulos O, Sklaviadis T. Prion protein gene polymorphisms in natural goat scrapie. Journal of General Virology. 2002;**83**;713–21. doi:10.1099/0022-1317-83-3-713

[81] Toumazos P, Alley MR. Scrapie in goats in Cyprus. New Zealand Veterinary Journal 1989;**37**(4):160–62. doi:10.1080/00480169.1989.35595

[82] Vaccari G, Panagiotidis CH, Acin C, Peletto S, Barillet F, Acutis P, Bossers A, Langeveld J, van Keulen L, Sklaviadis T, Badiola JJ, Andreéoletti O, Groschup MH, Agrimi U, Foster J, Goldmann W. State-of-the-art review of goat TSE in the European Union, with special emphasis on *PRNP* genetics and epidemiology. Veterinary Research. 2009;**40**(5):48. doi:10.1051/vetres/2009031

[83] Vaccari G, Di Bari MA, Morelli L, Nonno R, Chiappini B, Antonucci G, Marcon S, Esposito E, Fazzi P, Palazzini N, Troiano P, Petrella A, Di Guardo G, Agrimi U. Identification of an allelic variant of the goat PrP gene associated with resistance to scrapie. Journal of General Virology. 2006;**87**:1395–1402. doi:10.1099/vir.0.81485-0

[84] Acutis PL, Colussi S, Santagada G, Laurenza C, Maniaci MG, Riina MV, Peletto S, Goldmann W, Bossers A, Caramelli M, Cristoferi I, Maione S, Sacchi P, Rasero R. Genetic variability of the *PRNP* gene in goat breeds from northern and southern Italy. Journal of Applied Microbiology. 2008;**104**(6):1782–89. doi:10.1111/j.1365-2672.2007.03703.x

[85] Goldmann W, Perucchini M, Smith A, Hunter N. Genetic variability of the PrP gene in a goat herd in the UK. Veterinary Record. 2004;**155**:177–178.

[86] Goldmann W, Ryan K, Stewart P, Parnham D, Xicohtencatl R, Fernandez N, Saunders G, Windl O, González L, Bossers A, Foster J. Caprine prion gene polymorphisms are associated with decreased incidence of classical scrapie in goat herds in the United Kingdom. Veterinary Research. 2011;**42**:110. doi:10.1186/1297-9716-42-110

[87] Serrano C, Hammouchi M, Benomar A, Lyahyai J, Ranera B, Acín C, el Hamidi M, Monzón M, Badiola JJ, Tligui N, Zaragoza P, Martín-Burriel I. *PRNP* haplotype distribution in Moroccan goats. Animal Genetics. 2009;**40**(4):565–68. doi:10.1111/j.1365-2052.2009.01873.x

[88] Goldmann W, Martin T, Foster J, Hughes S, Smith G, Hughes K, Dawson M, Hunter N. Novel polymorphisms in the caprine PrP gene: A codon 142 mutation associated with scrapie incubation period. Journal of General Virology. 1996;**77**:2885–91. doi:10.1099/0022-1317-77-11-2885

[89] Barillet F, Mariat D, Amigues Y, Faugeras R, Caillat H, Moazami-Goudarzi K, Rupp R, Babilliot JM, Lacroux C, Lugan S, Schelcher F, Chartier C, Corbière F, Andréoletti O, Perrin-Chauvineau C. Identification of seven haplotypes of the caprine PrP gene at codons 127, 142, 154, 211, 222 and 240 in French alpine and saanen breeds and their association with classical scrapie. Journal of General Virology. 2009;**90**:769–76. doi:10.1099/vir.0.006114-0

[90] White SN, Reynolds JO, Waldron DF. Extended scrapie incubation time in goats singly heterozygous for *PRNP* S146 or K222. Gene. 2012;**501**:49–51. doi:10.1016/j.gene.2012.03.068

[91] Wopfner F, Weidenhöfer G, Schneider R, von Brunn A, Gilch S, Schwarz TF, Werner T, Schätzl HM. Analysis of 27 mammalian and 9 avian PrPs reveals high conservation of flexible regions of the prion protein. Journal of Molecular Biology. 1999;**289**(5):1163–78. doi:10.1006/jmbi.1999.2831

[92] Zhou RY, Li XL, Li LH, Wang HY, Lü JG. Polymorphism of the *PRNP* gene in the main breeds of indigenous Chinese goats. Archives of Virology. 2008;**153**:979–82. doi:10.1007/s00705-008-0074-1

[93] Acutis PL, Bossers A, Priem J, Riina MV, Peletto S, Mazza M, Casalone C, Forloni G, Ru G, Caramelli M. Identification of prion protein gene polymorphisms in goats from Italian scrapie outbreaks. The Journal of General Virology. 2006;87:1029–33. doi:10.1099/vir.0.81440-0

[94] Acutis PL, Martucci F, D'Angelo A, Peletto S, Colussi S, Maurella C, Porcario C, Iulini B, Mazza M, Dell'atti L, Zuccon F, Corona C, Martinelli N, Casalone C, Caramelli M, Lombardi G. Resistance to classical scrapie in experimentally challenged goats carrying mutation k222 of the prion protein gene. Veterinary Research. 2012;**1**:43–8. doi:10.1186/1297-9716-43-8

[95] Goldmann W, Chong A, Foster J, Hope J, Hunter N. The shortest known prion protein gene allele occurs in goats, has only three octapeptide repeats and is non-pathogenic. Journal of General Virology. 1998;**79**:3173–3176.

[96] Lan XY, Zhao HY, Li ZJ, Li AM, Lei CZ, Chen H, Pan CY. A novel 28-bp insertion–deletion polymorphism within goat *PRNP* gene and its association with production traits in Chinese native breeds. Genome. 2012;**55**(7):547–52. doi:10.1139/g2012-040

[97] Benestad SL, Sarradin P, Thu B, Schönheit J, Tranulis MA, Bratberg B. Cases of scrapie with unusual features in Norway and designation of a new type, Nor98. The Veterinary Record. 2003;**153**:202–8.

[98] Bruce ME, Nonno R, Foster J, Goldmann W, Di Bari M, Esposito E, Benestad SL, Hunter N, Agrimi U. Nor98-like sheep scrapie in the United Kingdom in 1989. Veterinary Record. 2007;**160**:665–66. doi:10.1136/vr.160.19.665

[99] Webb PR, Powell L, Denyer M, Marsh S, Weaver C, Simmons MM, Johns E, Sheehan J, Horsfield P, Lyth C, Wilson C, Long A, Cawthraw S, Saunders GC, Spencer YI. A retrospective immunohistochemical study reveals atypical scrapie has existed in the United Kingdom since at least 1987. Journal of Veterinary Diagnostic Investigation. 2009;**21**(6):826–29.

[100] Buschmann A, Biacabe A-G, Ziegler U, Bencsik A, Madec J-Y, Erhardt G, Lühken G, Baron T, Groschup MH. Atypical scrapie cases in Germany and France are identified by discrepant reaction patterns in BSE rapid tests. Journal of Virological Methods 2004;**117**(1):27–36. doi:10.1016/j.jviromet.2003.11.017

[101] Everest SJ, Thorne L, Barnicle DA, Edwards JC, Elliott H, Jackman R, Hope J. Atypical prion protein in sheep brain collected during the British scrapie-surveillance programme. Journal of General Virology. 2006;**87**:471–77. doi:10.1099/vir.0.81539-0

[102] Seuberlich T, Botteron C, Benestad SL, Brünisholz H, Wyss R, Kihm U, Schwermer H, Friess M, Nicolier A, Heim D, Zurbriggen A. Atypical scrapie in a Swiss goat and

implications for transmissible spongiform encephalopathy surveillance. Journal of Veterinary Diagnostic Investigation. 2007;**19**(1):2–8. doi:10.1177/10406387070 1900102

[103] Colussi S, Vaccari G, Maurella C, Bona C, Lorenzetti R, Troiano P, Casalinuovo F, Di Sarno A, Maniaci MG, Zuccon F, Nonno R, Casalone C, Mazza M, Ru G, Caramelli M, Agrimi U, Acutis PL. Histidine at codon 154 of the prion protein gene is a risk factor for Nor98 scrapie in goats. Journal of General Virology 2008;**89**:3173–76. doi:10.1099/vir.0.2008/004150-0

[104] Mitchell GB, O'Rourke KI, Harrington NP, Soutyrine A, Simmons MM, Dudas S, Zhuang D, Laude H, Balachandran A. Identification of atypical scrapie in Canadian Sheep. Journal of Veterinary Diagnostic Investigation. 2010;**22**(3):408–11. doi:10.1177/104063871002200310

[105] Kittelberger R, Chaplin MJ, Simmons MM, Ramirez-Villaescusa A, McIntyre L, MacDiarmid SC, Hannah MJ, Jenner J, Bueno R, Bayliss D, Black H, Pigott CJ, O'Keefe JS. Atypical scrapie/Nor98 in a sheep from New Zealand. Journal of Veterinary Diagnostic Investigation. 2010:**22**(6):863–75. doi:10.1177/10406387100220060

[106] Moum T, Olsaker I, Hopp P, Moldal T, Valheim M, Moum T, Benestad SL. Polymorphisms at codons 141 and 154 in the ovine prion protein gene are associated with scrapie Nor98 cases. Journal of General Virology. 2005;**86**(1):231–35. doi:10.1099/vir.0.80437-0

[107] Lühken G1, Buschmann A, Brandt H, Eiden M, Groschup MH, Erhardt G. Epidemiological and genetical differences between classical and atypical scrapie cases. Veterinary Research. 2007;**38**(1):65–80. doi:10.1006/geno.1993.1006

[108] Moreno CR, Moazami-Goudarzi K, Laurent P, Cazeau G, Andreoletti O, Chadi S, Elsen JM, Calavas D. Which prp haplotypes in a French sheep population are the most susceptible to atypical scrapie? Archives of Virology. 2007;**152**(6):1229–32. doi:10.1007/s00705-007-0956-7

[109] Arsac JN, Andreoletti O, Bilheude J-M, Lacroux C, Benestad SL, Taron T. Similar Biochemical signatures and prion protein genotypes in atypical scrapie and Nor98 cases, France and Norway. Emerging Infectious Diseases. 2007;**13**(1):58–65. doi:10.3201/eid1301.060393

[110] Wilesmith JW. Bovine Spongiform encephalopathy and related Diseases: An epidemiological overview. New Zealand Veterinary Journal. 1994;**42**(1):1–8. doi: 10.1080/00480169.1994.35774

[111] Ghani AC, Donnelly CA, Ferguson NM, Anderson RM. The transmission dynamics of BSE and vCJD. Comptes Rendus Biologies. 2002;**325**(1):37–47. doi:10.1016/S1631-0691(02)01389-6

[112] WHO "World Health Organization." World Health Organization WHO/CDS/CS (WHO Consultation on public health and animal TSEs epidemiology, risk and research requirements: 2000;1–47.

[113] Will RG, Ironside JW, Zeidler M, Estibeiro, Cousens SN, Smith PG, Alperovitch A, Poser S, Pocchiari M, Hofman M. A new variant of Creutzfeldt-Jakob disease in the UK. Lancet. 1996;**347**(9006):921–25. doi:10.5555/uri:pii:S0140673696914129

[114] Chazot G, Broussolle E, Lapras Cl, Blättler T, Aguzzi A, Kopp N. New variant of Creutzfeldt-Jakob disease in a 26-year-old French man. Lancet (London, England) 1996;**347**(9009):1181. doi:10.5555/uri:pii:S0140673696906388

[115] Will RG. Acquired prion disease: iatrogenic CJD, variant CJD, kuru. British Medical Bulletin. 2003;**66**:255–65. doi:10.1093/bmb/66.1.255

[116] Foster JD, Hope J, Fraser H. Transmission of bovine spongiform encephalopathy to sheep and goats. Veterinary Record. 1993;**133**(14):339–341. doi:10.1136/vr.133.14.339

[117] Foster JD, Parnham D, Chong A, Goldmann W, Hunter N. Clinical signs, histopathology and genetics of experimental transmission of BSE and natural scrapie to sheep and goats. Veterinary Record. 2001;**148**:165–71. doi:10.1136/vr.148.6.165

[118] Eloit M, Adjou K, Coulpier M, Fontaine JJ, Hamel R, Lilin T, Messiaen S, Andreoletti O, Baron T, Bencsik A, Biacabe AG, Beringue V, Laude H, Le Dur A, Vilotte JL, Comoy E, Deslys JP, Grassi J, Simon S, Lantier F, Sarradin P. BSE agent signatures in a goat. Veterinary Record. 2005;**156**(16):523–24.

[119] Spiropoulos J, Lockey R, Sallis RE, Terry LA, Thorne L, Holder TM, Beck KE, Simmons MM. Isolation of prion with BSE properties from farmed goat. Emerging Infectious Diseases. 2011;**17**(12):2253–61.

[120] Goldmann W, Hunter N, Martin T, Dawson M, Hope J. Different forms of the bovine PrP gene have five or six copies of a short, G-C-rich element within the protein-coding exon. Journal of General Virology. 1991b;**72:**201–204.

[121] Hunter N, Goldmann w, G Smith, Hope j. Frequencies of PrP gene variants in healthy cattle and cattle with BSE in Scotland. Veterinary Record. 1994;**135**(17):400–403.

[122] Hills D, Comincini S, Schlaepfer J, Dolf G, Ferretti L, Williams JL. Complete genomic sequence of the bovine prion gene (PRNP) and polymorphism in its promoter region. Animal Genetics. 2001;**32**(4):231–232. doi:10.1046/j.1365-2052.2001.0769a.x

[123] Hills D, Schlaepfer J, Comincini S, MacLean I, Dolf G, Ferretti L, Olsaker I, Williams JL. Sequence variation in the bovine and ovine *PRNP* genes. Animal Genetics. 2003;**34**(3):183–90. doi:10.1046/j.1365-2052.2003.00977.x

[124] Clawson ML, Heaton MP, Keele JW, Smith TP, Harhay GP, Laegreid WW. Prion gene haplotypes of U.S. Cattle. BMC Genetics. 2006;**7**:51. doi:10.1186/1471-2156-7-51

[125] Vernerova K, Tothova L, Mikova A, Vodrazka P, Simek B, Hanusova L, Citek J. BSE-associated polymorphisms in the prion protein gene : An investigation. Journal of Animal Breeding and Genetics. 2014;**131**(5):403–408. doi:10.1111/jbg.12090

[126] Biacabe AG, Laplanche JL, Ryder S, Baron T. Distinct molecular phenotypes in bovine prion diseases. EMBO Reports. 2004;**5**;110–15. doi:10.1038/sj.embor.7400054

[127] Casalone C, Zanusso G, Acutis P, Ferrari S, Capucci L, Tagliavini F, Monaco S, Caramelli M. Identification of a second bovine amyloidotic spongiform encephalopathy: Molecular similarities with sporadic Creutzfeldt-Jakob disease. Proceedings of the National Academy of Sciences of the United States of America. 2004;**101**(9):3065–70. doi:10.1073/pnas.0305777101

[128] Heaton MP, Keele JW, Harhay GP, Richt JA, Koohmaraie M, Wheeler TL, Shackelford SD, Casas E, King DA, Sonstegard TS, Van Tassell CP, Neibergs HL, Chase CC Jr, Kalbfleisch TS, Smith TP, Clawson ML, Laegreid WW. Prevalence of the prion protein gene E211K variant in U.S. Cattle. BMC Veterinary Research. 2008;**4**:25. doi:10.1186/1746-6148-4-25

[129] Richt JA, Mark Hall S. BSE with case associated prion protein gene mutation. PLoS Pathogens. 2008;**4**(9):e1000156. doi:10.1371/journal.ppat.1000156

[130] Nicholson EM, Brunelle BW, Richt JA, Kehrli ME Jr, Greenlee JJ. Identification of a heritable polymorphism in bovine *PRNP* associated with genetic transmissible spongiform encephalopathy: Evidence of heritable BSE. PloS One. 2008;**3**(8):e2912. doi:10.1371/journal.pone.0002912

[131] Clawson ML, Richt JA, Baron T, Biacabe AG, Czub S, Heaton MP, Smith TP, Laegreid WW. Association of a bovine prion gene haplotype with atypical BSE. PloS One. 2008;**3**(3):e1830. doi:10.1371/journal

[132] Gurgul A, Polak MP, Larska M, Słota E. *PRNP* and SPRN genes polymorphism in atypical bovine spongiform encephalopathy cases diagnosed in Polish Cattle. Journal of Applied Genetics. 2012;**53**(3):337–42. doi:10.1007/s13353-012-0102-4

[133] Greenlee JJ, Smith JD, West Greenlee MH, Nicholson EM. Clinical and pathologic features of H-type bovine spongiform encephalopathy associated with e211k prion protein polymorphism. PloS One. 2012;**7**(6):e38678. doi:10.1371/journal.pone. 0038678

[134] Anonymous. Agriculture statistics at regional level. [Internet]. 2015. http://ec.europa.eu/eurostat/statistics-explained/index.php/Agriculture_statistics_at_regional_level#Further_Eurostat_information [Accessed: 21.02.2015].

[135] Ru G, Maurella C, Maroni Ponti A, Ingravalle F, Caramelli M. Epidemiological study of the decline of BSE in Italy. Veterinary Record. 2007;**161**(15):511–14. doi:10.1136/vr.161.15.511

[136] Morley RS, Chen S, Rheault N. Assessment of the risk factors related to bovine spongiform encephalopathy. Revue scientifique et Technique. 2003;**22**(1):157–78.

[137] Di Guardo G. BSE in buffaloes. The Veterinary Record. 2014;174(19):485. doi:10.1136/vr.g3177

[138] Oztabak K, Ozkan E, Soysal I, Paya I, Un C. Detection of prion gene promoter and intron1 indel polymorphisms in Anatolian water buffalo (*Bubalus bubalis*). Journal of Animal Breeding and Genetics. 2009;**126**(6):463–67. doi:10.1111/j.1439-0388.2009.00821.x

[139] Imran M, Mahmood S, Babar ME, Hussain R, Yousaf MZ, Abid NB, Lone KP. *PRNP* gene variation in Pakistani cattle and buffaloes. Gene. 2012;**505**:180–85. doi:10.1016/j.gene.2012.05.038

[140] Kobak P, Sablik S, Zukiewicz A, Syczewski A, Lechowicz W. Analysis of indel polymorphism of the *PRNP* gene in water buffalo, *Bubalus bubalis*. Acta Scientiarum Polonorum Zootechnica. 2014;**13**(1):51–56.

[141] Yaman Y, Karadağ O, Ün C. Investigation of the prion protein gene (*PRNP)* polymorphisms in Anatolian, Murrah and crossbred water buffaloes (*Bubalus bubalis*). Tropical Animal Health and Production. doi:10.1007/s11250-016-1185-4

[142] Uchida L, Heriyanto A, Thongchai C, Hanh TT, Horiuchi M, Ishihara K, Tamura Y, Muramatsu Y. Genetic diversity in the prion protein gene (*PRNP*) of domestic cattle and water buffaloes in Vietnam, Indonesia and Thailand. Journal of Veterinary Medical Science. 2014;**76**(7):1001–8.

[143] Premzl M, Sangiorgio L, Strumbo B, Marshall Graves JA, Simonic T, Gready JE. Shadoo, a new protein highly conserved from fish to mammals and with similarity to prion protein. Gene. 2003;**314**:89–102. doi:10.1016/S0378-1119(03)00707-8

[144] Zhao H, Liu LL, Du SH, Wang SQ, Zhang YP. Comparative analysis of the shadoo gene between cattle and buffalo reveals significant differences. PloS One. 2012;**7**(10):e46601. doi:10.1371/journal.pone.0046601

[145] Zhang J, Wang F, Chatterjee S. Molecular dynamics studies on the buffalo prion protein. Journal of Biomolecular Structure & Dynamics. 2015;**34**(4):762–777. doi:10.1080/07391102.2015.1052849

Section 5

Modeling Prion In Silico and Neurobehavioral testing In Vitro

Chapter 9

Neurobehavioral Testing in Prion Disease Studies

Davis M. Seelig , Michael A. Benneyworth and
Damani N. Bryant

Additional information is available at the end of the chapter

http://dx.doi.org/10.5772/67520

Abstract

The prion diseases are neurodegenerative diseases characterized by progressive neurocognitive decline and terminal dementia. In this review, we will discuss the role of neurobehavioral testing in mammalian prion disease model systems, including (1) a review of the clinical phenotype of the major prion diseases in natural disease, (2) an evidence-based summary of the benefits and shortcomings of commonly used behavioral assays, and (3) a review of the neurobehavioral testing in rodent prion models. Based upon this review, and in light of the established importance of model systems in studies of prion pathogenesis and the proven role of behavioral testing in nonprion disease neurodegenerative diseases, it is vital that prion researchers consider the clinical consequences of prion infection so as to maximize the impact of their work.

Keywords: prion diseases, clinical signs, mouse models, behavioral testing, comparative neurosciences

1. Introduction

The prion diseases, or transmissible spongiform encephalopathies (TSEs), are a group of fatal neurodegenerative disorders resulting from the accumulation of a unique, nucleic-acid free/protein-only, infectious agent. Prion diseases affect both humans and nonhumans alike and include diseases that have genetic (familial or sporadic) or infectious causes. The pivotal and unifying event in prion pathogenesis is the posttranslational misfolding of the host-encoded, normal cellular prion protein (denoted PrP^{C}) into a misfolded variant (denoted PrP^{Sc} or PrP^{D}). Misfolding is characterized by increased β-sheet content, decreased α-helical content, and by conferred resistance to detergents, alcohol, formalin, proteases, boiling, autoclaving, and radiation [1]. The resulting PrP^{Sc} acts as a template for its self-propagation. In addition to their shared mechanism, prion diseases are united by their pathology, which includes amyloid deposition, vacuolization, synaptic dysfunction, glial-mediated neuroinflammation, and neuronal death.

INTECH
open science | open minds

Although the terminal pathologic event in prion disease is neuronal death and the terminal clinical event is neuronal death, the link between these is unclear. Historically, two competing hypotheses have been proposed, namely (1) a loss-of-function hypothesis or (2) a gain-of-function hypothesis. Based upon studies demonstrating that pre- and postnatal knockdown of PrP^{C} expression fails to replicate bona fide prion disease, it seems unlikely loss of function contributes significantly to prion pathogenesis [2–4]. However, while it is increasingly likely that an alternate isoform of PrP^{C} is responsible for prion toxicity, it is unclear whether this species presents a protease-sensitive or resistant form, a monomeric or oligomeric form, or if interactions with additional components are necessary. Lastly, while this model implicates PrP^{Sc} as a *necessary* player in the development of prion disease neurodegeneration, there is extensive work implicating that it is unlikely to be singularly *sufficient* to cause clinical prion disease. To this point, there are numerous studies demonstrating subclinical prion disease in which models accumulate often extensive amounts of PrP^{Sc} without developing clinical disease [5–10].

In a disease system rife with novelty, one of the most intriguing and clinically relevant aspects of prion disease biology is the existence of strains. Originally recognized in studies of sheep and goats with experimental scrapie, but the best characterized in scrapie-infected mice, the concept of strains reflects clinical, pathologic, and structural variants of prion disease [11]. Prion strains are unique isolates that demonstrate different phenotypical and biochemical differences when transmitted into identical hosts. Classically, these differences include pattern of PrP^{Sc} distribution (both within and outside of the CNS), PrP^{Sc} plaque morphology, vacuolar profile, incubation period, susceptibility to PK digestion, glycosylation profile, incubation period, and, most important for this article, clinical disease phenotype [12–14]. The biologic basis for strains is not entirely clear, but it is hypothesized that unique PrP^{Sc} confirmations and polymorphisms are significant contributors [15–17].

In a review of neurobehavioral testing in prion diseases, it is worth noting that there is not always a clear or proportional relationship between disease neuropathology (i.e., PrP^{Sc} accumulation, gliosis, and neuronal loss) and clinical phenotype. This is most dramatically represented in subclinical prion disease (i.e., measurable CNS PrP^{Sc} without clinical disease) and in prion-infected animals demonstrating significant clinical disease but lacking detectable PrP^{Sc} [7, 18, 19]. This lack of correlation between patterns of brain PrP^{Sc} deposition and clinical disease is well documented in many natural and experimentally infected TSE affected animals, including TSE-infected cattle, goats, and mice [18, 20–22]. In addition, a discordant relationship between neuronal loss and clinical signs is reported in BSE-infected cattle and between neuroinflammation and clinical signs in scrapie-infected sheep [23–27]. The cause(s) of this disparate relationship between PrP^{Sc} and prion disease are not completely clear, but the limited sensitivity of traditional PrP^{Sc} detection tools, the increasing recognition of the toxicity of protease-sensitive forms of misfolded PrP, and the complexity of the tissue response to misfolded prion protein likely contribute [27]. Finally, it is likely that shortcomings in behavioral testing have contributed to historical inabilities to document clinical disease in prion-infected animals, particularly those in which neurobehavioral deficits may be subtle. This is particularly likely in large animals, in which the vague and imprecise early clinical signs of TSE infection can mimic a number of nonprion infectious conditions.

2. Clinical phenotype of prion diseases

Despite their unifying cause, individual prion diseases demonstrate unique clinical presentations. This clinical heterogeneity not only applies between differing diseases (i.e., CJD vs. FFI) but also within a particular disease. The following section summarizes the major clinical features of the most common prion diseases of humans and domestic animals.

2.1. Creutzfeld-Jakob disease (CJD)

Creutzfeld-Jakob disease (CJD) is the most common form of human prion disease and can be divided into sporadic, hereditary (i.e., familial), iatrogenic, or variant forms. The hereditary form can be further subdivided into three distinct phenotypic subtypes, namely (1) Gerstmann-Straussler-Scheinker (GSS) disease, (2) fatal familial insomnia (FFI), and familial CJD (fCJD). Although the following section will review the unique clinical features of each of these forms, all variants of CJD are generally characterized by a rapid, progressive onset of dementia of unknown origin [28].

Sporadic CJD (sCJD) is the most common form of CJD, representing approximately 85% of cases [29]. Although six major variants of sCJD are recognized according to differences in molecular, genetic, and biochemical features, most CJD variants present a similar clinical phenotype [30, 31]. The common features of CJD are represented by progressive dementia with some combination of myoclonus, visual deficits, cerebellar disturbances, pyramidal or extrapyramidal symptoms (spasticity, hyperactive reflexes, muscle contractions, alterations in movement, tremor) or akinetic mutism (alertness with a lack of motor functions, including speech, gestures, and facial expression) [32]. However, notable clinically unique CJD subtypes include cerebellar (or ataxic subtypes), myoclonic CJD, thalamic CJD, and the Heidenhain variant (which manifests significant visual deficits) [33–36]. In addition to these variants, 41 distinct forms of inherited TSEs have been described in humans, each demonstrates unique clinical phenotypes unique point mutations or octapeptide insertion mutations [32].

Fatal familial insomnia (FFI) is a clinicopathologic variant of human prion disease considered to be a familiar variant of CJD. Genetically, FFI is characterized by a mutation at codon 178 of the prion protein gene (aspartic acid to asparagine) coupled to a methionine polymorphism at codon 129 on the corresponding abnormal allele. As the name indicates, FFI patients chiefly suffer from sleep disturbances—principally insomnia, but also including hypersomnia, restless sleep, and sleep attacks [37]. Beyond these, FFI patients demonstrate a range of clinical signs that are both similar to, and unique from classic CJD. Overlapping signs include cognitive deficits, spatial disorientation, ataxia, and hallucinations whereas clinical signs unique to FFI include weight loss, hyperhidrosis, and husky voice [38]. However, even among FFI patients, there are unique clinical syndromes that depend upon the codon 129 genotype. For example, it has been reported that hallucinations and myoclonus are more common in patients that are methionine homozygous (i.e., MM) at codon 129, whereas vegetative disturbances and nystagmus are more common in methionine heterozygous patients [37]. Interestingly, although the diagnosis of unique variants of prion disease based on clinical phenotype only is considered difficult, an algorithm of FFI specific and sensitive clinical signs has been developed which correctly identified 81% of patients during early disease stages [38].

Like FFI, Gerstmann-Straussler-Scheinker (GSS) is a mutational variant of CJD in which a number of differing prion protein gene point mutations have been identified, the most common of which is the P102L/129M variant [29]. There are two typical clinical phenotypes of P102L GSS, namely (1) a typical type with cerebellar ataxia and slow onset dementia and (2) a CJD-like form with acute dementia and myoclonus [29, 39].

2.2. Scrapie

Like other TSEs, scrapie is a clinically progressive disease that is most classically characterized by pruritus, altered behavior, and locomotion deficits [40]. However, like other prion diseases, the clinical phenotype of sheep scrapie varies somewhat according to strain and host characteristics. Accordingly, three profiles of clinical disease have been described, namely (1) a pruritic form, (2) a paralytic form (which lack pruritus), and (3) an atypical cerebellar (Nor98) form [41]. The neurologic signs of scrapie are wide-ranging, and include mentation abnormalities (e.g., hyperresponsiveness), motor deficits (e.g., incoordination, exaggerated gait, hypermetria, ataxia, tremors), visual deficits (including nystagmus and blindness), loss of the menace response, dysphagia, and dysphonia [42, 43]. Although not always the case, deficits in locomotion, including hypotonia, proprioceptive deficits, reduced withdrawal reflex, and ataxia, are reported to occur later in disease [27, 43]. Terminal sheep scrapie is characterized by depression, recumbency, and/or seizure activity. In addition to the classical form of the disease, an alternate strain of scrapie, denoted atypical or Nor98, has been described and is characterized clinically by motor deficits, including progressive ataxia and incoordination whereas pruritus is very uncommon [44]. Scrapie-infected goats demonstrate many of the same clinical signs as seen in sheep, including pruritus, restlessness, and terminal ataxia/recumbency [21]. Similar to sheep, discrete clinical phenotypes have been identified in goat scrapie, namely a "scratching syndrome" characterized principally by pruritus and a "drowsy syndrome" characterized by decreased activity and depression absent pruritus [21, 45, 46]. However additional features have been reported, including teeth grinding, irritability, and heightened alertness [42]. Additional noted differences between scrapie-infected sheep and goats include hyperesthesia in goats (as opposed to hypoesthesia in sheep) and nibbling of the body in goats (as opposed to rubbing of the body in sheep) [21].

2.3. Bovine spongiform encephalopathy (BSE)

In contrast to the prion diseases of nondomestic species, the clinical features of BSE-infected cattle are well described. Like other prion diseases, BSE infection in cattle is principally associated with progressive changes in behavior and locomotion. Early disease is dominated by changes in behavior, including increased alertness, nervousness, excitability, nervous ear/eye movements, and hypersensitivity to touch, sound, and visual stimuli, head shyness, panic-stricken response, reluctance to enter the milking parlor, and change in temperament [20, 47–49]. During this early phase, specific tests used to elicit hyperesthesia include: (1) the "flash test" (reactivity to a camera flash), (2) the "clipboard test" (reactivity to waving a clipboard towards the animal, (3) the "hand clap" (reactivity to clapping hands), and (4) the "stick test" (reactivity to a light touch of the hindlimbs with a flexible stick) [50]. As disease progresses, BSE-infected cattle develop deficits in locomotion include tremors, hypermetria, hindlimb and generalized ataxia, difficulty rising, spastic gait, and thermal recumbency [49]. Terminally, cattle may enter into a "dull" form of the disease characterized by loss of previous hyperesthesia and disinterest in surroundings [20]. Previous studies have shown that at least one, either apprehension, hyper-reactivity, or ataxia, is found in 97% of cattle with BSE [51].

Outside of cattle, there is sparse information on BSE infection in other species. In BSE-infected goats, hyperesthesia, pruritus, head tossing, or shaking, overreactivity to touch of the hindlimbs, and hypermetria are reported [21]. There are conflicting reports on the clinical phenotype of BSE-infected sheep, which may reflect route of inoculation, age of infected sheep, or intensity of clinical monitoring. In one report, BSE-infected sheep demonstrate a uniform clinical disease characterized by early pruritus with late locomotion deficits [41]. Whereas, other studies suggest that sudden-onset ataxia is common in BSE-infected sheep [52].

In addition to classical BSE (C-BSE), two unique strains of BSE have been described. These strains denoted by H-BSE and L-BSE according to their biochemical characteristics and migration profile of the proteinase-resistant fragments on Western blot, demonstrate some clinical features unique from C-BSE. Similar to C-BSE, cattle experimentally infected with either H-BSE or L-BSE demonstrate both hyperesthesia and dullness, however the magnitude of hyperresponsiveness is reported to be higher in C-BSE [20]. While no consistent differences were noted when the clinical phenotype of H- and L-type BSE were compared, cattle with either of these two forms of atypical BSE did not progress to permanent recumbency and failed to demonstrate tremors, which contrasts with C-BSE [20].

2.4. Chronic wasting disease (CWD)

Chronic wasting disease (CWD) is an endemic prion disease of cervids, affecting white-tailed deer, mule deer, elk, moose, red deer, sika deer, muntjac, and reindeer. The two most recognized clinical signs of natural CWD are behavioral changes and loss of body mass. Not surprisingly, the behavioral phenotype of CWD in wild, naturally infected animals is not well-described, but work with captive (both naturally and experimentally infected) animals has provided some descriptive insights. Like other ruminant TSEs, CWD is a progressive disease. Early in the progression of CWD, the behavioral abnormalities in CWD are considered subtle and best appreciated by those who are in repeated contact with infected animals. Early clinical signs include alterations in patterns of interaction with humans (either increased or decreased contact), fixed gaze, repetitive behaviors (head tossing, exaggerated lifting of the legs), diminished alertness, prolonged periods of somnolence, and aggressive behavior which, late in disease, progresses to motor deficits (incoordination, trembling, and stumbling) [42, 53, 54]. Although distinct strains of CWD have been identified, as reflected by incubation period and neuropathologic differences, their neurobehavioral characteristics have not been reported [55, 56].

3. The basic toolkit of behavioral phenotyping

Behavioral research in laboratory rodent species has progressed for decades, largely with the aim of understanding the biological basis of normal behavior and brain function. When properly utilized, behavioral analysis has the potential to be both explanatory of the *in vivo* impact of underlying molecular changes and by suggesting novel areas of dysfunction. With the advent of gene targeting, focus has begun to shift toward the utility of behavioral analysis within the context of disease modeling and drug development. This disease focused behavioral research can be looked at assays as falling into three gross categories [57]; behavioral models of a disease state (e.g., self-administration of cocaine by rodents as an addiction model), behavioral bioassays of specific neural activity (e.g., stereotyped head twitch responses to drugs targeting serotonin 2A subtype receptors), or screening tools to assess the impact of biological manipulations (chemical/pharmacological, genetic, or neurological). It is in this last category that most of the present discussion falls where we will look at some of the tools that are widely used in behavioral phenotyping analysis. For simplicity, the tools are broken down into three broad categories of behavior: neuromotor function, learning and memory, and anxiety and depression-related behavior.

3.1. Neuromotor function

One of the first classes of behaviors that is often looked at in phenotyping studies, is the effect of the manipulation on neuromotor function, e.g., general activity, coordination, strength. A wide array of assays is available to assess the diverse aspects of neuromotor function. All of these assays are very approachable and several are amenable to automated scoring systems (for further review see Pierce and Kalivas and Wahlsten) [58, 59]. The main differences to note in the assessment of these tests are the aspect of motor function being examined, the context of the test environment, and the motivational drive for movement.

Open field locomotion test. Animals are placed in a novel, open test arena and distance traveled is determined for anywhere from 10 to 120 min, depending on the goals of the testing. The test arena can be almost any shape, but square is most common. Automated scoring is achieved through either beam breaks of a photocell grid or by video-based tracking of animal position. Exploration of the open field is driven by the novelty of the test arena. As such, with additional time (or repeated exposures) activity levels decline. Repeated testing can be used to assess habituation learning. Data in this test is generally binned to look at changes in activity over time, or presented as a single measurement of distance traveled during the test.

Home cage running wheel activity. While open field locomotion provides a rapid way to assess general activity, it does present a limitation by measuring activity in a foreign environment. So, activity level can be confounded by anxiety/stress responses in unexpected ways. Measurement of activity in the home cage overcomes this limitation, and additionally provides the opportunity to measure activity over long periods of time. Computer-tracked wheel running systems are used to count rotations. Critical to the use of these systems is the understanding that it can take several days for a mouse to figure out the running wheel, and begin high rates of running. It is also noteworthy that activity follows a robust circadian pattern, with running

http://dx.doi.org/10.5772/67520

activity ramping up during the dark-phase. With studies of home-cage wheel running, investigations can simply look at the magnitude of activity, degree of entrainment to light cycle, or alterations in the free-running cycle observed in the absence of external light cycle. In addition to running wheels, photocell grids can be placed around the home-cage to measure horizontal movement. This affords the ability to measure normal home cage ambulation, but it is unclear if such studies display the same robust circadian rhythms in activity as mice may spend much of their active time digging and grooming as opposed to ambulating. An unavoidable source of confound in these home-cage activity studies is the need to single-house the mice which can have dramatic, if not variable, effects on behavior.

Rotarod. More a test of coordination and balance than general activity, the rotarod assesses the ability to walk on a continually (often accelerating) rotating rod, where the aversion to falling motivates the mice to keep walking. Animals are placed on the rotating rod and the latency to fall is determined in multiple trials across 3–4 days of testing. The repeated testing days gives an assessment of motor learning that is not easily achieved by other measures. The accelerating rotarod protocol is a task fairly sensitive to motor impairments, as the increasing speed becomes a fairly difficult task for mice, and is well suited to longitudinal studies. The confounders in this test are few, but two behaviors can emerge that can affect the validity of the data: (1) mice decide that falling is not aversive and (2) mice develop the ability to grasp onto the rod and rotate instead of walking on the rod. Both of these confounding behaviors present the investigator with a decision of whether to exclude data or, in the case of the later situation, manually stop a trial. With logically applied criterion, these confounds can be minimized and the task can retain its high sensitivity to motor deficits.

Balance beam test. The balance beam test simply consists of training mice to walk across a balance beam, from a brightly lit start position to a dark enclosure at the end of the beam [60]. Training takes 2 or 3 days, then the mice are tested on beams of differing diameters (10–25 mm) and shapes (square vs. round). The basic data measure is latency to cross the beam and the number of hindpaw slips that are observed. Both time and footslips are sensitive to subtle impairments. The apparatus for this test is easy to construct and scoring is done by a trained observer, making this a fairly easy assay to set up in any lab. Additionally, we have found this assay to be useful in longitudinal test designs, as the mice retain the initial training and do not often need as much follow-up training.

Gait analysis. Gait analysis can be performed in mice using paw-inking methods or through the use of more sophisticated video-based paw tracking software. The latter method employs a high speed camera mounted below a transparent walkway or treadmill and computer-assisted tracking of individual paws. The software for these systems is capable of tracking numerous metrics about stride characteristics (swing, breaking, propulsion), as well as providing information about stance width and paw placement angles. Though quite useful in terms of the variety of information, these systems can be expensive, require significant user review of the paw tracking analysis, and significant amount of research into the various domains in the gait analysis to understand their utility.

Grip strength. Various apparatus have been developed to assess grip (muscle) strength in mice. Very simple tests using inverted screens or wire can be used to assess hanging duration, or the ability to hang on to objects of varying weight can be timed [61]. These timing-based measures are very simple to employ but may not offer the sensitivity or accuracy of more sophisticated tools using force sensors to measure the strength of an animal to hold onto a grid or rod (in response to an opposing force applied by the experimenter). These metric are largely devoid of the motivational confound in other tests and provide complementary information.

3.2. Learning and memory

Another broad category of behavior that is regularly looked at is learning and memory (cognitive function). Assessing cognitive function can take many forms as there are multiple domains of cognitive function. Some of the basic domains include spatial navigation learning, working memory, and conditioning can be readily studied in mouse models without complicated and prolonged training. Additionally, each of these tests measures very different functions that involve different neural circuitry.

Spontaneous alternation tasks. For measuring spatial working memory via spontaneous alternation task, one of two variants (T- or Y-maze) can be used. The T-maze task is a very simple way to assess working memory function, utilizing a T-shaped maze that consists of a start box and two choice arms. This task is based upon optimizing foraging strategies suggesting that the animal will alternate entries into choice arms, so as to avoid arm previously explored. Animals will typically display ~70% spontaneous alternation. The use of a start box in T-maze task allows for discrete trials and control of intertrial intervals. Varying the intertrial interval can modulate the working memory load on the mice and alter the "difficulty" of the task. Rewarded versions of this task are often utilized that would allow an investigator to drive performance above 85% alternation, providing higher detection window for deficits. Also, the rewarded version can be utilized for repeated testing to observe the effects of manipulations during testing in the same mice. A continuous performance version of this task, the Y-maze, is often used and presents an animal with a radially symmetrical maze where all arms are in effect choice and start positions, which offers an investigator an opportunity to observe exploration continuously without external interruptions.

Spatial navigation tasks: Morris Water Maze (MWM) and Barnes Maze (BM). These are widely employed tests of hippocampal-based spatial navigation learning. The MWM involves placing the test subjects in a large (<1 m diameter) water tank, where the subjects must find the escape platform that is hidden just beneath the water surface. Using distal, extra-maze visual cues that remain in a fixed position relative to the escape platform, acquisition of the task can take anywhere from 4 to 10 days. Subsequently spatial memory is assessed in a "probe trial," during which time there is no escape platform and the memory for the platform position is determined. The major metrics of memory include, exploration bias (typically a quadrant analysis of exploration of the tank), average proximity to or number of crosses of the platform location, or latency to first approach the platform location. Analysis is effectively performed by commercially available video-based tracking software. While this test has become widely adopted, it is not without confounds, notably confounding swim strategies such as floating and thigmotaxis. Often a response to the stress of the test, these behaviors can complicate the use of any of the time-dependent (including exploration bias) measures.

http://dx.doi.org/10.5772/67520

Additionally, this test can be very sensitive to, and negatively impacted by, motor impairments and/or sensitivity to effects of water exposure on body temperature. The Barnes Maze is a dry-land version of the water maze, originally developed for rats as a way to avoid some of the motivational confounds of other tests that utilized strongly aversive stimuli. Subsequent studies adapted the procedure for mice [62]. The BM involves an elevated circular platform, with numerous (e.g., 20) holes located on the perimeter of the apparatus, one of these holes leads to an escape box. The maze is lit from above and the combination of the light and openness serve as a motivator to encourage mice to escape from the maze to a small, dark enclosure, to be then returned to their home cage. Just as in the MWM, extra-maze cues are used to navigate to the escape hole and software can be used to analyze behavior. In addition to the mentioned advantages over MWM, the lack of a water tank and the use of a collapsible test platform make the BM a great choice for space constrained investigators/facilities in need of tests that confer a high degree of modularity to a test space with a minimal amount of setup, breakdown, and cleanup.

Fear learning. Fear learning tasks involve the assessment of a behavioral response to cues associated with an electric shock. In avoidance tasks (e.g., two-way active avoidance) the subject learns to shuttle between the two sides of a chamber in response to predictive cues (tones or lights), as such an avoidance response prevents or terminates the shock. Retention of the conditioning in tested in a subsequent test session. This procedure actually involves two interacting forms of learning, classical, and operant conditioning [63]. The classical conditioning involves association of the predictive cue (conditioned stimulus) and the shock (unconditioned stimulus), leading to the enhancement of an innate fear response. Subsequently, operant conditioning occurs whereby the animal develops an escape response as it learns that this operant response leads to termination or avoidance of the shock. As a result the neural circuitry involved in this test is more complicated than behavioral tests where the only classical or operant conditioning is utilized. To some degree the conditioned fear (often resulting in freezing) is also at odds with the avoidance behavior, so clear interpretations of slower escape latencies can be unclear if the mice are quick to display a freezing response. As an alternative to avoidance tasks, conditioned freezing procedures that exclusively utilize classical (Pavlovian) conditioning can be utilized. Multiple procedural variants have been developed that present an inescapable shock in combination (or not) with discrete cues. The animals adopt a freezing response to both the context in which the testing takes place, as well as to the cues. In one of the most widely used variants, delay fear conditioning, the brief footshock is presented in cotermination with the cue (sounds and/or light), and the predictive association that forms between the discrete cues and the shocks can drive a long-lasting fear response. The fear that develops to the cues is suggested to involve neural processes involving the amygdala, while information about the test environment (context) also takes on fear-inducing qualities related to hippocampal function [64]. Variants of this task can be employed to selectively look at contextual fear (no paired cues) or time intervals can be utilized in between the termination of the cue and the presentation of the shock in so-called trace fear conditioning tests [65]. This variation of adding the trace interval alters the circuitry involved in memory formation so involve a more complex circuitry that involves the hippocampus and prefrontal cortex [66].

3.3. Anxiety and depression-related behavior

This is an area of research typified by some very approachable tests that are useful in their own right to study the impact of manipulations on anxiety and depression-related behavior [67, 68]. These assays are also important tools to use as controls for altered motivation in cognitive assays [69]. These assays are often fairly easy to employ, but can be easily impacted by uncontrolled external variabilities, and many times subject to misinterpretation/overinterpretation of data. Critical to effectively using these behavioral tests is an understanding their test validity, be it construct, face, or predictive [70]. Also, as there is some inherent fallibility in interpreting these behaviors as they relate to affective and mood disorders, it is important to utilize multiple tests in combination for a thorough evaluation.

Exploratory conflict tests: elevated plus maze (EPM) and the open field test (OFT). The EPM test offers the animal an opportunity to explore two distinct zones, closed arms and open arms, of a plus-shaped maze. The open arms are the more aversive environment as they are more brightly lit than the closed arms and do not contain the side wall enclosure. Aversion to the open arms can be modulated, to a degree, by altering the open arm light levels. Additionally the test platform is elevated (~1 m) to enhance the aversive nature of the open arm and deter a possible escape route (i.e., jumping off the maze). In assessing exploration, the preferred metric is to look at open arm time as a function of total arm exploration time. This measure avoids confounds of interpreting data collected while the mouse is in the center zone of the maze, where indecisive exploration of the arm openings is apparent. Data in this task is fairly resistant to hyper/hypoactivity confounds and has been shown on numerous occasions to be responsive to proven anxiolytic drugs (i.e., predictive validity) [71, 72]. The OFT is simpler to run, though perhaps the more difficult to interpret. The OFT looks for anxiety by assessing the pattern of exploration of a novel arena. In this assay, changes in the exploration of the center zone (e.g., 40 × 40 cm) of a large arena (e.g., 50 × 50 cm) examined as a measure of anxiety. This test is conceptually similar to the EPM test in the exploration conflict and attempting to quantify the same aversion to open spaces. However, this test can easily show false positives (e.g., psychomotor stimulants) and in our hands has not consistently shown to be sensitive to benzodiazepine anxiolytics.

Stress-induced hyperthermia assay (SIH) and social interaction test. Two nonexploration-based tasks that are sensitive to changes in anxiety are the SIH assay and social interaction test. SIH measures the physiological response to stress (increase in body temperature) that is shared across warm-blooded animals [73]. This measure is particularly effective at identifying anxiolysis, and as such is a good screening tool for novel anxiolytic drugs. The social interaction test is an observer scored assay that scores the interaction of two freely moving mice in a novel test environment. Elevations in anxiety levels of a test subject are thought to be reflected as a decrease in affiliative responses (grooming, sniffing, etc.) to a novel social partner. Beyond anxiety, this assay is also utilized in the neuropsychiatry literature in models of diseases where social deficits are present, e.g., autism and schizophrenia.

Forced swim test (FST) and the tail suspension test (TST). FST and TST are tests of stress-coping responses. These tests look at the behavioral response of subjects to an inescapable stressor. FST puts mice in an inescapable water tank, while in the TST mice are inverted and suspended by their tails. Both tests are fairly brief (5–6 min) and look to quantify the level of immobility, viewed as the adaptive response that develops during the test. Automated analysis of these behaviors has proven quite effective for scoring large numbers of test subjects. In some variants of the FST, investigators will use long exposures to swim stress prior to the actual testing, in order to precipitate a stronger immobility response.

Two-bottle sucrose preference test (SPT). Anhedonia is specifically a symptom of depression which is characterized by a lack of pleasure seeking. In rodents, there are multiple ways to assess this, but the most readily utilized measure is the SPT, which compares consumption of a sucrose solution to normal water in a home cage setting over a several day period, with increasing sucrose concentrations resulting in an increased preference. Anhedonia is observed as a reduction in preferred consumption of sucrose as compared to water.

This discussion of behavioral testing has mostly focused on individual tests, what they are, how they work, what is the utility and what the confounds are to their use. However, at this point it is important to discuss the use of combinations of tests into so-called "test batteries." The idea of a broad-based analysis of behavior is at the heart of behavioral phenotyping efforts that have grown in response to advances in murine genetics and increasing emphasis on disease modeling research (for review see Crawley) [74, 75]. The construction of a proper test battery is not a trivial or even standardized operation. Test batteries can be designed to be intentionally broad with an emphasis on observation and characterization as is often done with gene knockout studies. Such designs tend to take a relatively agnostic approach to hypotheses about phenotype and may use an initial screen to suggest more detailed behavioral analysis or follow-up mechanistic studies. Another way to design a screen is with investigation of a very specific endpoint in mind (e.g., cognitive deficit). In this case supplemental tests may be chosen to satisfy controls for confounding behavioral deficits (motor dysfunction, sensory deficit, or changes in motivation). In all situations it is advisable to at least consider the use of multiple tests within the same behavioral domain that utilize different outputs or behavioral abilities to complete the test.

4. Behavior assays used in mouse models of prion disease

The adjective insidious is commonly used to describe the prion diseases because there are no obvious outward symptoms to alert the public to infection and progression. This presents a problem to those seeking to provide a therapeutic intervention. A common theme in medicine is the idea that early intervention in disease progression is more likely to lead to a better prognosis. Thus, the conundrum with prion diseases is that since this disease progresses silently, how are we to be alerted to its progression in order to intervene? Luckily for us, prion diseases are neurological diseases and there is an expansive literature on brain—behavior relationships. Thus, behavioral testing using experimental animal model systems allows for sufficient control of variables to rigorously test specific hypotheses about the impact of prion disease progression on behavior. As such, there have been a number of studies that have attempted to use behavior assays to document the progression of prion diseases.

Although this chapter focuses on the utility of behavior analysis for understanding prion diseases, it is interesting that early studies used scrapie to understand brain-behavior relationships. Savage and Field used the open field test to measure emotionality (at various dpi) in mice that were intracerebrally (IC) inoculated with scrapie (third passage from sheep) [76]. Their data indicate that disease progression is correlated with a decline in emotionality, but not ambulation. A subsequent study used 263 K scrapie inoculum to unilaterally ablate the striatum in golden hamsters [77]. Striatal destruction was verified using the apomorphine stimulated rotation task. The authors suggest that scrapie might be a useful tool for studying other brain regions such as the basal ganglia.

Clinical signs of disease progression in IC inoculated scrapie mouse model systems are observed around 23 weeks or 161 days post inoculation [78, 79]. By this time, the disease has progressed to the point where no therapeutic intervention will succeed. Mice at this stage of the disease show reduced mobility, hunched posture and lack of grooming [78, 79]. Heitzman and Corp wanted to determine if they could detect behavioral symptoms of scrapie prior to the then current standard of 16 weeks post inoculation [80]. They tested mice that were IC inoculated with scrapie using the open field test and the emergence test. Although they did not observe any effect of early disease progression on the open field test, they did observe a statistically significant effect of scrapie on the emergence test at 6 weeks post inoculation. This data suggests that scrapie inoculated mice show reduced exploratory behavior or increased anxiety. More importantly, this data also indicates that it is possible to observe changes in behavior 9 weeks prior to the onset of clinical symptoms in scrapie-inoculated mice.

Outram put forth several "to be met" criteria required for scrapie-behavior correlations [81]. (1) The behavior change must be a consequence of scrapie. (2) One should determine whether the change in behavior is correlated with altered central or peripheral nervous system activity. (3) The behavioral assay itself should not modify disease progression. (4) The behavior assayed and its neural bases should be well characterized. With these criteria in mind Outram demonstrated that drinking behavior is altered in IC inoculated scrapie mice [81]. Declines in drinking behavior were observed approximately 7 weeks post inoculation using a number of fluids, including sucrose, water, and glucose + saline. This finding was seen in mice that were IC or IP inoculated with several scrapie strains including ME7, 22A, 79A. This effect was also observed in several mouse strains, including C57BL, A2G, VL, and VM mice.

Subsequent work by McFarland et al. found that both mouse strain and scrapie strain affected the open field and Y maze performance [82]. In Nya:NYLAR, C57/10J, and ICR mice that were IC inoculated with Chandler scrapie, only ICR mice showed a statistically significant reduction in spontaneous alternation in the y-maze task. Moreover, Y-maze performance was diminished in the Nya:NYLAR and ICR mice, but not C57 mice. In the second experiment Nya:NYLAR mice were IC inoculated with one of three scrapie strains: 22C, ME7, and 79-A and tested at 95–103 dpi. The 22-C inoculated mice exhibited a statistically significant decrease in activity, but 79-A mice exhibited a statistically significant increase in activity. Moreover, only the ME-7 and 79-A strains resulted in a reduced entry into the center field. Although there was no effect of scrapie strain on y-maze spontaneous alternation, 79-A inoculated mice exhibited an increased number of arm entries. The strain specificity of prion clinical phenotype was further demonstrated by a study examining behavioral effects on C57BL/6 mice IC inoculated with either the scrapie strains 139A or ME7 or the mouse adapted BSE strain 301C [83]. Mice inoculated with 301C were generally less active during the dark phase of the light-dark cycle than control or scrapie inoculated mice. In contrast, ME7 inoculated mice also showed a decline in activity during the dark phase, although not to the same extent as 301C inoculated mice. Statistically significant scrapie strain effects were observed in measures of the duration of several open field behaviors including, rearing, wall rearing, sniffing, grooming, and walking [83]. Scrapie inoculated mice did show a decline in water consumption around 10 weeks post inoculation, consistent with data published by Outram [81]. All mice exhibited similar scrapie induced neuropathological changes [83]. Taken together, these studies indicate that scrapie strain and mouse strain may impact the outcome of behavioral assays.

More recently, a battery of behavioral tests has been successfully used to visualize the progression of prion disease across several scrapie strains [61, 78, 79, 84–86]. Based on their work over the years, the aforementioned authors have elucidated the timing of behaviors that are affected. Nesting and affective behaviors (glucose consumption and burrowing) are first to be affected. Motor, strength, and coordination deficits appear subsequently. Finally, mice show decreased activity and prototypical clinical signs of scrapie. Betmouni et al. took advantage of evidence that the ME7 scrapie strain apparently targets the hippocampus, in order to determine if behavioral testing is useful for detecting early, subtle, hippocampal deficits in scrapie inoculated mice [78, 79]. Hippocampal deficits have been associated with hyperactivity and deficits at passive avoidance tasks. The authors observed increased locomotor activity and impaired retention of a multitrial passive avoidance task in scrapie inoculated mice around 12–14 weeks post inoculation. The authors also observed motor function impairments on the inverted screen and horizontal bar tests before the onset of known clinical signs of scrapie. A subsequent study examined the behavioral correlates of scrapie progression using a similar battery of tests [87]. Burrowing of food in the home cage was found to be inversely proportional to disease progression in scrapie inoculated mice. Consistent with other studies there was a decline in spontaneous alternation, beginning around 10 weeks post inoculation and there was a statistically significant reduction in glucose consumption in scrapie inoculated mice during weeks 15–19. A statistically significant effect of group was also observed in the horizontal bar test, which tests motor coordination [84]. The authors did not observe any statistically significant differences between groups in the rotarod or the inverted screen test. In sum, the development of a battery of behavioral assays is a boon for science in that it facilitates the comparison of experimental findings across investigators.

As previously discussed, early studies provide evidence that both scrapie and mouse strain may impact on the outcome of behavior assays. Cunningham et al. examined the behavioral progression of scrapie in C57BL/6J mice inoculated with one of the following strains: ME7, 79A, 22L, and 22A [86]. All mice were intrahippocampally inoculated with one of the aforementioned scrapie strains or normal brain homogenate. After recovery mice were subjected to the battery of behavioral tests described above. A similar disease progression was observed in all scrapie inoculated mice, except those that were inoculated with 22A. These mice exhibited a delayed disease progression. ME7 inoculated mice were the first to show decreased glucose consumption around 10 weeks post inoculation, followed by 79A and 22L at 12 weeks post inoculation. In these mice, although the progression of scrapie was generally similar, there were differences in end stage neuropathology. Although all scrapie inoculated mice showed microglial activation, the degree of activation appeared to be less in the 22L inoculated mice. There were strain differences in vacuolation in the hippocampus, septum, and thalamus. Although all scrapie inoculated mice showed widespread PrP^{SC} staining, there were also strain-dependent differences in the density of scrapie with some strains showing more diffuse immunoreactivity and others show plaques or punctate immunoreactivity. Neuron loss was fairly similar in all scrapie inoculated mice. One striking finding was that there was a lack of hippocampal cell death in 22L or 22A inoculated mice, despite the fact that all scrapie inoculated mice received an intrahippocampal injection. The authors note that this is consistent with the idea that variables other than site of exposure contribute to PrP^{SC} spread and neuropathology.

Taken together this brief review of the literature indicates that it is possible to use behavioral testing as a proxy to monitor the progression of prion disease in mouse model systems. An important caveat, however, is that investigators must carefully consider scrapie strain effects, mouse strain effects or interactions between the two. Although this is an important variable to consider, there are exceptions to this generalization. For instance, Asuni et al. noted that their previous studies used C57BL/6J mice from Harlan laboratories, a mouse strain that was subsequently shown to have a spontaneous deletion of alpha synuclein [88]. The authors were concerned that the absence of alpha synuclein represented a potential confound with data that correlate synaptic loss with prion disease progression. A comparison of C57 mice with and without alpha synuclein revealed no impact of alpha synuclein on the progression of scrapie as assayed by behavioral testing.

4.1. Behavioral studies in transgenic mouse models

4.1.1. Behavior assays have been used to validate prion knockout mice

As mentioned earlier, our current understanding of prion disease is that it is a consequence of misfolded PrP^{C}. However, the function of PrP^{C} is not wholly known. To further understanding of its function, a number of groups have developed PrP^{C} knockout (PrP^{KO}) mice. As part of these studies, behavior assays have been used to assess the impact of PrP ablation. The first PrP^{KO} mouse, also known as the *Zurich 1* line was generated in 1992 [2]. This first KO mouse was highly anticipated and a number of behavioral tests were performed across several studies in order to elucidate the normal biological function of PrP^{C}. Surprisingly, Bueler et al. reported that the mice did not show any gross anatomical or immunological abnormalities [2]. These mice did not show any deficits in spatial navigation on the water maze test even after 2 years [89]. These mice also failed to show any deficits in the y-maze discrimination test, or the two-way active avoidance test. These data suggested that the mice did not have any deficits in hippocampal-dependent spatial learning and memory, problem solving strategy and hippocampal-dependent associative and nonassociative learning.

However, other researchers have found that *Zurich 1* mice do demonstrate behavioral deficits, including altered circadian locomotor behavior, increased number of crossing in an open field test, and a decreased in latency to step down (i.e., memory impairment) in reference [90–92]. The memory impairment of the PrP^{KO} mice appeared to be more prominent on long-term memory (24 h retention) than short term memory (90 min retention), though this difference is likely related to the poor memory retention of the control mice in the short-term memory test.

http://dx.doi.org/10.5772/67520

Additionally, *Zurich 1* mice have been shown to have impaired swimming capacity, the magnitude of which increased as the task difficulty increased [93].

Meotti et al. used a number of thermal and chemical nociception tests, to determine whether PrP^C has a role in pain detection [94]. *Zurich 1* mice also show an increased latency to remove the tail during the tail flick test, an assay of thermal nociception and a transient increase in the number of abdominal constrictions in response to IP injection of acetic acid, which is a visceral nociception test [94]. *Zurich 1* mice also show olfactory deficits, as assayed by the buried food test [95]. Lastly, *Zurich 1* mice have been shown to have increased aggressive behavior relative to wild-type controls as measured by the resident intruder test, which measures aggression in males in response to novel intruder males [96, 97]. In addition to prion protein ablation, the impact of PrP^C overexpression has been examined. Lobao-Soares et al. examined a number of behaviors including locomotor, exploration, and anxiety using the rotarod, open field and elevated plus maze, respectively, in PrP^C overexpressing mice [98]. Their data indicate that PrP^C overexpression was associated with better performance on all tasks [98].

5. Future directions

This review of the behavioral effects of prion disease has attempted to demonstrate the dramatic, host, agent, and disease-specific heterogeneity in natural and experimental systems. While these differences are recognized, the reasons underlying them are not known. As much as this unknown reflects uncertainties regarding the mechanisms of prion neurotoxicity, it also demonstrates the limited body of work that has systematically cataloged and characterized the clinical deficits these systems. Due to this knowledge gap, in concert with a growing understanding of the scientific importance of behavioral testing, it is important that prion researchers continue to consider clinical phenotype in future *in vivo* prion investigations.

Author details

Davis M. Seelig[1]*, Michael A. Benneyworth[2] and Damani N. Bryant[1]

*Address all correspondence to: dseelig@umn.edu

1 Veterinary Clinical Sciences Department, University of Minnesota, Saint Paul, MN, USA

2 Department of Neuroscience, University of Minnesota, Minneapolis, MN, USA

References

[1] Pan KM, Baldwin M, Nguyen J, et al. Conversion of alpha-helices into beta-sheets features in the formation of the scrapie prion proteins. *Proc Natl Acad Sci USA* 1993;90: 10962–10966.

[2] Bueler H, Fischer M, Lang Y, et al. Normal development and behaviour of mice lacking the neuronal cell-surface PrP protein. *Nature* 1992;356:577–582.

[3] Bueler H, Aguzzi A, Sailer A, et al. Mice devoid of PrP are resistant to scrapie. *Cell* 1993;73:1339–1347.

[4] Mallucci GR, Ratte S, Asante EA, et al. Post-natal knockout of prion protein alters hippocampal CA1 properties, but does not result in neurodegeneration. *EMBO J* 2002;21:202–210.

[5] Haley NJ, Mathiason CK, Zabel MD, et al. Detection of sub-clinical CWD infection in conventional test-negative deer long after oral exposure to urine and feces from CWD+ deer. *PLoS One* 2009;4:e7990.

[6] Castilla J, Gutierrez-Adan A, Brun A, et al. Subclinical bovine spongiform encephalopathy infection in transgenic mice expressing porcine prion protein. *J Neurosci* 2004;24:5063–5069.

[7] Hill AF, Collinge J. Subclinical prion infection. *Trends Microbiol* 2003;11:578–584.

[8] Ersdal C, Ulvund MJ, Benestad SL, et al. Accumulation of pathogenic prion protein (PrPSc) in nervous and lymphoid tissues of sheep with subclinical scrapie. *Vet Pathol* 2003;40:164–174.

[9] Thackray AM, Klein MA, Aguzzi A, et al. Chronic subclinical prion disease induced by low-dose inoculum. *J Virol* 2002;76:2510–2517.

[10] Race R, Meade-White K, Raines A, et al. Subclinical scrapie infection in a resistant species: persistence, replication, and adaptation of infectivity during four passages. *J Infect Dis* 2002;186 Suppl 2:S166–170.

[11] Fraser H, Dickinson AG. Scrapie in mice. Agent-strain differences in the distribution and intensity of grey matter vacuolation. *J Comp Pathol* 1973;83:29–40.

[12] Langevin C, Andreoletti O, Le Dur A, et al. Marked influence of the route of infection on prion strain apparent phenotype in a scrapie transgenic mouse model. *Neurobiol Dis* 2011;41:219–225.

[13] Aguzzi A, Sigurdson C, Heikenwaelder M. Molecular mechanisms of prion pathogenesis. *Annu Rev Pathol* 2008;3:11–40.

[14] Collinge J, Clarke AR. A general model of prion strains and their pathogenicity. *Science* 2007;318:930–936.

[15] Safar J, Wille H, Itri V, et al. Eight prion strains have PrP(Sc) molecules with different conformations. *Nat Med* 1998;4:1157–1165.

[16] Goldfarb LG, Petersen RB, Tabaton M, et al. Fatal familial insomnia and familial Creutzfeldt-Jakob disease: disease phenotype determined by a DNA polymorphism. *Science* 1992;258:806–808.

[17] Dickinson AG, Meikle VM. Host-genotype and agent effects in scrapie incubation: change in allelic interaction with different strains of agent. *Mol Gen Genet* 1971;112:73–79.

[18] Lasmezas CI, Deslys JP, Robain O, et al. Transmission of the BSE agent to mice in the absence of detectable abnormal prion protein. *Science* 1997;275:402–405.

[19] Collinge J, Owen F, Poulter M, et al. Prion dementia without characteristic pathology. *Lancet* 1990;336:7–9.

[20] Konold T, Bone GE, Clifford D, et al. Experimental H-type and L-type bovine spongiform encephalopathy in cattle: observation of two clinical syndromes and diagnostic challenges. *BMC Vet Res* 2012;8:22.

[21] Konold T, Bone GE, Phelan LJ, et al. Monitoring of clinical signs in goats with transmissible spongiform encephalopathies. *BMC Vet Res* 2010;6:13.

[22] Konold T, Lee YH, Stack MJ, et al. Different prion disease phenotypes result from inoculation of cattle with two temporally separated sources of sheep scrapie from Great Britain. *BMC Vet Res* 2006;2:31.

[23] Jeffrey M, Halliday WG. Numbers of neurons in vacuolated and non-vacuolated neuroanatomical nuclei in bovine spongiform encephalopathy-affected brains. *J Comp Pathol* 1994;110:287–293.

[24] Jeffrey M, Halliday WG, Goodsir CM. A morphometric and immunohistochemical study of the vestibular nuclear complex in bovine spongiform encephalopathy. *Acta Neuropathol* 1992;84:651–657.

[25] Austin AR, Meek S, Webster S, et al. Heart rate variability in BSE. *Vet Rec* 1996;139:631.

[26] Mackenzie A. Immunohistochemical demonstration of glial fibrillary acidic protein in scrapie. *J Comp Pathol* 1983;93:251–259.

[27] Jeffrey M, Gonzalez L. Classical sheep transmissible spongiform encephalopathies: pathogenesis, pathological phenotypes and clinical disease. *Neuropathol Appl Neurobiol* 2007;33:373–394.

[28] Manix M, Kalakoti P, Henry M, et al. Creutzfeldt-Jakob disease: updated diagnostic criteria, treatment algorithm, and the utility of brain biopsy. *Neurosurg Focus* 2015;39:E2.

[29] Ironside JW, Ghetti B, Head MW, et al. Prion diseases In: Love S, Louis DN,Ellison DW, eds. *Greenfield's Neuropathology.* 8th ed. London: Hodder Arnold, 2008;1197–1273.

[30] Parchi P, Saverioni D. Molecular pathology, classification, and diagnosis of sporadic human prion disease variants. *Folia Neuropathol* 2012;50:20–45.

[31] Parchi P, Giese A, Capellari S, et al. Classification of sporadic Creutzfeldt-Jakob disease based on molecular and phenotypic analysis of 300 subjects. *Ann Neurol* 1999;46:224–233.

[32] Brown P, Brunk C, Budka H, et al. *WHO Manual for surveillance of human transmissible spongiform encephalopathies including variant Cretuzfeldt-Jakob disease.* Geneva: World Health Organization; 2003.

[33] Cali I, Castellani R, Yuan J, et al. Classification of sporadic Creutzfeldt-Jakob disease revisited. *Brain* 2006;129:2266–2277.

[34] Baiardi S, Capellari S, Ladogana A, et al. Revisiting the heidenhain variant of Creutzfeldt-Jakob disease: evidence for prion type variability influencing clinical course and laboratory findings. *J Alzheimers Dis* 2015;50:465–476.

[35] Grant MP, Cohen M, Petersen RB, et al. Abnormal eye movements in Creutzfeldt-Jakob disease. *Ann Neurol* 1993;34:192–197.

[36] Alema G, Bignami A. Subacute degenerative presenile polioencephalopathy with akinetic stupor and decorticate rigidity with myoclonus ("myoclonic" variety of the Jakob-Creutzfeld disease). *Riv Sper Freniatr Med Leg Alien Ment* 1959;83 Suppl 4: 1485–1623.

[37] Krasnianski A, Bartl M, Sanchez Juan PJ, et al. Fatal familial insomnia: Clinical features and early identification. *Ann Neurol* 2008;63:658–661.

[38] Krasnianski A, Sanchez Juan P, Ponto C, et al. A proposal of new diagnostic pathway for fatal familial insomnia. *J Neurol Neurosurg Psychiatry* 2014;85:654–659.

[39] Iwasaki Y, Mori K, Ito M, et al. Gerstmann-Straeussler-Scheinker disease with P102L prion protein gene mutation presenting with rapidly progressive clinical course. *Clin Neuropathol* 2014;33:344–353.

[40] Parry HB, Oppenheimer DR. *Scrapie disease in sheep: historical, clinical, epidemiological, pathological, and practical aspects of the natural disease*. London; New York: Academic Press; 1983.

[41] Konold T, Bone G, Vidal-Diez A, et al. Pruritus is a common feature in sheep infected with the BSE agent. *BMC Vet Res* 2008;4:16.

[42] Imran M, Mahmood S. An overview of animal prion diseases. *Virol J* 2011;8:493.

[43] Healy AM, Weavers E, McElroy M, et al. The clinical neurology of scrapie in Irish sheep. *J Vet Intern Med* 2003;17:908–916.

[44] Benestad SL, Sarradin P, Thu B, et al. Cases of scrapie with unusual features in Norway and designation of a new type, Nor98. *Vet Rec* 2003;153:202–208.

[45] Pattison IH, Millson GC. Scrapie produced experimentally in goats with special reference to the clinical syndrome. *J Comp Pathol* 1961;71:101–109.

[46] Pattison IH, Millson GC. Further observations on the experimental production of scrapie in goats and sheep. *J Comp Pathol* 1960;70:182–193.

[47] Saegerman C, Speybroeck N, Roels S, et al. Decision support tools for clinical diagnosis of disease in cows with suspected bovine spongiform encephalopathy. *J Clin Microbiol* 2004;42:172–178.

[48] Braun U, Schicker E, Hornlimann B. Diagnostic reliability of clinical signs in cows with suspected bovine spongiform encephalopathy. *Vet Rec* 1998;143:101–105.

[49] Konold T, Bone G, Ryder S, et al. Clinical findings in 78 suspected cases of bovine spongiform encephalopathy in Great Britain. *Vet Rec* 2004;155:659–666.

[50] Konold T, Sivam SK, Ryan J, et al. Analysis of clinical signs associated with bovine spongiform encephalopathy in casualty slaughter cattle. *Vet J* 2006;171:438–444.

[51] Wilesmith JW, Hoinville LJ, Ryan JB, et al. Bovine spongiform encephalopathy: aspects of the clinical picture and analyses of possible changes 1986–1990. *Vet Rec* 1992;130:197–201.

[52] Houston EF, Gravenor MB. Clinical signs in sheep experimentally infected with scrapie and BSE. *Vet Rec* 2003;152:333–334.

[53] Mathiason CK, Hays SA, Powers J, et al. Infectious prions in pre-clinical deer and transmission of chronic wasting disease solely by environmental exposure. *PLoS One* 2009;4:e5916.

[54] Williams ES, Miller MW, Kreeger TJ, et al. Chronic wasting disease of deer and elk: a review with recommendations for management. *Journal of Wildlife Management* 2002;66:551–563.

[55] Angers RC, Kang HE, Napier D, et al. Prion strain mutation determined by prion protein conformational compatibility and primary structure. *Science* 2010;328:1154–1158.

[56] Raymond GJ, Raymond LD, Meade-White KD, et al. Transmission and adaptation of chronic wasting disease to hamsters and transgenic mice: evidence for strains. *J Virol* 2007;81:4305–4314.

[57] Tecott LH, Nestler EJ. Neurobehavioral assessment in the information age. *Nat Neurosci* 2004;7:462–466.

[58] Pierce RC, Kalivas PW. Locomotor behavior. *Curr Protoc Neurosci* 2007;Chapter 8:Unit 8 1.

[59] Wahlsten D. *Mouse behavioral testing: how to use mice in behavioral neuroscience*. 1st ed. London; Burlington, VT: Academic, 2011.

[60] Luong TN, Carlisle HJ, Southwell A, et al. Assessment of motor balance and coordination in mice using the balance beam. *J Vis Exp* 2011;49:1–3.

[61] Deacon RM. Measuring the strength of mice. *J Vis Exp* 2013;76:1–4.

[62] Pompl PN, Mullan MJ, Bjugstad K, et al. Adaptation of the circular platform spatial memory task for mice: use in detecting cognitive impairment in the APP(SW) transgenic mouse model for Alzheimer's disease. *J Neurosci Methods* 1999;87:87–95.

[63] Mowrer OH, Lamoreaux RR. Fear as an intervening variable in avoidance conditioning. *J Comp Psychol* 1946;39:29–50.

[64] Phillips RG, LeDoux JE. Differential contribution of amygdala and hippocampus to cued and contextual fear conditioning. *Behav Neurosci* 1992;106:274–285.

[65] Fanselow MS. Contextual fear, gestalt memories, and the hippocampus. *Behav Brain Res* 2000;110:73–81.

[66] Raybuck JD, Lattal KM. Bridging the interval: theory and neurobiology of trace conditioning. *Behav Processes* 2014;101:103–111.

[67] File SE, Lippa AS, Beer B, et al. Animal tests of anxiety. *Curr Protoc Neurosci* 2004;Chapter 8:Unit 8 3.

[68] Cryan JF, Holmes A. The ascent of mouse: advances in modelling human depression and anxiety. *Nat Rev Drug Discov* 2005;4:775–790.

[69] Hunsaker MR. The importance of considering all attributes of memory in behavioral endophenotyping of mouse models of genetic disease. *Behav Neurosci* 2012;126:371–380.

[70] Davis KL. American College of Neuropsychopharmacology. *Neuropsychopharmacology: the fifth generation of progress: an official publication of the American College of Neuropsychopharmacology.* Philadelphia: Lippincott Williams & Wilkins, 2002.

[71] Griebel G, Belzung C, Perrault G, et al. Differences in anxiety-related behaviours and in sensitivity to diazepam in inbred and outbred strains of mice. *Psychopharmacology (Berl)* 2000;148:164–170.

[72] Mathiasen LS, Mirza NR, Rodgers RJ. Strain- and model-dependent effects of chlordiazepoxide, L-838,417 and zolpidem on anxiety-like behaviours in laboratory mice. *Pharmacol Biochem Behav* 2008;90:19–36.

[73] Groenink L, Vinkers C, van Oorschot R, et al. Models of anxiety: stress-induced hyperthermia (SIH) in singly housed mice. *Curr Protoc Pharmacol* 2009;Chapter 5:Unit 5 16.

[74] Crawley JN. Behavioral phenotyping strategies for mutant mice. *Neuron* 2008;57:809–818.

[75] Crawley JN. *What's wrong with my mouse? Behavioral phenotyping of transgenic and knockout mice.* 2nd ed. Hoboken, NJ: Wiley-Interscience, 2007.

[76] Savage RD, Field EJ. Brain damage and emotional behaviour: the effects of scrapie on the emotional responses of mice. *Anim Behav* 1965;13:443–446.

[77] Gorde JM, Bert J, Gambarelli D, et al. Apomorphine-induced circling behaviour in hamsters following unilateral injection of scrapie gent in the striatum. *Neurosci Lett* 1981;22:201–204.

[78] Betmouni S, Perry VH. The acute inflammatory response in CNS following injection of prion brain homogenate or normal brain homogenate. *Neuropathol Appl Neurobiol* 1999;25:20–28.

[79] Betmouni S, Clements J, Perry VH. Vacuolation in murine prion disease: an informative artifact. *Curr Biol* 1999;9:R677–679.

[80] Heitzman RJ, Corp CR. Behaviour in emergence and open-field tests of normal and scrapie mice. *Res Vet Sci* 1968;9:600–601.

[81] Outram GW. Early reduction of drinking in mice with scrapie. *Lancet* 1971;1:397.

[82] McFarland DJ, Baker FD, Hotchin J. Host and viral genetic determinants of the behavioral effects of scrapie encephalopathy. *Physiol Behav* 1980;24:911–914.

[83] Dell'Omo G, Vannoni E, Vyssotski AL, et al. Early behavioural changes in mice infected with BSE and scrapie: automated home cage monitoring reveals prion strain differences. *Eur J Neurosci* 2002;16:735–742.

[84] Deacon RM. Measuring motor coordination in mice. *J Vis Exp* 2013:e2609;75:1–8.

[85] Guenther K, Deacon RM, Perry VH, et al. Early behavioural changes in scrapie-affected mice and the influence of dapsone. *Eur J Neurosci* 2001;14:401–409.

[86] Cunningham C, Deacon RM, Chan K, et al. Neuropathologically distinct prion strains give rise to similar temporal profiles of behavioral deficits. *Neurobiol Dis* 2005;18:258–269.

[87] Deacon RM, Raley JM, Perry VH, et al. Burrowing into prion disease. *Neuroreport* 2001;12:2053–2057.

[88] Asuni AA, Hilton K, Siskova Z, et al. Alpha-synuclein deficiency in the C57BL/6JOlaHsd strain does not modify disease progression in the ME7-model of prion disease. *Neuroscience* 2010;165:662–674.

[89] Lipp HP, Stagliar-Bozicevic M, Fischer M, et al. A 2-year longitudinal study of swimming navigation in mice devoid of the prion protein: no evidence for neurological anomalies or spatial learning impairments. *Behav Brain Res* 1998;95:47–54.

[90] Coitinho AS, Freitas AR, Lopes MH, et al. The interaction between prion protein and laminin modulates memory consolidation. *Eur J Neurosci* 2006;24:3255–3264.

[91] Tobler I, Gaus SE, Deboer T, et al. Altered circadian activity rhythms and sleep in mice devoid of prion protein. *Nature* 1996;380:639–642.

[92] Roesler R, Walz R, Quevedo J, et al. Normal inhibitory avoidance learning and anxiety, but increased locomotor activity in mice devoid of PrP(C). *Brain Res Mol Brain Res* 1999;71:349–353.

[93] Nico PB, Lobao-Soares B, Landemberger MC, et al. Impaired exercise capacity, but unaltered mitochondrial respiration in skeletal or cardiac muscle of mice lacking cellular prion protein. *Neurosci Lett* 2005;388:21–26.

[94] Meotti FC, Carqueja CL, Gadotti Vde M, et al. Involvement of cellular prion protein in the nociceptive response in mice. *Brain Res* 2007;1151:84–90.

[95] Le Pichon CE, Valley MT, Polymenidou M, et al. Olfactory behavior and physiology are disrupted in prion protein knockout mice. *Nat Neurosci* 2009;12:60–69.

[96] Budefeld T, Majer A, Jerin A, et al. Deletion of the prion gene Prnp affects offensive aggression in mice. *Behav Brain Res* 2014;266:216–221.

[97] Koolhaas JM, Coppens CM, de Boer SF, et al. The resident-intruder paradigm: a standardized test for aggression, violence and social stress. *J Vis Exp* 2013:e4367;77:1–7.

[98] Lobao-Soares B, Walz R, Carlotti CG, Jr., et al. Cellular prion protein regulates the motor behaviour performance and anxiety-induced responses in genetically modified mice. *Behav Brain Res* 2007;183:87–94.

Chapter 10

Mathematical Modeling of Prion Disease

Suzanne S. Sindi

Additional information is available at the end of the chapter

http://dx.doi.org/10.5772/66917

Abstract

The prion hypothesis, once a heretical violation of the central dogma of molecular biology, has become an accepted mechanism used to explain a host of progressive neurodegenerative diseases in mammals and heritable phenotypes in yeast. From the beginning, mathematical models have been an essential tool in studying prion and other protein misfolding/aggregation processes. In this work, we review some of the major mathematical studies that have contributed to our understanding of prion disease and discuss trends in current and future studies.

Keywords: protein misfolding, mathematical modeling, differential equations, aggregation, fragmentation

1. Introduction

In the past century, the use of mathematical models to study biological phenomena has gone from an occasional dalliance of a theoretical mathematician to an established field of its own. Today, mathematics has impacted virtually every area in biology—from evolution (e.g., Fisher's Fundamental Theorem of Natural Selection) to biochemistry (e.g., Michaelis-Menten Kinetics) [1]. But, the impact of biology on mathematics has been just as transformative and biology itself has served to motivate the development of novel mathematics [2].

In the latter part of the twentieth century, both biologists and mathematicians worked to identify and characterize mechanisms to explain a host of fatal neurodegenerative diseases in mammals ranging from scrapie—an infectious diseases observed in sheep—to fatal familial insomnia—a genetic disorder in humans. Initially, much of the focus of these studies centered on first the identification of the infectious agent of these diseases. The discovery of the prion—a proteinaceous infectious particle—originally represented a fundamental contradiction in the central dogma of molecular biology. But today there is increasing acceptance of protein-only-inheritance (see **Figure 1**) not only for mammalian diseases but also for heritable phenotypes in yeast. At present, mammalian prion diseases are untreatable and continued experimental, mathematical and interdisciplinary research offers the promise for identification of regulatory mechanisms and therapeutic targets.

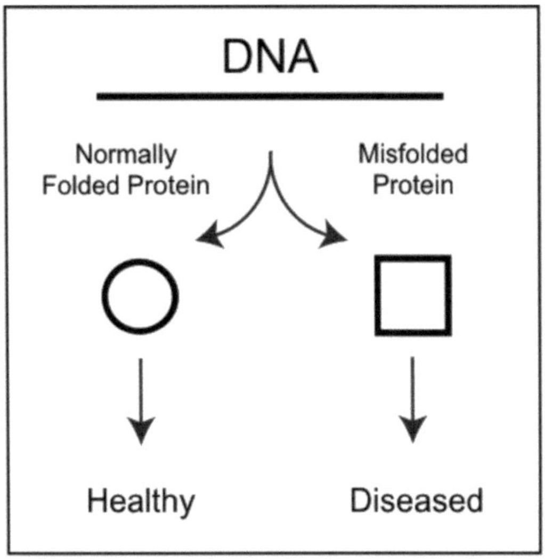

Figure 1. Prion and protein-only inheritance. The central dogma of molecular biology stipulated that genotype (DNA) encodes phenotype (visible traits). However, prion proteins represent an important departure from this rule where inheritance may arise from proteins alone. Through adopting a stable misfolded conformation (square) a protein can go from harmless to capable of conferring a number of fatal, progressive neurodegenerative diseases.

Prion diseases offer a particularly intriguing biological phenomenon for mathematical analysis because such diseases cover many different systems and time scales. At the level of a population, such as a herd of sheep or population of deer, prion disease can be studied as a classical epidemic model where infections are spread among an initially uninfected (susceptible population). Prion disease can also be studied as a genetic disease whose phenotype is caused by a gain of function mutation in the gene coding for Prp. While the age of disease onset and death appear to be heritable, linking genotype to phenotype remains challenging [3]. Spontaneous prion disease is thought to be nucleation limited, with the formation of a stable minimal size aggregate (nucleus) of misfolded protein serving as the rate-limiting step in the appearance of prion diseases. All prion diseases are characterized by aggregates of misfolded protein serving as templates to convert normally folded protein and amplifying through fragmentation. As such, many mathematical formulations have focused primarily on the dynamics of the aggregates themselves through modeling either discrete or continuous sizes using ordinary differential equations (ODEs) or partial differential equations (PDEs), respectively. Finally, in order to model the loss or reversal of the prion phenotype in certain experimental systems, prion dynamics are modeled as a stochastic process.

This chapter reviews the application of mathematical models to the study of prions. Our goal is to serve as a tool for both mathematicians and biologists interested in interdisciplinary research in prion disease. We first describe the time before the identification of the prion, when the work of mathematician Griffiths was central to proposing a protein-only disease process. We next overview mathematical formulations focusing on the dynamics of prion disease through modeling the kinetics protein misfolding and aggregation as well as the coagulation and fragmentation dynamics of the misfolded aggregates themselves. We close by discussing recent advances and ongoing work in mathematical modeling of prions that are serving to further our understanding and motivate experimental studies and present some open questions.

2. Mysterious mammalian diseases, heritable yeast phenotypes and the mathematical origins of the prion hypothesis

No discussion of prion disease would be complete without discussion of the field prior to the establishment of the prion hypothesis, which stipulates that protein, rather than virus or bacteria, is the infectious agent of the prion disease. Here we give an overview of historical observations linking a variety of diseases in mammals, leading to the formulation of the prion hypothesis by Griffith [4], subsequent experimental validation by Prusiner [5] and discovery of prions in fungi. (For a more complete history of prion diseases refer to any of these reviews [6–10].)

Scrapie is likely the first prion disease to be observed with reports dating back to the 1500s [7, 11]. The first publication describing scrapie appeared in 1759 [12] and because scrapie was reported to be an infectious "distemper" from which sheep could never recover, shepherds of the time were advised to separate any animal observing symptoms from the rest of the flock. Publications at this time discussed and debated possible modes of transmission for this disease; ideas were wide ranging from inbreeding [13], humidity of the sheep pen [14] and even atmospheric events [15]. By the late nineteenth century, it was strongly believed that scrapie was a hereditary disease, but some reports noted spontaneous occurrences leading some to believe there was two forms of scrapie: hereditary and non-hereditary [7].

In 1913, Sir Steward Stockman published "Scrapie: An Obscure Disease of Sheep" [16], which served as both a historical record of the disease as well as analysis of its symptoms and progression. In particular, he notes that scrapie has a long incubation time of 2–3 years. Research on the method of transmission of scrapie continued and by the early 1960s, it had been established that scrapie could spread through indirect contact between sheep (grazing in a field that had been occupied by an infected herd) [17], could transmit either as an infectious or heritable disease [18], could be transmitted through serum as when a vaccine for another disease (Louping-ill) was prepared from sheep infected with scrapie [19] and could transmit between species (from sheep to goat [20] and sheep to mouse [21]). In combination, these observations suggested that scrapie did not behave as any previously observed disease-causing agent.

Scrapie was not the only prion disease studied in the mid-twentieth century. Around the same time that cross-species infectivity of scrapie was demonstrated, researchers were studying kuru, a progressive neurodegenerative disease that appeared in Papua New Guinea. The disease was first reported in the scientific literature when anthropologists [22] and pediatricians [23] reported a deadly disease among the Fore people called kuru. The disease had an unusual distribution by sex and age; among children, both male and female could have the disease, but among adults incidence was nearly always limited to females [9]. It was also observed that the pathology of kuru was similar to a Cruzfeld-Jacob disease, a very rare neurological disorder [24].

Researchers continued to conduct experiments to uncover the method by which scrapie and kuru were transmitted. In 1959, a critical connection was made between these seemingly separate disorders; Hadlow, a veterinarian, attended an exhibit at the Wellcome Medical Museum in London featuring images of neurological tissue from the brains of individuals who died from kuru. He noted the patterns and appearance of damage was extremely similar to what he had seen in scrapie. The similar pathology, combined with the apparent ability of kuru and scrapie diseases to be acquired or hereditary caused him to conjecture that a similar mechanism could be responsible for both diseases and advised researchers to see experiment with transmission of kuru from humans to other mammals (as had been done for scrapie) [25]. Indeed, soon after Hadlow's publication it was shown that, like scrapie, kuru could be transmitted to other mammals [26, 27].

While linking diseases such as scrapie, kuru and Cruzfeld-Jacob was significant in formulating the prion hypothesis, it did not directly address the question of the infectious unit of the disease. In 1966, Alper and colleagues used radiation and filtration experiments on brains from mice scrapie and determined the infectious agent of scrapie appeared to be able to self-replicate but without a nucleic acid code; they conclude by indicating the scrapie agent "is likely to be of an unusual nature" [28].

In 1967, Griffiths, a mathematician at Bedford College in London took the observations from Alper [28] and Pattison [29] and suggested the infectious agent of scrapie was "probably a protein without nucleic acid" [4]. While precise mathematical formulations were not given, Griffiths used the same type of reasoning that goes into the development of mathematical models to pose three possible mechanisms by which a host-encoded protein could act as an infectious agent. Namely, he worked within the known rules of the underlying biological processes to pose hypotheses, which could then act to motivate further experimental design. It is precisely this form of interplay between the mathematical and biological sciences that serve to drive discovery.

It is worth noting that Griffith's proposed mechanisms for a protein infectious unit involved three distinct biological processes: gene regulation, protein aggregation and immune response. Because his second mechanism is closest to what we believe to be correct today, we postpone its discussion. First, he suggested a process by a gene encoding the prion protein was typically in the "OFF" state. If the prion protein was capable of acting as an inducer to this gene (i.e., turning it "ON"), then the introduction of prion protein would act infectiously by turning the gene "ON" and further production of the protein would maintain the gene in the "ON" state. As such a prion disease could occur spontaneously if the gene were perturbed to the "ON" state in an individual or be acquired through consumption of a protein. His third mechanism was one where the immune response (antibody) was itself equivalent to the foreign body (antigen) and thus prion disease could be the hosts immunity backfiring.

Remarkably, his second proposal quite closely depicts the dynamics of protein aggregation and fragmentation that today we believe was that of protein aggregation and fragmentation. He posed a simple model where proteins could exist as monomer, dimer, trimer and tetramer. Increase in size could occur through monomer addition and tetramers could split into two dimers. If the reaction to create a dimer from two monomers was itself required the catalytic influence of a dimer, the all-monomer state would persist stably unless a dimer were introduced. Such a system he noted would be capable of self-propagating as long as there were monomer (which could be produced by the host) and an initial infectious unit (a dimer, trimer, or tetramer).

Griffith's proposed "protein-only" method of disease transmission spurred further experimental studies. Finally, in 1982, Prusiner demonstrated through several distinct lines of evidence (including sensitivity to proteases) that the infectious agent was a protein and coined the term "prion" to mean proteinaceous infectious particle [5]. Not long after, a team of researchers discovered the host gene coding for the prion protein, named PrP for prion protein, in mammals [30].

While mammalian disease was the driving force behind the investigations so far discussed, mammals are not the only organisms that today we know to exhibit protein-only inheritance. In 1994, Wickner was investigating a heritable phenotype in yeast that did not appear to have a chromosomal determinant, but was associated with an altered form of a yeast protein Ure2p [31]; he proposed that this phenotype could be prion based. Thus, the prion hypothesis could plausibly explain a number of non-Mendialian phenotypes discovered and studied by Cox [32]. The facility of yeast as an experimental system has spurred the identification of nearly a dozen prion proteins in yeast each of which is linked with a seemingly harmless phenotype [6, 33]. Thus, this opens the possibility that protein-only inheritance may well have evolved as a regulatory mechanism.

While today there remain some scientists that reject the notion that a host-encoded protein could be the infectious agent, increasingly sophisticated experimental studies continue to support the prion hypothesis. For example, in 2013 Zhang and colleagues demonstrated that prion diseases could be induced in mammals from recombinant prion protein produced in bacteria [34]. As such, the prion hypothesis has become the accepted view for both mammalian prion diseases and heritable yeast phenotypes.

Today we understand that proteins capable of propagating through a protein-only mechanism do so by adopting an abnormal folded-state (conformation) and forming aggregates each of which may act as a template to induce further misfolding among normally folded protein. (Note that we use the term "prion phenotype" to encompass both the concept of mammalian prion disease and harmless prion phenotypes in yeast.) Indeed, there are multiple possible prion phenotypes (in mammals these correspond to distinct incubation periods for disease symptoms) each of which corresponds to a distinct conformation typically called a prion strain. Finally, while all known mammalian prion phenotypes correspond to the same protein PrP, in fungi there are a number of prion proteins each linked to distinct phenotypes [6, 33].

However, as we will detail further, identification of this infectious agent is only the beginning in characterizing these processes.

3. Establishing a mathematical framework of prion aggregate dynamics

In this section, we discuss contributions of mathematical modeling in understanding the dynamics associated with prion disease (more generally phenotype). Because prion phenotypes can be either spontaneous or acquired, a distinction is often made between **nucleation**, the spontaneous appearance of an initially infectious unit and **propagation** of the infectious unit. However, since both phases involve aggregation of misfolded protein, similar mathematical formulations have been applied to both processes. Indeed both processes are also fundamental to other protein aggregation processes and disorders such as Alzheimer's and Parkinson's diseases. Because several reviews exist on mathematical models of aggregation in more general biological processes [35, 36], in this work we focus on mathematical methods of appearance and propagation as specifically applied to the *in vivo* dynamics of prion phenotypes. Although in spontaneous prion disease, nucleation occurs first, we will begin our discussion with propagation as this step has been better characterized.

Propagation. The first mathematical formulation of the autocatalytic propagation of prion aggregates was published by Eigen in 1996 [37] where, inspired by the dimerization process expressed in Griffiths' third hypothesis [4] and observations from by Prusiner [38] and Lansbury [39–41], he developed systems of differential equations to analyze two theories on protein-only amplification. Through his mathematical analysis, Eigen was able to demonstrate support for the idea that prion aggregates are themselves the infectious agent of prion disease but, as Eigen writes "aggregation of the prionic form is most probably a necessary, but not possibly sufficient, prerequisite of infection".

In Eigen's first model, he explores the possibility suggested by Prusiner [38] that heterodimers act to template misfolding. He considers a system with two-protein species: A, normal conformation and B, prion conformation; proteins of type A are capable of forming heterodimers with proteins of type B and through that interaction are irreversibly converted to type B. The resulting homodimer of B would then resolve creating two proteins of state B, each of which may then act to template further conversion events. (Note that in this model the capacity of the system to convert protein from state A to state B depends linearly on the total concentration of B.)

The mathematical model resulting from these assumptions consists of two coupled differential equations. Eigen performed steady-state analysis to determine the possible asymptotic concentrations of each protein species and how the local stability of each depended on the underlying kinetic values. He found two types of asymptotic behavior were possible and the one the system would converge to depended on the ratio of two kinetic parameters: the catalytic conversion rate and the death/decay rate of the prion conformation of the protein. If the death rate exceeded the conversion rate, the asymptotic concentration of prion proteins (type B) approaches 0 and nearly all the protein will be in then normal conformation (type A). When the conversion rate exceeds the death rate, the reverse happens, namely the amount of protein in the prion conformation (type B) will grow exponentially and most of the protein present is in the prion conformation. Since neither of these possibilities was consistent with the true behavior of prion disease, namely that the vast majority of individuals have primarily healthy protein and, even in the few individuals that do have prion diseases, still have detectable levels of normal protein. As such, Eigen concluded that a model where the conversion capacity was linear with the concentration of misfolded protein was not possible [37].

Eigen's second model, considered two mechanisms where the infectious agents were not individual misfolded protein monomers: a cooperative auto-catalytic mechanism, which generalized his first model and aggregates of misfolded protein, in accordance with a proposed aggregation mechanism from Lansbury [39–41]. These assumptions result in their own—more complicated—sets of differential equations, but as for the previous model, steady-state analysis revealed important properties of the asymptotic dynamics. Both models exhibited a "threshold" effect, that is, if the concentration of prion protein were low enough, the healthy state was maintained but the introduction of prion protein exceeding a threshold would cause the exponential growth of prion protein. While the results of Eigen's work did not definitively detail all necessary steps in the propagation of prion phenotypes, nor did he demonstrate global asymptotic stability of the prion phenotype, his work demonstrated that mathematical modeling—in particular systems of deterministic ODEs—could be used to theoretically interrogate biological hypotheses on prion dynamics. In particular, Eigen's analysis demonstrated that "aggregation is necessarily involved" [37] in prion propagation.

In 1998, Nowak and colleagues built upon Eigen's seminal work by incorporating additional experimental observations, in particular work demonstrating sensitivity of distinct Prp strains to protease cleavage. Their mathematical framework of prion infection dynamics was based on having prion aggregates act in two ways; first (as in Eigen's model) they would template additional misfolding, but now aggregates themselves could increase fragmentation [42]. Because this model forms the basis of most subsequent mathematical models on prion dynamics, we discuss its formulation in some detail. In this mathematical formulation, the state of the system at time t, is the concentration of proteins in the normal conformation, $x(t)$ and prion aggregates of every discrete size i, $y_i(t)$. They assume protein in the normal conformation is created at rate λ and decays at rate d, aggregates of all sizes decay at rate a. Conversion occurs through contact between aggregates and normal conformers at a rate depending on the size of the aggregate, β_i. Finally, the total number of aggregates increases through fragmentation; in their most general formulation they specify the rate that aggregates of size j fragment to create an aggregate of size i as $b_{j,i}$ and that during fragmentation no mass is lost (i.e., if an aggregate of size j is always fragmented into two aggregates of size i and $(j–i)$). Translating these biochemical kinetic assumptions into a set of differential equations results in the following infinite system:

$$\frac{dx}{dt} = \lambda - dx(t) - \sum_{i=1}^{\infty} \beta_i x(t) y_i(t), \tag{1}$$

$$\frac{dy_i}{dt} = \beta_{i-1} x(t) y_{i-1}(t) - \beta_i x(t) y_i(t) - a y_i(t) + \sum_{j=i+1}^{\infty} (b_{j,i} + b_{j,i-j}) y_j(t) - \sum_{j=1}^{i-1} b_{i,j} y_i(t), \tag{2}$$

for $i = 1, 2, \ldots$, etc. While the model allows for quite general dynamics, under the simple assumptions that the conversion rate is independent of aggregate size, that fragmentation increases linearly with aggregate size and that fragmentation is equally likely between any two adjacent monomers in an aggregate, this infinite system of differential equations reduces to the following three-dimensional system:

$$\frac{dx}{dt} = \lambda - dx(t) - \beta x(t)Y(t) \tag{3}$$

$$\frac{dY}{dt} = bZ(t) - (a+b)Y(t) \tag{4}$$

$$\frac{dZ}{dt} = \beta x(t)Y(t) - aZ(t) \tag{5}$$

where $Y(t) = \sum_{i=1}^{\infty} y_i(t)$ represents the total number of aggregates and $Z(t) = \sum_{i=1}^{\infty} iy_i(t)$ is the total amount of prion protein. We note that mathematically $Y(t)$ and $Z(t)$ correspond to the zeroth and first moments of the distribution of aggregate sizes and, as such, this demonstrates a moment closure of the aggregate size distribution. That is, the time-evolution of the complete aggregate size distribution under these kinetic simplifications is determined by purely the zeroth and first moments. Nowak and colleagues remarked this reduced formulation was mathematically equivalent to prior viral models studied in mathematical epidemiology and derived an expression for the basic reproductive number of a prion aggregate. The basic reproductive number, or R_0 as is commonly denoted in the epidemic community, specifies the number of secondary infections (in this case infectious aggregate) created by an infection aggregate during its lifetime. In the case that $R_0 > 1$, we expect exponential growth of disease in a purely susceptible population and, as such, prion aggregate to persist stably. If $R_0 < 1$, we expect the infectious elements, in this case prion aggregates, to exponentially decay and ultimately be lost from the system. In this case the R_0 was shown to be a ratio of the underlying kinetic parameters: $R_0 = \frac{\beta\lambda b}{da(a+b)}$. As such, the stability of prion phenotypes was now shown to be explicitly a function of biochemical properties offering the promise to interpret results in this new context.

Nowak and colleagues [42] were also the first to formalize what today is considered to be the standard prion aggregate kinetics, the **nucleated polymerization model (NPM)**. In this model, the infectious units are aggregates above a critical size. Below this critical size, aggregates of the misfolded prion form of the protein are presumed to be highly unstable and are rapidly resolved into monomers (see **Figure 2**). (It is this nucleation process that forms the rate-limiting step in the establishment of prion phenotypes and we discuss this extensively in the next section.) The dynamics of the NPM are similar to those presented in Nowak's first model; however, the minimal nucleus size modifies the resulting equations slightly. First, the quantities $Y(t)$ and $Z(t)$ now represent the aggregates above this critical minimal size, n_0. That is,

$$Y(t) = \sum_{i=n_0}^{\infty} y_i(t) \text{ and } Z(t) = \sum_{i=n_0}^{\infty} i\, y_i(t). \tag{6}$$

Under the previous simplifications on kinetic rates, this changes the resulting moment closure of the infinite system of ODEs to the following three-dimensional system of ODEs:

http://dx.doi.org/10.5772/66917

$$\frac{dx}{dt} = \lambda - dx(t) - \beta x(t)Y(t) + b(n_0)(n_0 - 1)Y(t), \tag{7}$$

$$\frac{dY}{dt} = bZ(t) - (a + b(2n_0 - 1))Y(t), \tag{8}$$

$$\frac{dZ}{dt} = \beta x(t)Y(t) - aZ(t) - b(n_0)(n_0 - 1)Y(t). \tag{9}$$

In this new formulation the basic reproductive number of a prion aggregate now also depends on the minimal nucleus size n_0. This form of the NPM has become the standard approach for modeling prion aggregate dynamics and inspired many future mathematical studies.

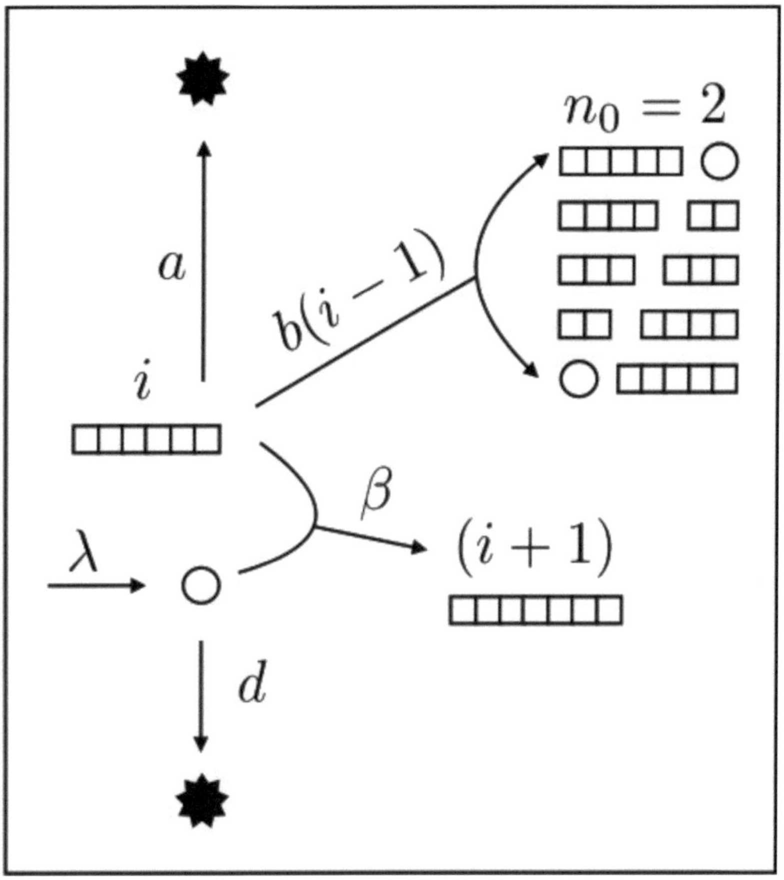

Figure 2. Nucleated polymerization model of prion dynamics. This demonstrates the key steps in the nucleated polymerization model (NPM) of prion aggregate dynamics. (The description of the kinetic parameters is in the text.) This model is characterized by prion aggregates below a critical size $n_0 = 2$ (the nucleus size) resolving to protein monomers in the normal folded state.

In 1999 Masel, Jensen and Nowak conducted an extensive analysis of the NPM [43]. In particular, they sought to link experimental observations on the time to appearance of prion disease symptoms with the kinetic parameters of the NPM. Among other contributions, Masel and colleagues determined a viable range of minimal nucleus sizes, n_0. Overall, there was remarkable consistency between parameters predicted from different experimental data sets analyzed providing support at the time for this mathematical formulation. In addition, Masel et al. [43] (and then Greer and colleagues with a generalization [44]) demonstrated that the dynamics of aggregates under the NPM are consistent with the long-incubation time observed for prion phenotypes. If prion disease begins with the introduction of a small amount of prion protein (in the form of aggregates) those aggregates will first have to increase in size until there are enough fragmentation sites to permit aggregate amplification through fragmentation.

In early twenty-first century, mathematicians continued formalizing the NPM. Prüss and colleagues [45] demonstrated that the prion phenotypes were globally asymptotically stable and not merely locally stable, through deriving a Lyapunov function. Engler et al. [46] analyzed the well-posedness of the generalization of the NPM where aggregate sizes were continuous, instead of discrete. As such, rather than an infinite system of ordinary differential equations, the system consisted of a single ODE for protein in the normal configuration and a PDE specifying the distribution of aggregate sizes. While this formulation departs from the physically discrete nature of aggregates, in the limit of large aggregate sizes these formalisms are provably equivalent [47] and the use of PDEs permits a wider array of mathematical techniques. Most notably, the continuous relaxation on aggregate sizes has permitted determination of the explicit asymptotic density [44, 46]. (In comparison, the asymptotic density for the aggregate model with discrete aggregate sizes, while first approximated in 2003 by Pöschel et al. [48], was derived only recently by Davis and Sindi and required special functions [49].)

While today mathematical models of prion aggregate dynamics have been formulated under many more general kinetic assumptions (see [47, 50–52] for example) most of these models have been compared to only *in vitro* aggregation studies. For yeast, *in vivo* comparisons have been made for the Sup35/[*PSI*$^+$] prion system [53–55], but linking experimental outcomes uniquely to specific kinetic parameters remains challenging.

Nucleation. As mentioned in the previous section, the rate-limiting step in prion phenotypes is thought to be the time to the appearance of stable nucleus, that is, an aggregate of misfolded protein that persists stably. (It is typically thought that this nucleus corresponds to a misfolded aggregate of a minimal stable size [42, 43].) The self-assembly of particles into aggregates is fundamental to many physical, chemical and biological processes. Such a process is referred to in statistical physics as nucleation and mathematical models of nucleation have been studied for nearly a century [56]. In contrast to other biochemical models of protein aggregation, the spontaneous appearance of a prion nucleus is thought to be rare [57, 58]. As such, mathematical models of prion appearance are often framed as first-passage processes; that is, these models focus on determining the amount of time until a critical event occurs, in this case the appearance of a prion nucleus.

One of the earliest models of self-assembly of particles was proposed by in 1916 by Smoluchowski [59]. He considered the evolution of the density of clusters of discrete particle sizes under the assumption that clusters of any size could join together (coagulation). In 1935, Becker and Döring introduced kinetic equations for a similar process but where clusters could only change in size through monomer addition or removal [60]. More generally, models of particle self-assembly are distinguished by their associated set of biochemical equations governing the evolution of cluster sizes. As such, the problem of prion nucleus appearance can be framed as: given a set of biochemical equations governing misfolded protein aggregate formation, determine the time it takes for a critical sized nucleus to form [61].

Broadly speaking, two mathematical formulations have been used to describe the time to nucleus formation: deterministic and stochastic. In a deterministic mathematical model, the predictions or model output is always the same for a given input. In such a formulation, the Law of Mass Action is used to convert the set of biochemical equations to a system of ordinary differential equations (ODEs) [62]. For the standard aggregation processes, like the Becker-Döring process, systems of ODEs have been extensively studied [60, 63, 64]. In these ODEs, the mathematical model output is a continuously varying quantity approximating the concentration or number of aggregates of each possible size. The time to nucleation would then be specified as the time at which the value associated with the critical nucleus size exceeds a threshold value. When the number of total proteins present is large, a deterministic formulation describes the dynamics well; however, when the number of proteins is small, random effects begin to dominate and to capture these effects a stochastic formulation is required [65]. (We note that for *in vitro* experiments of prion aggregation, when the concentration of proteins far exceeds physiological settings, deterministic models have proven to be consistent with observed quantities [66, 67].)

Stochastic mathematical models allow for the possibility of the same input to produce different output. In this case, the state of the system is given not as a deterministic quantity, but a random variable that can take on different values [68]. For example, given a coin with two sides (heads and tails), the number of times a coin must be flipped until heads appears is a random variable; one might attain heads on the first try or require many trials before heads appears. Because the observed output can change, the quantity of interest is not the specific output but rather its properties. To continue our example, we might wish to know either what the **mean** (average) number of flips will be required from a fair coin to produce heads and possibly the **variance** in that quantity. Alternatively, we might wish to know the probability associated with observing any possible outcome (i.e., what is the probability we flip the coin k times before observing a head); this corresponds to a **probability density function**. For our example of the coin, the number of flips required before heads appears is given as a geometric probability distribution. That is, the probability that k coin flips are required before the first heads is observed is given by: $(1-p)^{k-1}p$ where p is the probability of heads on any given trial. For all but simple systems, such as our coin flip example, it is not possible to obtain an explicit formula for our random variable in question. As such, an increasingly sophisticated set of mathematical and computational tools have been employed to aid in such processes.

We note that for nucleation problems, we are interested not in the state of our protein molecules at any particular time, but the first-arrival time of the nucleus. That is, the time at which the first aggregate of minimal stable size appears. Below we refer to misfolded protein aggregates smaller than the critical nucleus as **proto-nuclei** and any aggregate larger than the nucleus size as a **propagon**. (We note this is consistent with the definition of a propagon as being a prion aggregate capable of transmitting the prion phenotype upon transmission to an environment with normally folded protein [33, 69].)

We will first frame this problem as a continuous-time stochastic process and then discuss how statistical properties of the first-arrival time may be computed. (For a detailed discussion of stochastic processes and first arrival times in biological systems, refer to [61, 68].) For simplicity, let us assume that our system consists of a total number of m molecules of our protein in question and that this number remains constant (i.e., no synthesis or degradation). In this case, if we observe the system at any particular time the state of the system consists of the number of protein aggregates of each possible size. If $n_i(t)$ is the total number of aggregates of each size i at time t ($i = 1$ corresponds to monomer), then for all time we have:

$$\sum_{i=1}^{m} i\, n_i(t) = m. \tag{10}$$

We use Ω to denote set of all possible molecular configurations and observe that the size of this space increases exponentially in m but, because there is no synthesis or degradation, Ω is finite. We distinguish between two sets of configurations in Ω; A: those configurations with only proto-nuclei and $A^C = \Omega$: those where the system has at least one propagon. While not required, it is often assumed that the system begins in the all-monomer state (i.e., $n_1(0) = m$, $n_i(i) = 0$ for all $i > 1$) [61, 70]. At any given time, aggregates of any size may increase or decrease in time through dynamics such as monomer addition, fragmentation and/or coagulation as allowed by the biochemical assumptions (for example, the Smoluchowski [59] or Becker-Döring [60] assumptions). Refer to **Figure 3** for a visualization of the stochastic model. The first-arrival time is the time that the stochastic process reaches any configuration in A^C.

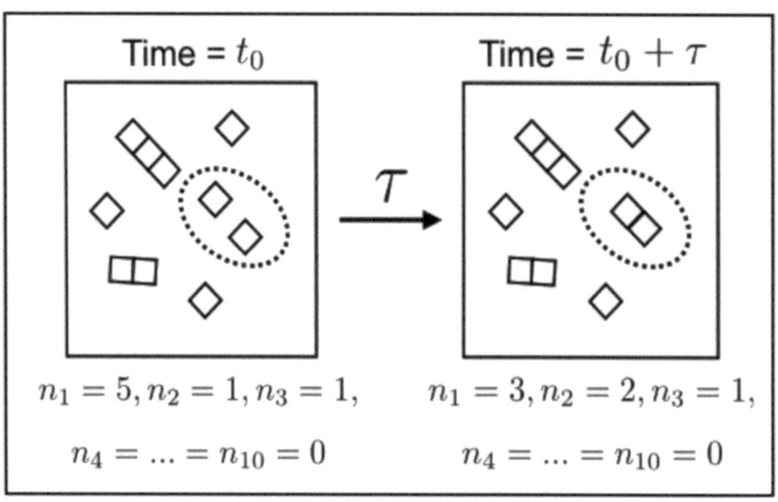

Figure 3. Stochastic model for prion nucleus appearance. The rate-limiting step in the appearance of prion phenotypes is thought to be the waiting-time until the appearance of a nucleus, an aggregate of misfolded prion protein that exceeds a critical size. In a stochastic formulation, the number of prion subunits of each size is tracked in time. As detailed in the text, we are considering a reduced system where the total number of protein molecules (m) remains fixed in time.

http://dx.doi.org/10.5772/66917

There are three methods for computing first-arrival times and their associated moments (mean, variance, etc.) in this stochastic formulation. First, these quantities may be defined directly by analyzing solutions of the chemical master equation (CME). The CME is the first-order linear differential equation that describes the time-evolution of the probability of the system to occupy any particular configuration [68, 71–74]. Because the size of the state-space is exponential in the number of monomers, the CME is computationally intractable for all but very simple systems. Second, computational simulations representing individual realizations of the nucleation process are generated *in silico*; the mean and moments of the first-passage times are then calculated from these empirical results [75, 76]. While Monte Carlo approaches are typically easy to code and highly parallelizable, they suffer from slow convergence and in the case of rare events, like nucleation, individual realizations may take arbitrarily long to terminate [77]. Third, heuristics may be used to simplify the dynamics in particular regimes. For example, in a series of studies Chou and colleagues [65, 78–80] approximated the mean first-arrival time to a critical nucleus for the Becker-Döring model (only monomer growth or detachment) in for two parameter regimes (strong growth and weak growth) by computing the arrival time for the dominant pathway from the all-monomer state to the appearance of the first aggregate of a minimal stable size. While dominant path approaches are readily apparent for some models of aggregation, like Becker-Döring, they are difficult to determine for more general sets of reactions. Further, because these results rely on particular parameter combinations, the approximations pose challenges to parameter inference—where we want to determine the kinetic parameters that best match available data.

We note that beyond the mathematical challenges in modeling nucleation there remain many practical challenges. Experimentally, it is typically not possible to separate the spontaneous appearance of a propagon, an initial infectious aggregate, from the prion phenotype itself. Finally, critical events in the underlying biochemical kinetics of nucleus formation in prion disease are unknown. In our formulation above, we described protein subunits, but the protein itself is only capable of aggregating when in a particular conformational state. As such, an accurate predictive model of spontaneous nucleation must also include a model of protein misfolding. While it is clear that particular prion variants (distinct conformations) are favored under particular experimental conditions [81], the connection between nucleus formation and conformation has yet to be fully explored. As such, nucleation remains a challenge on experimental, mathematical and computational fronts.

4. Present state and challenges in prion disease modeling

As described above, a combination of mathematical and experimental studies over the past few decades have led to the formulation of a protein-only form of inheritance associated with prion phenotypes. We first summarize our present knowledge and then remark on present day studies and challenges that remain in modeling prion disease. Today we believe that prion phenotypes are established through two distinct phases, nucleation and amplification. Once an initial nucleus—prion aggregate above a critical size—is introduced to a host, four steps are required for successful *in vivo* propagation of prion phenotypes (see **Figure 4**). First, normal folded protein must be continuously created. Second, aggregates of the misfolded form of the protein act as templates by converting normally folded protein to the same misfolded state. Third, the total number of templates increases through fragmentation where a single aggregate is split into two (or more) smaller aggregates. Finally, misfolded protein must spread through other cells. For yeast, this transfer of misfolded protein occurs through cell division where for mammals this likely involves extracellular diffusion [33].

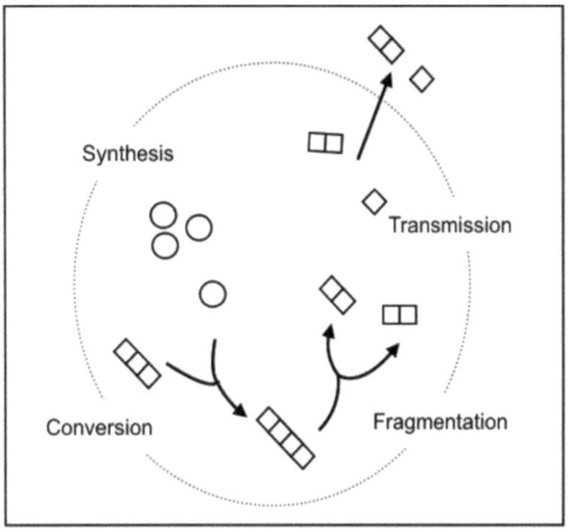

Figure 4. *In vivo* prion propagation. The infectious agent of prion disease is aggregates of misfolded proteins (squares). Four steps are essential to stable propagation of the prion form of the protein: (1) new normally folded protein must be created, (2) prion aggregates act as templates to convert normally folded protein to the misfolded state, (3) prion aggregates are fragmented into smaller aggregates each of which may be capable of acting as a template, and (4) prion infectious units must spread through other cells. In the case of yeast prions, this transmission occurs through the normal process of cell division while for mammalian disease transmission corresponds to diffusion and transport through tissue.

However, beyond this basic understanding remain many challenges, both mathematical and biological. We briefly outline some open questions in prion biology we believe are amenable to interdisciplinary approaches.

Consideration of the cellular environment. Prion phenotypes are established through protein misfolding, but protein misfolding itself is not rare. Eukaryotic cells have developed a complex network of molecular chaperones and protein degradation factors that act continuously to identify and clear misfolded proteins [33]. As such, understanding the *in vivo* propagation of prion phenotypes requires considering the environment in which they appear. In the case of yeast prions, the molecular chaperone Hsp104 has been shown to be essential for the propagation of [*PSI*$^+$] prion phenotype in yeast. While comparatively few mathematical studies have considered the role of Hsp104 as enzyme catalyzing fragmentation [55, 82], the results from these studies have resolved previously unsupported results on shifts in aggregate size distributions and (as we will discuss further below) rates of loss (curing) of specific [*PSI*$^+$] strain phenotypes.

Spread of prion aggregates. A major open question in prion biology amenable to mathematical analysis is how prion aggregates spread between cells either through cell division (yeast prion phenotypes) or within a mammalian tissue. Although this question was first explored when Nowak and colleagues [42] presented simulations of their NPM where prion aggregates could move between distinct cells in a population and when Payne and Krakauer [83] considered prions spreading in tissue as a traveling wave, our understanding of the spread of prion aggregates is still incomplete. Because the long incubation period and complicated physical domains involved in mammalian prion disease will pose significant experimental and mathematical challenges, yeast prion phenotypes may provide a useful tool in this question. While stochastic models have been developed for yeast, which link cellular levels of prion aggregates with computational simulations [55], formulations amenable to analytical treatment need to be developed to allow for a more systematic characterization of the spread of prion aggregates.

Reversing prion phenotypes. Mammalian prion diseases remain untreatable and ultimately fatal and as such the identification of clinical treatments and methods of early detection remain important scientific and technical challenges. Of particular challenge may be that drugs which act to promote aggregate fragmentation, with the goal of causing all aggregate to drop below the critical nucleus size, may in fact promote prion amplification at low doses when they would merely act to accelerate the exponential growth of prion aggregates [84].

A promising avenue toward finding approaches to manage prion diseases in mammals, might be to more clearly understand the biochemical processes responsible for a number of reversible prion phenotypes in yeast [33]. As was demonstrated by Derdowski et al. [55], a combination of enzyme-limited fragmentation and aggregate-size transmission bias appeared to be responsible for the observed natural rates of curing for the [PSI^{+}] weak phenotype. In addition, for yeast treatment with GdnHCl has been shown to significantly slow aggregate fragmentation leading to a natural reversal of prion phenotypes by dilution of the aggregate during cell division [69, 85–88].

Further, biological and mathematical researchers should consider mechanisms of curing prion disease through studying mutations in prion proteins, which are known to slow or halt the disease progression. Such mutations are known to exist in mammals [89] and yeast [90].

Evolvability of prions. While prions were originally implicated in mammalian disease, the fact that they persist as a number of harmless heritable phenotypes in yeast raises intriguing questions about how and why prions may have evolved [57, 91, 92]. Because the yeast phenotype [PSI^{+}] is associated with a decreased efficiency in stop-codon recognition, it is thought to serve as an evolutionary capacitor by promoting the generation of novel transcripts [57]. More recently, a combination of mathematical and experimental studies have demonstrated that smaller [PSI^{+}] aggregates still retain function associated with the normal Sup35 conformation offering the possibility this system evolved to tune stop-codon recognition [54]. While we are still far from understanding the forces behind prion phenotype evolution, the evidence continues to mount for possible beneficial examples of prion-like mechanisms [93].

5. Conclusion

Many questions remain about prion phenotypes and it is essential once again for scientists with different backgrounds to utilize their disciplinary expertise and methods to address these questions. As we have discussed, two critical points in the history of prion disease came from researchers that were not primarily biologists, namely the mathematician Griffith [4] and the veterinarian Hadlow [25]. If the past is any predictor, future studies in prion phenotypes will continue to benefit from an interdisciplinary approach.

Author details

Suzanne S. Sindi

Address all correspondence to: ssindi@ucmerced.edu

Applied Mathematics, University of California, Merced, California, United States of America

References

[1] Jungck, J.R., Ten equations that changed biology: mathematics in problem-solving biology curricula. Bioscene, 1997. **23**(1): 11–36.

[2] Reed, M.C., Mathematical biology is good for mathematics. Notices of the AMS, 2015. **62** (10): 1172–6.

[3] Webb, T., et al., Age of onset and death in inherited prion disease are heritable. American Journal of Medical Genetics Part B: Neuropsychiatric Genetics, 2009. **150**(4): 496–501.

[4] Griffith, J.S., Self-replication and scrapie. Nature, 1967. **215**(5105): 1043–4.

[5] Prusiner, S.B., Novel proteinaceous infectious particles cause scrapie. Science, 1982. **216** (4542): 136–44.

[6] Tuite, M.F. and T.R. Serio, The prion hypothesis: from biological anomaly to basic regulatory mechanism. Nature Reviews Molecular Cell Biology, 2010. **11**(12): 823–33.

[7] Schneider, K., et al., The early history of the transmissible spongiform encephalopathies exemplified by scrapie. Brain Research Bulletin, 2008. **77**(6): 343–55.

[8] Poser, C.M., Notes on the history of the prion diseases. Part II. Clinical Neurology and Neurosurgery, 2002. **104**(2): 77–86.

[9] Poser, C.M., Notes on the history of the prion diseases. Part I. Clinical Neurology and Neurosurgery, 2002. **104**(1): 1–9.

[10] Goldfarb, L.G., Kuru: the old epidemic in a new mirror. Microbes and Infection, 2002. **4** (8): 875–82.

[11] Brown, D.R., Neurodegeneration and Prion Disease. 2005: Springer Science & Business Media, New York, NY, USA.

[12] Leopoldt J.G., Useful Introduction to Agriculture Based on Experience. volume 5, Christian Friedrich Günthern, Glogau, Berlin, 1759.

[13] May G., The sheep: its wool, races, breeding, nutrition, and use, as well as its diseases: First Edition in 2 vol, Eduard Trewendt, Breslau, 1868.

[14] Richter, F., Compilation of the observations made by me concerning the troubles or gnubber's disease with regard to their symptoms, the causative organism. Momente, Weiterverbreitung, Verhütung und Heilung. Magazin für die gesamte Thierheilkunde, 1841. **7**: 198–209.

[15] Ribbe, J., Thoughts, and remarks concerning the sheep, and some diseases peculiar to this animal race, and especially the trotting, which is now so frequently evident. Oekonomische Neuigkeiten und Verhandlungen, 1826. **50**: 397–99.

[16] Stockman, S., Scrapie: an obscure disease of sheep. Journal of Comparative Pathology and Therapeutics, 1913. **26**: 317–27.

[17] Greig, R., *Scrapie.* Transactions of the Highland and Agricultural Society of Scotland, 1940. **52**: 71–9.

[18] Cuillé, J. and P.-L. Chelle, The so-called trembling disease of the sheep is inoculable. Comptes Rendus de l'Académie des Sciences, 1936. **203**: 1552–4.

[19] Gordon, W., Louping ill, tickborne fever and scrapie. The Veterinary Record, 1946. **58**: 516–25.

[20] Pattison, I., Transmission of scrapie to the goat. The Lancet, 1957. **272**: 104–5.

[21] Chandler, R., Encephalopathy in mice produced by inoculation with scrapie brain material. The Lancet, 1961. **277**(7191): 1378–9.

[22] Berndt, R.M., Reaction to contact in the Eastern Highlands of New Guinea. Oceania, 1954. **24**(3): 190–228.

[23] Gajdusek, D.C. and J.E. Smadel, Correspondence on the Discovery and Original Investigations on Kuru: Smadel-Gajdusek Correspondence 1955-1958. DHEW Publication No. (NIH) 76–1168. 1976: US Department of Health, Education and Welfare.

[24] Klatzo, I., D.C. Gajdusek and V. Zigas, Pathology of kuru. Laboratory Investigation, 1959. **8**(4): 799.

[25] Hadlow, W.J., Scrapie and kuru. The Lancet, 1959. **274**(7097): 289–90.

[26] Gajdusek, D.C., et al., Transmission of experimental kuru to the spider monkey (Ateles geoffreyi). Science, 1968. **162**(3854): 693–94.

[27] Gajdusek, D.C., C. Gibbs Jr and M. Alpers, Experimental transmission of a kuril-like syndrome to chimpanzees. Nature, 1966. **209**: 794–6.

[28] Alper, T., D. Haig and M. Clarke, The exceptionally small size of the scrapie agent. Biochemical and Biophysical Research Communications, 1966. **22**(3): 278–84.

[29] Pattison, I. and K.M. Jones, The possible nature of the transmissible agent of scrapie. Veterinary Record, 1967. **80**(1): 2–9.

[30] Oesch, B., et al., A cellular gene encodes scrapie PrP 27-30 protein. Cell, 1985. **40**(4): 735–46.

[31] Wickner, R.B., [URE3] as an altered URE2 protein: evidence for a prion analog in Saccharomyces cerevisiae. Science, 1994. **264**(5158): 566–9.

[32] Cox, B., Cytoplasmic inheritance. Prion-like factors in yeast. Current Biology, 1994. **4**(8): 744–8.

[33] Sindi, S.S. and T.R. Serio, Prion dynamics and the quest for the genetic determinant in protein-only inheritance. Current Opinion in Microbiology, 2009. **12**(6): 623–30.

[34] Zhang, Z., et al., De novo generation of infectious prions with bacterially expressed recombinant prion protein. The FASEB Journal, 2013. **27**(12): 4768–75.

[35] Cohen, S.I., et al., From macroscopic measurements to microscopic mechanisms of protein aggregation. Journal of Molecular Biology, 2012. **421**(2): 160–71.

[36] Morris, A.M., M.A. Watzky and R.G. Finke, Protein aggregation kinetics, mechanism and curve-fitting: a review of the literature. Biochimica et Biophysica Acta (BBA)-Proteins and Proteomics, 2009. **1794**(3): 375–97.

[37] Eigen, M., Prionics or the kinetic basis of prion diseases. Biophysical Chemistry, 1996. **63** (1): A1–18.

[38] Prusiner, S.B., Molecular biology of prion diseases. Science, 1991. **252**(5012): 1515–22.

[39] Caughey, B., et al., Aggregates of scrapie-associated prion protein induce the cell-free conversion of protease-sensitive prion protein to the protease-resistant state. Chemistry & Biology, 1995. **2**(12): 807–17.

[40] Come, J.H., P.E. Fraser and P.T. Lansbury, Jr., A kinetic model for amyloid formation in the prion diseases: importance of seeding. Proceedings of the National Academy of Sciences of the United States of America, 1993. **90**(13): 5959–63.

[41] Lansbury, P.T., Jr. and B. Caughey, The chemistry of scrapie infection: implications of the 'ice 9' metaphor. Chemistry & Biology, 1995. **2**(1): 1–5.

[42] Nowak, M.A., et al., Prion infection dynamics. Integrative Biology Issues News and Reviews, 1998. **1**(1): 3–15.

[43] Masel, J., V.A. Jansen and M.A. Nowak, Quantifying the kinetic parameters of prion replication. Biophysical Chemistry, 1999. **77**(2): 139–52.

[44] Greer, M.L., L. Pujo-Menjouet and G.F. Webb, A mathematical analysis of the dynamics of prion proliferation. Journal of Theoretical Biology, 2006. **242**(3): 598–606.

[45] Prüss, J., et al., Analysis of a model for the dynamics of prions. Discrete and Continuous Dynamical Systems–Series B, 2006. **6**(1): 225–35.

[46] Engler, J., J. Pruss and G.F. Webb, Analysis of a model for the dynamics of prions II. Journal of Mathematical Analysis and Applications, 2006. **324**(1): 98–117.

[47] Doumic, M., et al., Scaling limit of a discrete prion dynamics model. Communications in Mathematical Sciences, 2009. **7**(4): 839–65.

[48] Pöschel, T., N.V. Brilliantov and C. Frömmel, Kinetics of prion growth. Biophysical Journal, 2003. **85**(6): 3460–74.

[49] Davis, J.K. and S.S. Sindi, A study in nucleated polymerization models of protein aggregation. Applied Mathematics Letters, 2015. **40**: 97–101.

[50] Calvez, V., et al., Prion dynamics with size dependency-strain phenomena. Journal of Biological Dynamics, 2010. **4**(1): 28–42.

[51] Calvez, V., et al., Size distribution dependence of prion aggregates infectivity. Mathematical Biosciences, 2009. **217**(1): 88–99.

[52] Doumic, M. and P. Gabriel, Eigenelements of a general aggregation-fragmentation model. Mathematical Models and Methods in Applied Sciences, 2010. **20**(05): 757–83.

[53] Tanaka, M., et al., The physical basis of how prion conformations determine strain phenotypes. Nature, 2006. **442**(7102): 585–9.

[54] Pezza, J.A., et al., Amyloid-associated activity contributes to the severity and toxicity of a prion phenotype. Nature Communications, 2014. **5**: 4384.

[55] Derdowski, A., et al., A size threshold limits prion transmission and establishes phenotypic diversity. Science, 2010. **330**(6004): 680–83.

[56] Wattis, J.A., An introduction to mathematical models of coagulation–fragmentation processes: a discrete deterministic mean-field approach. Physica D: Nonlinear Phenomena, 2006. **222**(1): 1–20.

[57] Lancaster, A.K., et al., The spontaneous appearance rate of the yeast prion [PSI+] and its implications for the evolution of the evolvability properties of the [PSI+] system. Genetics, 2010. **184**(2): 393–400.

[58] Belay, E.D. and L.B. Schonberger, The public health impact of prion diseases 1. Annual Review of Public Health, 2005. **26**: 191–212.

[59] Von Smoluchowski, M., Three lectures on diffusion. Brownian motion and coagulation of colloid particles. Zeitschrift für Physik, 1916. **17**: 557–85.

[60] Becker, R. and W. Döring, Kinetic treatment of nucleation in saturated steam. Annalen der Physik, 1935. **416**(8): 719–52.

[61] Chou, T. and M.R. D'Orsogna, First passage problems in biology. In S. Redner, R. Metzler & G. Oshanin (Eds.) First-Passage Phenomena and Their Applications. Hackensack, NJ: World Scientific, 2014. 306–345.

[62] Edelstein-Keshet, L. (1998) Mathematical Models in Biology. Philadelphia, PA: SIAM.

[63] Ball, J., J. Carr and O. Penrose, The Becker-Döring cluster equations: basic properties and asymptotic behaviour of solutions. Communications in Mathematical Physics, 1986. **104** (4): 657–92.

[64] Ball, J. and J. Carr, The discrete coagulation-fragmentation equations: existence, uniqueness and density conservation. Journal of Statistical Physics, 1990. **61**(1–2): 203–34.

[65] D'Orsogna, M., G. Lakatos and T. Chou, Stochastic self-assembly of incommensurate clusters. The Journal of Chemical Physics, 2012. **136**(8): 084110.

[66] Knowles, T.P., et al., An analytical solution to the kinetics of breakable filament assembly. Science, 2009. **326**(5959): 1533–7.

[67] Xue, W.-F., S.W. Homans and S.E. Radford, Systematic analysis of nucleation-dependent polymerization reveals new insights into the mechanism of amyloid self-assembly. Proceedings of the National Academy of Sciencesof the United States of America, 2008. **105** (26): 8926–31.

[68] Allen, L., An Introduction to Stochastic Processes with Applications to Biology 2003: Pearson/Prentice Hall. Boca Raton, FL, USA.

[69] Byrne, L.J., et al., The number and transmission of [PSI+] prion seeds (Propagons) in the yeast Saccharomyces cerevisiae. PLoS One, 2009. **4**(3): e4670.

[70] Davis, J.K. and S.S. Sindi, Initial condition of stochastic self-assembly. Physical Review E, 2016. **93**(2): 022109.

[71] Van Kampen, N.G., Stochastic Processes in Physics and Chemistry. Vol. 1. 1992: Elsevier. Amsterdam, The Netherlands.

[72] Durrett, R., Essentials of Stochastic Processes. 1999: Springer, New York, NY, USA.

[73] Doob, J.L., Stochastic Processes. Vol. 101. 1953: New York: Wiley.

[74] Van Kampen, N.G., Stochastic Processes in Physics and Chemistry. 1981, Amsterdam: North-Holland Publishing Company. 419 p.

[75] Gillespie, D.T., Stochastic simulation of chemical kinetics. Annual Review of Physical Chemistry, 2007. **58**: 35–55.

[76] Gillespie, D., Exact stochastic simulation of coupled chemical reactions. The Journal of Physical Chemistry, 1977. **81**(25): 2430–61.

[77] Hammersley, J., Monte Carlo Methods. 2013: Springer Science & Business Media. New York, NY, USA.

[78] Yvinec, R., M.R. D'Orsogna and T. Chou, First passage times in homogeneous nucleation and self-assembly. The Journal of Chemical Physics, 2012. **137**(24): 244107.

[79] D'Orsogna, M.R., Zhao, B., Berenji, B., & Chou, T. Combinatoric analysis of heterogeneous stochastic self-assembly. The Journal of Chemical Physics, 2013, **139**(12), 121918.

[80] D'Orsogna, M.R., Q. Lei and T. Chou, First assembly times and equilibration in stochastic coagulation-fragmentation. The Journal of Chemical Physics, 2015. **143**(1): 014112.

[81] Sharma, J. and S.W. Liebman, Exploring the basis of [PIN(+)] variant differences in [PSI (+)] induction. Journal of Molecular Biology, 2013. **425**(17): 3046–59.

[82] Davis, J.K. and S.S. Sindi, A mathematical model of the dynamics of prion aggregates with chaperone-mediated fragmentation. Journal of Mathematical Biology, 2016. **72**(6): 1555–78.

[83] Payne, R.J. and D.C. Krakauer, The spatial dynamics of prion disease. Proceedings of the Royal Society B: Biological Sciences, 1998. **265**(1412): 2341–6.

[84] Masel, J. and V.A. Jansen, Designing drugs to stop the formation of prion aggregates and other amyloids. Biophysical Chemistry, 2000. **88**(1–3): 47–59.

[85] Ridout, M.S., Computational methods for yeast prion curing curves. Mathematical Biosciences, 2008. **215**(2): 152–7.

[86] Ridout, M., et al., Modelling prion dynamics in yeast. Int. Statistical Inst.: Proc. 58th World Statistical Congress, Dublin (Session IPS020), 2011.

[87] Palmer, K., M. Ridout and B. Morgan, Kinetic models of guanidine hydrochloride-induced curing of the yeast [PSI^+] prion. Journal of Theoretical Biology, 2011. **274**(1): 1–11.

[88] Olofsson, P., S.S. Sindi and others, A Crump-Mode-Jagers branching process model of prion loss in yeast. Journal of Applied Probability, 2014. **51**(2): 453–65.

[89] Hunter, N., PrP genetics in sheep and the implications for scrapie and BSE. Trends in Microbiology, 1997. **5**(8): 331–34.

[90] DiSalvo, S., et al., Dominant prion mutants induce curing through pathways that promote chaperone-mediated disaggregation. Nature Structural & Molecular Biology, 2011. **18**(4): 486–92.

[91] Griswold, C.K. and J. Masel, Complex adaptations can drive the evolution of the capacitor [PSI], even with realistic rates of yeast sex. PLoS Genetics, 2009. **5**(6): e1000517.

[92] Masel, J. and A. Bergman, The evolution of the evolvability properties of the yeast prion [PSI+]. Evolution, 2003. **57**(7): 1498–512.

[93] Newby, G.A. and S. Lindquist, Blessings in disguise: biological benefits of prion-like mechanisms. Trends in Cell Biology, 2013. **23**(6): 251–9.